The Book of
Herbal
Wisdom

The Book of

Herbal
Wisdom

MATTHEW WOOD

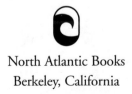

North Atlantic Books
Berkeley, California

The Book of Herbal Wisdom

Published by
North Atlantic Books
P.O. Box 12327
Berkeley, California 94712

Cover and book design by Andrea DuFlon
Cover photo by Ninon Sullivan

Printed in the United States of America

Distributed to the book trade by Publishers Group West

The Book of Herbal Wisdom is sponsored by the Society for the Study of Native Arts and Sciences, a nonprofit educational corporation whose goals are to develop an educational and crosscultural perspective linking various scientific, social, and artistic fields; to nurture a holistic view of arts, sciences, humanities, and healing; and to publish and distribute literature on the relationship of mind, body, and nature.

Library of Congress Cataloging-in-Publication Data
Wood, Matthew, 1954–
    The Book of herbal wisdom: using plants as medicine / Matthew Wood.
        p.   cm.
    Includes bibliographical references and index.
    ISBN 1-55643-232-1
    1. Herbs–Therapeutic use.   I. Title.
RM666.H33W655 1997
615'.321—dc21   96-49794
                                                                         CIP

        3   4   5   6   7   8   9   /   04   03   02   01   00

Dedication

To Dr. Frances Hole and Mr. Charles W. Brunelle

Also in memory of the late Ninon Sullivan

Contents

Foreword

When I was about nine, my family traveled to Wausau, Wisconsin, to attend "Northern Half Yearly Meeting." That's the Quaker get-together in the Upper Midwest. In those days the train still ran from Minneapolis to Wausau. It was an adventure. The meeting was held at the Marathon County Historical Society—the county where they grow all the Ginseng. It was an old Victorian mansion full of curios and artifacts. For years afterwards I played with the facsimile Confederate money I bought in the gift shop; it reminded me of that wonderful weekend. Over the years, many of my significant dreams—where ancient and profound truths are revealed—were set in old Victorian mansions.

First Day School, the Quaker version of Sunday School, was taught by an animated fellow named Francis Hole. He was a Soil Science professor at the University of Wisconsin. He took our class up on top of Rib Mountain, an old chunk of weathered volcanic core, worn down by eons of silent erosion; it constitutes the geological substratum of the Badger state. There was a fire tower on top. The air sparkled. I don't remember everything Francis taught us, but a feeling came out of him. "Nature is alive, Nature is alive." That feeling sank into me and conjoined with the core of my being. It was an initiation into the invisible, spiritual life which resides inside the material husk of Mother Nature.

Years later, on a trip through Wisconsin, I stopped and visited Francis at his home near the Yahara River, on the isthmus which comprises the old city of Madison. I thanked him for the insights he brought me. "Ah, yes," he mused, "that was a magical weekend." I showed him my first book, *Seven Herbs, Plants as Teachers* (1987). I explained how I was trying to get across the idea, the feeling, that Nature is a living being, an entity full of life, awareness, and treasures of the spirit. "People crave that knowledge," he commented. "It is life itself and they can't live a happy life without it." Francis understood. I said good-bye and headed on to Minnesota.

For me, this revelation of the life of Nature began to manifest as an interest in herbal medicine. I felt that the plants were living representatives of this hidden world. They are like letters of the alphabet in the language of life. They were both healers and teachers of wisdom. They led me on to discover more about the unseen life behind the world.

What Francis began was expanded upon for me many years later. I met a woman in northern Minnesota whose grandfather had been a famous medicine man. Again, I felt a transmission of knowledge. It was at this time I learned that the living intelligence of Nature is articulated into seven simple lessons which form a beautiful and complete harmony. What I had previously experienced as a field of life or energy was now concisely defined. I now felt that I had completed something deeply significant. I have described these lessons in my previous book, *Seven Herbs, Plants As Teachers.*

To feel the living spirit and intelligence of Nature is the true foundation for developing a knowledge of herbal medicine. The people up north have an extensive tradition, but it is their own, and they are not particularly interested in teaching outsiders. The rest of my journey involved "filling in the gaps." That means understanding how plants work *from the perspective of Nature,* not the perspective imposed on Nature by humanity. Every plant personifies some lesson about the operation of body, soul, life force, spirit or Nature. It took time to gain a perspective on such an enormous body of knowledge. The task is never done, each person has their own wisdom to assimilate, but the time came when I could share some of what I had learned.

When we learn to think as does Nature, we think in a different fashion from our custom. Nature has constructed patterns and whole units, such as "wolf," "carrot," "diamond," "heart." Scientific knowledge of nature and medicine is based upon a material, rational, reductive model, which emphasizes the pieces, not the whole, and assumes that Nature has no inherent logic.

Patterns, wholes and holism are constantly observed in Nature. We see lessons of this holism expressed in folk-medicine, in some of the alternative medical movements which have been shunned by modern science, and especially in the system of natural medicine practiced by the Indian people. It is unfortunate that this kind of wisdom is not respected. We have lost ninety-nine per cent of it. But there are still a lot of people who are working to remind us about Natural wisdom.

Through the years I have learned from a variety of teachers, practitioners, colleagues, and the plants themselves. In addition, I have learned from the steady stream of sick folk who have come to my door over the years. They were the final evidence of whether the herbs work or not. Among these many people, there is one who stands out from the rest.

I first got to know Susan when she came into Present Moment Herbs in Minneapolis, where I used to work. She was seeking help for a terminal illness. I have never met anybody who has been through as many near-fatal experiences as Susan, and over the years she came to be a constant source of medical experience for me. She became something like the "archetypal patient," as well as a friend.

Susan is a sharp little spitfire, about five feet two, eighty-four pounds, with black eyes like knifeblades and a vocabulary to match. When I first got to know her she was working for a box company—"all boxed up," I thought. Ten years later she is an accomplished healer herself.

The first aim of *The Book of Herbal Wisdom* is to show that herbal medicines are agents of both healing and wisdom. The realm of Dame Nature is a book about life. The leaves of this book are the plants, animals, people, and minerals which populate the natural landscape. Each species is alive with an inner life, a flash of energy from the Divine fiat, which is the guiding rule, the life, the purpose of that organism. Each of them represents a lesson, an awareness, a piece of ancient wisdom which we can perceive and learn from, enriching our lives and giving us meaning. The conjunction of their essence with our own brings us knowledge, life, and healing.

The second and more practical aim of *The Book of Herbal Wisdom* is to bring before the reader a useful catalog of medicine plants. Studying them, one learns how to see into the mysteries of the human organism, how to approach health problems, and how to use medicinal herbs in a careful and successful manner.

In order to understand a medicinal agent, it is often necessary to understand the historical context which gave birth to its medical use. Not only does this give us insight into the plant itself, but it allows us to respect the people who have gone before, who have learned about the properties of the plant, who brought it into use. This is the approach of a civilized people, with a long memory. Unfortunately, the difficulties through which we herbalists have had to pass in the last several hundred years have caused us to lose some of our history. I have tried to restore this context wherever possible.

The herbs described in this book come to us from a variety of sources including folk doctors, allopathic medicine, homeopathy, and flower essence practitioners. I hope that *The Book of Herbal Wisdom* will show how the medicinal properties of an herb shine forth, no matter which school originally brought foreword the knowledge. Herbal properties do not change with the method of preparation or philosophy of application, but ray forth from a deeper level at the root of Nature, beneath the philosophical contortions of human beings. Thus, I hope that this book will serve people of several different schools, especially homeopathy and herbal medicine.

The appearance of the second edition has allowed me to make some changes in the text. I also have the opportunity to pack in one more story. It seemed most appropriate as it involved a return to those Quaker roots.

I am, alas, rarely seen at Quaker functions these days, but recently I attended a dinner. Sitting down next to an older woman I'd known since childhood, I was surprised by her first comment. "Did you hear about the miracle cure your book caused?" I mumbled something over my plate of pot-luck. Her ex-husband had kidney failure, was all hooked up with shunts for dialysis ("you'll have to come in every week for the rest of your life"), when their daughter brought him some Nettle tea. The kidney function quickly picked up and a month later the doctors removed the shunts. "We made peace," my friend continued. "Then the old what-do-ya-call-him lived!"

Matthew Wood
Sunnyfield Herb Farm
Minnetrista, Minnesota

Summer Solstice, 1998

Herbalism and the Wisdom of Nature

Give me truths;
For I am weary of the surfaces,
And die of inanition. If I knew
Only the herbs and simples of the wood,
Rue, cinquefoil, gill, vervain and agrimony....

RALPH WALDO EMERSON

Within this fantastic circle stands a Lamp, and it
typifies the Light of Nature. This is the Secret Candle
of God, which He hath tinned in the elements:
it burns and is not seen, for it shines in a dark place.

THOMAS VAUGHAN

Herbs, Healing, and Wisdom

From the most ancient times, human beings have had a primal belief that plants contain healing powers. Herbs have also been seen as a source of wisdom. The herbalist versed in herbal lore has been looked up to (or persecuted, sometimes) as a person who sees into the inner secrets of Nature. Such ideas are so universally entertained by different cultures and peoples as to constitute a bedrock feature of folklore and myth.

At times, the dominant religion in the Western world has been threatened by this belief. By this I mean not just Christianity, but modern science. The lowly herbalist has been persecuted, as if he or she were some sort of heretic. I speak from experience, having supported myself as a professional herbalist for most of my adult life. We survive despite the threat of legal action against us and without the billions of dollars lavished on conventional medical research. As I write, one of my friends is being prosecuted by the state Attorney General.

There is no rational foundation upon which to base a defense of this deeply held belief in healing power and wisdom concentrated in our green friends. Although it is possible to prove that herbs have certain properties or that some traditional uses are valid, science cannot give us the reasons why people around the world look to plants as sources of medicine and understanding. The origins of herbalism and medicine lie in the mythopoetic universe of the imagination. Modern science cuts us off from this level of our being, where we find satisfaction and truth. The modern approach to science and medicine does not approach the spirit,

3

the soul, the imagination and intuition, the strange productions of folk-culture. It keeps us on a safe, but not a healthy surface where our spirits wither.

As to why herbs should occupy a position which, to judge from the opposition of religion and science, places them on a level with gods and goddesses, is difficult to explain. I believe it is built into the fabric of the world we live in. The herbs live in and adapt to environmental stresses and niches which correspond to our own problems. The excesses of climate they experience are like the excesses of life situations which we too must face. The triumphs of their life force over the adversities of Nature are etched into their genetic makeup, and these correspond with our own challenges. Thus, the herbs become our medicines. They are also reference points for understanding the world around us.

I have not attempted to construct this book of herbal knowledge upon a modern scientific scaffold. That has been done before and will be done again. What I have found is that a deeper understanding of the herbs brings us into a weirdly magical world which goes beyond the modern scientific foundation.

The plants in fact seem to have their own story to tell. From what I have learned, their story would begin in the hidden depths of the earth, in the unknown light of a place called the Underworld. From this source of mystery and power, the healing power and wisdom of the herbs ray out like a light, into our world. They never lose the magic that is innate to the inhabitants of a world of mystery, and in order to understand them as they are, we must adapt ourselves to their happy, mysterious selves. People try to press herbs into a rational, scientific box. This is not only entirely foreign to them, it kills their spirit and does not make ours soar.

While we must emphasize the mysterious, magical heritage of medicine plants, we must also understand how to use them. Otherwise, we are still stuck in a place where we are outsiders looking in, wishing for a connection but not making it. Using them as medicines provides us with the opportunity to learn wisdom about ourselves and Nature in a slowly unfolding manner. We can never know it all—only a fraction in fact—but the herbs are capable of constantly drawing us into a deeper understanding of ourselves as they heal us and we understand them.

Medicine plants have been subjected to many different cultural

665914

207 967 5272

CUSTOMER'S ORDER NO.		DEPARTMENT		DATE 4/13/02	

NAME
Chantal Bergeron

ADDRESS
93 R Wildes Distr Rd

CITY, STATE, ZIP
Kennebunkport, Me. 04046.

SOLD BY		CASH	C.O.D.	CHARGE	ON ACCT.	MDSE RETD	PAID OUT

QUANTITY	DESCRIPTION		PRICE	AMOUNT	
1					
2	1 "The Living Energy"			21	95
3	by Schwartz			3	00
4					
5	Ship↑			24	95
6					
7					
8					
9					
10					
11					
12					
13					
14					
15					
16					
17	*Homeopathic Educational Services*				
18	*2124 Kittredge St.*				
19	*Berkeley, CA 94704*				
20	*510-649-0294*				
RECEIVED BY					

a adams
5805

KEEP THIS SLIP FOR REFERENCE

interpretations, classification schemes, and analytical methods. In order to understand medicine plants, we need to understand some of the perspectives used to study them. These perspectives range from the magical journey of the shaman to the light of the rational scientist. In order to help us, the herbs have to pass from their home in dreamtime through layers such as these, to help us in our home in the rational world. Thus, I have written some introductory accounts of different systems and approaches to herbal knowledge.

On a basic level, this herbal should serve as a book of useful information about medicinal plants for the practicing homeopath and herbalist. The approach I take in my writing, as in my practice, does not differentiate between these two schools. I see them as divided by an artificial, man-made gulf. The emphasis of the homeopath on bringing forth the pattern in the symptoms to match the pattern in the medicine points us to the core personality of the plant. The knowledge of the herbalist is more empirical, based on traditional uses and experience in the field and at the bedside, but it also points one ultimately towards the medicinal essence.

In order to understand how the herbs fit into the context of the human organism, it has been necessary for me to adopt a perspective which is "energetic," as people would say today. The herbs do not fit the modern approach to pathology in medicine. They are suited to patterns in the organism, based on simple natural changes, such as hot and cold, dry and damp. They treat simple imbalances within the human frame, not the viruses and bacteria which settle into these imbalanced environments. Thus, I have had to adopt many concepts from Traditional Chinese Medicine and other systems based on patterns. At the same time, I have attempted to show how these intuitive ideas of pattern fit in with modern understanding about the organism. The herbs help me in this endeavor, because they personify different patterns. They teach us about Nature and ourselves.

Medicine is the daughter of dream.

IAMBLICHUS

Herbalism and Dreamtime

egend tells us of a great tree which stands at the foundation of the world. It is variously described as an Ash, a Fir, an Apple, among others. In the Norse sagas the world tree reaches fabulous proportions. In Indian country, up north, they say the Tree of Life, a fir or cedar, rises up from the back of an enormous turtle. And in the legends of many cultures, an eagle is pictured in the top branches of the tree.

This remarkable tree is generally said to penetrate through three worlds or dimensions, binding them together. According to the northern European version, the middle world (or "Middle Earth") is the familiar world we live in. The light of this world is the light of our waking hours. The upper world is described as a Heaven or Overworld. It is here where we customarily direct our prayers and look for directions from divine and higher sources. The lower world is spoken of in hushed tones. It is called the Underworld, a dimension apart from ordinary consciousness. Here, if we entertain the old tales, the root essence of each creature is found in its unblemished origin and potency.

The Underworld is a most important place from the standpoint of ancient and traditional herbalism, for it is here that the shaman/herbalist/physician must journey, in order to get to know the regenerative power of nature, the healing virtues of the medicine plants, and the vital energy which runs the human organism. Here at the knee of Mother Nature the secrets are imparted, the tools handed out, the virtues made known.

This realm is not just an abstract place where archetypes reside, waiting for our conscious mind to alight upon them. Rather, it is a living world populated by beings sentient in their own dimension. These inhabitants are, as it were, the primal persons behind the virtues. In that world they have their life and communicate among themselves and with us.

This otherworldly dimension is a thorough shift away from what we are used to, yet it has its own light of consciousness, as does our world. This glow in the Underworld has been called the light inside the earth or the light of Nature. It is a living light, yet hidden. This is the light within which Adam stood at the beginning of days, when he named all the creatures from their source in Paradise.

The alchemical version of our story says that the tree has three roots. One descends into the *primordia,* from which all possible paths of destiny are woven. Another extends into the *materia,* the material world, in which hardball experience takes place. The third conjoins with the *potentia,* the life substance which gives rise to all lifeforms.

The root which extends into the *primordia* of destiny is said to be divided into three again, representing the Three Fates. These are the ones who weave the destinies of all people. One of them is like the Ancient of Days, a fountain gurgling forth from the beginning of time down to the present. All things which have ever happened reside within the compass of this power. Another is our friend, the Eternal Now. These two together, they say, create the third. This is not the future—as one might expect—because the future is not an actual thing for us. Rather, it is the result or Destiny, because what is happening in our life is the fruition of our past and present. They are engulfingly total and in any given moment we are swept to the Destiny which is the natural unfolding of our decisions past and present.

Sometimes the number of trees multiply, so that there are two or three. In the Book of Genesis, at the beginning of the Hebrew Bible, we find the Tree of Life, standing in the center of the Garden of Eden. The exact nature of this tree is not clearly described in this story, but we may guess that it is the same tree found in the other myths and legends around the world. It is the great trunk from which all lifeforms spring, binding them together into the all-life. It is at the center of the garden and is the life of that place, so that when Adam and Eve are cut off from the tree, they are exiled from the garden itself.

While Adam is living in the garden which belongs to this tree, his central occupation was to name all living beings. After he named them, Adam became lonely. A rather anthropomorphic God saw his loneliness directly and fashioned a companion for him. Adam, still in the naming mode, called her Eve.

In the original Hebrew, the transparency of the names is more evident. The word *adam* means "humanity," not an individual man *(ish),* while *chavah* or Eve means "life," not an individual woman *(ishah).* We are not hearing about individuals, but about massive archetypes which loom giant over a mythological landscape.

In Adam we see the human archetype, and therefore he is also capable of naming things, or seeing the archetype in other things. Ancient lore says that he is the primal archetype, encompassing all the rest, because he names them all. With Eve we move to life; she is called "the mother of all living things." With her we move from the rather arid plane of the pure archetype to the level of the living. Things get much more interesting, and with that, more dangerous.

Now a more fascinating motif appears in the garden, around which much revolves. This is the "tree of the knowledge of good and evil," that fateful tree which represents the opportunity for separation from the garden, the Creator, and all the other lifeforms. It is by virtue of this tree that freewill is possible, but also the necessity for repercussions. Good and evil enter the picture for the first time. Although paradise is lost, something else takes its place. We might call this new thing "the world we live in." The story is a readout from the land of the imagination, giving a picture of our history and make-up.

A third tree is found in the stormy Book of Revelation at the end of the Christian Bible. This is the tree which gives eternal life after the torments which follow the exercise of freewill in the cauldron of good and evil. The leaves of this tree are "for the healing of the nations."

In the Underworld tradition of northern Europe, there are three trees: the "Oak, Ash, and Thorn." The Ash represents the great tree which stands at the foundation of the world, hidden deep someplace inaccessible. It is the power found in the depths of the Underworld, the living realm of Nature, from which all life springs. As the source of life, it is the source of all gifts, talents, skills, and separate qualities. The Hawthorn (one of the darlings of the herbalists) represents the opportunity for experience. It is found any place where it is possible to prick one's finger and fall, pell-mell, headfirst into experience—that is to say, something beyond oneself. The stern Oak relates to the guardian who tests all aspirants hoping to gain something traversing the byways of a magical world. Spiritual gifts are not given lightly, not without a price. This is the tree of ultimate responsibility.

The individual life of a human being is composed of these diverse elements. We are citizens of different simultaneous worlds. We have life and a connection to the spiritual insights and gifts which emanate from the all-life. We also have the gift of experience, pain, alienation, and exile from this tree to our kingdom in the material world. Then we have the quest, the test, the doom; whether or not we lived out a full and meaningful destiny during the passage of our life. We are born to a world of boring material thoughts but also a magical world. Whether or not we can round up the different facets of our nature depends upon the strength of the questing urge within us, the peculiarities of our destiny and our fortitude to persevere to the end.

Whether we have a happy life or not is another issue. It is a "revolutionary act," as physician/clown Patch Adams likes to say. Happiness does not originate in the stick-in-the-mud boring material world to which we are born, but is interjected by surprise from another dimension. Humor, art, and true medicine come from this other/magical place. The contrary, clown, trickster, poet, artist, crazy person, shaman, physician, steals a fleck of light from that world and brings it to this world, where it works its liberating, healing, happy-making, regenerating ferment. The bringer is wounded in the process.

The laughter of the youngest child and the wisdom of the oldest sage are messages from that other world. They rise in spite of, in the face of conventional religion, science, art, and medicine. The myth of the contrary stealing the light from the magical world in order to bring it to our habitation and being punished for it, is timeless. In some legends, the Creator himself is said to be crucified hanging on the tree of the all-life, in order to bring this knowledge to our world.

Each leaf upon the tree of the all-life is a separate life form, a species, a personality. As such, it is a little window opening into a play setting or theater, illustrating a spiritual lesson which is the peculiarity of that creature to manifest in the great symphony of life. The green leaves incarnate as organic beings in the material world, to provide us with living examples of spiritual visions, lessons, and quests. They dance thus, available, directly in front of our eyes. They are stones, vegetables, animals, and people.

Each medicine plant is a leaf from the tree, from the book of Mother Nature. In the Underworld, these leaves have their existence as conscious beings, just as we have our conscious lives in the material world. We may travel to this world and converse with these archetypal individuals directly, as person to person. These interior virtues reflect outwardly into the material world, where we can detect them with our intuitive and imaginative eye. These material reflections are the signatures or marks, which tell us what the plants are for.

The Vision Quest

The oldest method of acquiring herbal wisdom is the shamanic journey, which takes us directly into dreamtime for education and training. This is still the primary method of medicine used by American Indian doctors. Young aspirants after knowledge go out alone to fast, pray, and cry out for a vision. Sometimes they are rewarded. Others do not seek a vision, but it comes to them unsolicited. Such people become friends with the spirits, who help them and others seeking their advice. Out of the journey into the other world comes the knowledge of medicine. Very often, medicine people are taught in the dream world by an animal or spirit person about a plant or plants. At the same time, they are also taught about plants by the animals using them in the regular world. When people come to the medicine people for help, they generally ask the spirits, the ancestors for help regarding the sick person and they receive advice directly about medicines, changes in lifestyle, or problems in the environment.

As Elliot Cowan points out in *Plant Spirit Medicine* (1995), the plant will often show the shaman journeying to meet it, an animal, person, or spirit who explains the properties of the plant.

There is, however, another class of practitioners in Indian society who are more what we would recognize as herbalists. They are apprenticed out at a young age with an elder. They learn about herb lore which has been collected down through the generations—from watching animals, medical experiences, or visions. When people come to them they carefully observe their condition, as seen in the complexion and sometimes the pulse. They question them carefully and ascertain the nature of the disease. Very often, this form of practice owes a lot to dreamtime, but the therapy itself does not depend on an immediate interface with the spirits.

Over the generations, knowledge about medicine and life was gathered up and organized into a body which could be passed on. It must not be thought that there was only one religion among the Indian people in the old days. There were many societies and belief systems competing for interest. Among the Indian people living in my region, the Grand Medicine Society is one of the most powerful. Knowledge is graded into several ranks and many deep secrets of medicine and occultism are preserved and passed on. By no means is the Society or Medicine Lodge a completely altruistic affair. Some of its members are feared, while others are loved for their wisdom and help. Let us, however, dwell on the happier aspects of medicine knowledge.

The medicine knowledge of the elders is often arranged around the principal plants and animals native to the region. These become reference points for inner and outer experience. The large, important animals of the area—eagle, wolf, bear, turtle, deer—become the major symbols around which knowledge is coalesced. Very often, this knowledge is derived directly by watching these animals in the wild, or in dreamtime, over many generations. An elaborate, yet simple and effective system of medicine and knowledge is derived from the environment and distilled through dreamtime as well as medical experience.

The bear is a particularly important animal for the native herbalist. This omnivorous animal digs up roots, tears off barks, and collects berries with its claws. By watching the bear, the Indian people learned about plants for medicine and food. They enriched this knowledge by watching other animals, but the bear is the representative or totem animal for the healer. To dream of the bear brings empowerment in healing and work with plants. The native healers had a preference for roots and barks, because these were the forms in which the bear used plants.

If we look at the pharmacopoeia of Western herbalism we find that many of the medicines we use as roots and barks come to us from the American Indian heritage (Black Cohosh, Blue Cohosh, Goldenseal, Blue Flag, Bayberry, Sassafras, Prickly Ash, Echinacea, Blood Root, etc.). By comparison, the flowers, leaves, seeds, or aerial parts of plants were preferred in the European tradition (Calendula, Vervain, Chamomile, St. John's Wort, Lady's Mantle). In the south of Europe, plants rich in volatile oils were particularly favored (Sage, Thyme, Dill, Marjoram, Hyssop, etc.) Sometimes we see the contrast directly. For instance,

Linden flowers are used in Europe, but when its American cousin Basswood is used, the bark is preferred by Indians—yet, the properties are the same. There are, of course, many exceptions to this generalization.

The bear also represents the idea of taking care of people. The mother bear guards her cubs ferociously. One of my friends saw an adult grizzly bear run away from a black bear with her cubs! When a young Indian man was old enough to marry he went out hunting and hoped to come back with a bear, because the bear skin was large enough to serve as a blanket for him and his wife in the winter. This was particularly appropriate, since the bear slept through the long winter. The hibernation of the bear also pointed to its relationship to medicine plants which reactivate digestion and metabolism. The people watched the bear in the spring, to see what it first went out to eat. These plants are called Bear Medicines (Osha Root, Lomatium, and Balsam Root). Each of these sends up parts which look like furry brown paws and contains resins which stir up fats and oils, stimulate circulation, and remove mucus. Generally, Bear Medicines work on the lungs, heart, and liver—the aeration, circulation, and metabolism of the body.

The wolf, on the other hand, is related to boundary lines; the wolf pack is highly conscious of the confines of its hunting territory. The pack organizes the animals within that region. A trapper said to me, "Once you know where the wolves are, you know where everything else is." They are the commanders of the other animals because they prey on them all, from the mouse to the moose. This keeps them separated from the others by an invisible boundary line. For human beings, the wolf represents the absolutely wild, as opposed to the tame or domesticated, i.e., the dog.

As a representative of things medicinal, the wolf is most closely related to the animal instincts which reside in the solar plexus, the digestive tract to which it gives enervation, and the gallbladder, which is tied so closely to it by nerve reflexes. Wolves are known for their voracious hunger.

On a psychological level, wolf relates to the conscious ego, which dominates, organizes, rules, and sets boundaries. Yet, wolf also represents the ability to cross the boundaries, transform and move into something completely outside of known experience. Wolf Medicines usually show

13

evidence of right angles, which represent change, and act strongly on the digestion, stomach, gallbladder, or articulations (Werewolf Root, Solomon's Seal, Agrimony, St. John's Wort).

Turtle Medicine is very powerful. The old people say that the lessons of the Medicine Lodge are inscribed on the back of a turtle shell. "Everything there is to know" is already there to be seen on the shell before anyone is initiated into the Society. Let us pick up this shell and look at it carefully.

The upper, outward side is hard and protective. This represents the outward, material realm of Nature, the world in which we live, as opposed to the inward, living creature or realm. It also represents the outer wall of the Medicine Lodge, closed to the outside world, within which the mysteries take place. Upon this hard shell are engraved little circles or "eyes" which are separated from each other by lines. Each of these "eyes" represents a mystery, story, or stage setting, which tells about the history and meaning of the world, from the beginning of time down to the present. Grandfather Turtle is the repository and guardian of that history.

On the under side of the shell we see an X-ray picture of the body of the turtle within the shell. (What light made that X-ray?) Pick up a turtle shell and look at this image. (There is no replacement for experience.) This represents the soft underside of the creation, in which we see the signatures of the inner world impressed upon the outer. Grandfather Turtle is the teacher of hidden wisdom.

Then there is the body of the turtle inside the shell. This represents the living reality, Mother Nature, alive inside the material garment of the outer world. Here we meet the inhabitants, the denizens of that magical fairy land. Grandfather Turtle is alive.

Just as the great sea turtle rose out of the great water in the beginning of time to form the basis for the earth, so do the Turtle Medicines correlate with the separation and cooperation between liquids and solids in the body. This function relates particularly to the kidneys, but also to the spleen-lymphatics, through which the flesh of the body is built up by the assimilation of food out of the watery lymph. Turtle Medicine is very ancient, quiet, and powerful. Gravel Root is the only medicine I can place here.

The Purification Fast

Like the American Indians, the ancient Greeks also believed that medical knowledge grew out of experience in dreamtime. Ancient Greece was dotted with temples where people went for renewal and cure. Like the Indians, they fasted and prayed for a dream or vision. It was understood that fasting was conducive to dreaming. At the temples there were priests and priestesses who knew how to interpret dreams and help people understand their experience. It was in this milieu that the foundational therapeutic doctrine of Hippocratic medicine arose.

Hippocrates was a semi-legendary physician at a healing temple on the Island of Cos in the Aegean Sea. A school of followers gathered around him and they generated a corpus of writings which bear evidence of different hands but which also show common themes. These have come down to us as the "Hippocratic writings."

Some of the Hippocratic writers reasoned essentially as follows: we cannot understand what is going on in the hidden interior of the body, we cannot understand the action of medicinal plants, and we cannot understand the nature of disease. How then are we going to cure people? The solution they proposed is that we need one basic technique that will cure all people, all the time, regardless of the constitution or the disease. How is such a thing possible? A simple solution is suggested: fast a person on a moderate diet until the body is able to detoxify itself.

This is the single, universal healing method around which the corpus of Hippocratic medical knowledge developed. When a person is fasted, the body is given a chance to release encumbrances, usually after about four to seven days. At this point, symptoms begin to appear. Discharges, commonly of mucus or diarrhea, set in. The Hippocratic doctors referred to this event as the "healing crisis." At this time the disease is unmasked and now, for the first time, the physician can read the symptoms and understand what is going on. This is also the point at which the condition, fully manifested, can be understood and a prognosis given for the patient and his or her relatives. The physician assesses, from the nature of the discharges, whether the fast is "complete" and the toxins have been discharged, or whether some remain, calling for a fast at a later date.

We can now understand why there is an entire book in the Hippocratic corpus on prognostication. This places the emphasis on "what will happen," not what is wrong, as would diagnosis. Such an orientation would seem foreign to the modern doctor. Medical historians have thought this treatise showed an unfortunate bow to superstition, because sick people want answers, want to know "how it is going to turn out," or "am I going to live?" Historians of medicine lost the thread of the Hippocratic tradition. They did not understand that a technique which brings on a healing crisis engenders a need for prognosis, not diagnosis. It has also been said that the Hippocratic doctors taught "hygiene." This is also a misunderstanding. They taught an active, interventive technique which would provoke the healing power of the body.

The Hippocratic doctors coined the word *physis,* meaning the healing power of nature, and the term *physician,* meaning a person who assists or encourages this power. They believed that the natural healing ability within the body, when freed of impediments, would rectify the imbalance and return the person to health.

The "detoxification fast," as Hakim G. M. Chishti describes it in *The Traditional Healer* (1988) is still actively used in Arabic or *Tibb* medicine, complete with the Hippocratic guidelines for prognosis.

After this system had been forgotten in the West, it was rediscovered by the founders of naturopathy. Dr. Henry Lindlahr, who specialized in fasting as a therapeutic method, pointed out the connection. He also came to respect the fine points of the Hippocratic system, including the law of the healing crisis. Ironically, while he could appreciate the teachings of Hippocrates, his allopathic brethren were incapable of understanding either his approach or that of the "father of medicine." The preservation and use of this ancient and simple teaching was reserved for medical heretics.

Good Medicine, Bad Medicine

An herbalism based on mythology and the imagination is not all beauty and elegance. In the ancient and medieval literature of Western herbalism we find that one of the principal uses of herbs is to get rid of demons and witches. At the same time, herbs and plants came to be associated with witchcraft.

This is not just a byproduct of Christian propaganda. The use of herbs to make or break enchantment appears in pagan literature and in many non-Christian societies around the world. Indeed, in many cultures one of the most important uses of medicine plants is to protect against witchcraft. This function is well documented in American Indian medicine. Wherever there are shape-shifters and tent-shakers there are sorcerers and witches.

I've taken flack from some white people for using the word witch in a pejorative fashion. They maintain that it originally referred to a person who was wise in pagan times; later it was changed by the church to have an evil connotation. Finally, as we know, thousands of people were burned as witches.

I have continually had white people tell me that Indians have a negative attitude towards witches that they picked up from Christian missionaries. As far as I know, none of the people who say this grew up on an Indian reservation. I did. I am trying to represent here, not only my own experiences and understanding of this phenomena, but that of traditional Indian people.

Many people do not believe that there is any such thing as witchcraft. Either they don't believe in evil or they don't believe in a nonmaterial universe in which psychic manipulation and abuse takes place. Some people are capable of believing that an ill-disposed person can "bad vibe" or "psychially attack" a person, but this still does not begin to touch upon the Indian concept of witchcraft.

In Indian society the full-fledged witch is not seen as someone who merely bad vibes people. I'm sorry to be a cynic, but this is what all of us do a lot of the time! No, the witch operates in the level of dreamtime, beyond the medium of psychic and psychological manipulation. The witch has the ability to grasp the strands of destiny which are woven to create a person's future. In order to do this it is necessary, in fact, for them not to be swayed by strong emotions. They have the ability to weave these strands so that accidents occur, children are lost and destroyed, valuable possessions are stolen or lost, and in short, *the most precious things in one's life are damaged.*

Imagine what it would feel like if your life was going along fine, you felt you were fulfilling your spiritual calling and making a living at it, you were in a happy relationship with someone who felt like the "right person", and your children were healthy and doing well in school, when all of a sudden, odd, threatening little things began to happen. You left your checkbook in the restaurant. You felt an impulse to turn the wrong way down a one way street. The dog got hit by a car. Your children started to act malicious and run with a bad crowd. Uncountable frictions entered into your marital relationship. Your very destiny, what seems "right" in your life, is disappearing. Hopefully you become aware that "something is not right" before too much damage is done.

What would your reaction be? I can describe what mine has been: biological fear and revulsion. This kind of meddling in other people's lives feels like an insidious perversion and it needs to be rebuked absolutely.

It is customary for traditional Indian people to treat the religion of other people with respect. When it comes to witchcraft, however, many Indian people react with biological fear and revulsion. Many elders do not understand that some younger white people have adopted the term witch as their religious identity. I knew of a well-liked young white man who attended ceremonies and was long considered a friend. One evening, he mentioned that he was marrying a woman who was wiccan, a witch. He was told to leave immediately and never come back, on pain of injury. While he told me this he was crying. I have also seen what happens when the person came back!

For myself, I am intolerant of the use of words in ways which promote ambiguity about spiritual evil. People do this with many different words. I obstinately continue to use the word "witch," even if it makes me "politically incorrect."

One night a friend and I were driving to a ceremony at an Indian community in rural Minnesota. All of a sudden we saw a black liquid form move across the sky in front of us. We were so shocked we stopped the car. Later I was told by an Indian man that the witches lived in the dark spots in the night sky. Imagine, however, the horror of one of my friends. She was camping alone by herself in the woods. This time the liquid blackness came down out of the night sky and landed in the top of a nearby tree. It jumped closer and closer, tree by tree, then it pounced on her with a blood-curdling screaming laugh, as if to say: I have you now. "The hell you do," my friend retorted. "God will protect me." And it was gone. My friend commented, "If I was a cartoon character, every organ in my body would have jumped out of every orifice."

The Magical Uses of Medicine Plants

If we were to ignore the magical level of our herbal tradition, we would be throwing away a great portion of our literature, whether we are speaking of European or Native American or some other kind of lore. In herbal tradition, medicine plants have long been associated with magic. What does magic mean? Do herbs really act on this level? How can we understand and use them on this plane? And should we?

I always used to say, "Herbs work on the physical, emotional, mental, and spiritual levels of existence." Later I came to understand that they also work on the magical level. What this means is that they do not just change our person but that they can transform the environment around us. They can actually cause events to occur. Ultimately, what makes an event magical is that it is unexpected. So, in other words, the herbs seem to get a step ahead of us and create an event which we did not foresee, but which corrects or enriches our lives.

Medicine plants are capable of operating on the level of dreamtime. Indeed, I think we should call this their natural home. Through this level of existence they have the ability to restore people to their spiritual sacredness, core, or path. At the same time, they act on the mental and emotional level to rectify psychological misunderstandings and problems. Finally, descending to the physical level, they operate on physical health problems.

In the western Christian culture there is a taboo against attempting to influence the course of events around oneself or another person. People who attempted to work on this level were almost always, as a matter of fact, called witches! Considering this, we are going to have to rehabilitate the name after all! At any rate, this taboo generally did not exist in the pre-Columbian world of the Indian people. Here the idea was rather that people are always subject to the pressure of people and things attempting to influence the course of their lives. Therefore, we "two-leggeds" have the right to defend and actualize ourselves in the face of this hidden onslaught of dreamtime influences. Medicine plants are fully capable of helping us, as well as randomly influencing us. For the Indian doctor the magical level is often the main station through which medicine plants are seen to be operating.

By magically changing our lives, our little green friends restore physical health, psychological happiness, and spiritual purpose. A little miracle occurs when the magical level clicks in, in fact, whenever an herb cures in a real and radical way. This is the sign that something great and new has come in from a different world to enrich and develop our lives to their fullest potential.

Within the infant rind of this small flower
Poison hath residence, and medicine power.

WILLIAM SHAKESPEARE

Signatures, Similars, and Patterns

We have seen how people, as they emerge out of dreamtime, arrange knowledge into an orderly system. One group of plants are designated Bear Medicines, another are Wolf Medicines. After a while, a corpus of knowledge is collected which can be communicated to an apprentice. Medicine still remains on the level of dreamtime—the student still was expected to have had the dream or vision making them a candidate for medical knowledge.

Even in this organized state, knowledge still continues to be passed along in dreamtime. Members of a family, clan, or tribe have dreams or visions, from generation to generation, about animals, spirits, and plants their family has gained as helpers. There is also, of course, a pragmatic set of skills and knowledge which needs to be transmitted through regular training.

As medicine emerges out of dreamtime, the first doctrine which appears as an organizing construct is what is usually called the "doctrine of signatures." This is the idea that a plant resembles the disease, organ, or person for which it is remedial. *Scrophularia* roots look like swollen glands, hence it was used for swollen glands and hemorrhoids. The orange-yellow sap of *Chelidonium* indicates that it is for the bile. *Agrimonia* bristles with tension, and is an important medicine for tension.

The logic behind this procedure is not in alignment with contemporary science, but it is still a valid approach. Signatures represent configurations of energy or patterns in plants and these correspond to

21

similar patterns in people. We are not looking here for a superficial resemblance, but for one that operates on the level of essence.

In my previous book, *The Magical Staff* (1993), I quoted two Renaissance writers to give examples of the right and wrong ways to look for signatures. Agrippa von Nettesheim and Paracelsus both studied under the same teacher (Trithemus), in the early sixteenth century, but they each came away with different lessons. Agrippa speaks of treating the left eye of a man with the left eye of a frog, the right foot with the right foot of a turtle, etc. "Brain helps the brain, and lungs the lungs," he says. "As foot to foot, hand to hand, right to right, left to left." This is incorrect because these are literal, material resemblances. In contrast to this we have Paracelsus, who says, "Not spleen of a cow, not the brain of a swine to the brain of man, but the brain—that is, the external brain to man's internal brain." In other words, the plant with the signature of the brain is medicine from the external world for the brain of an individual.

Admittedly, this kind of thinking is based on subjective criteria, and could easily lead one into absurd conclusions. What defense can be offered in return? If the life force and Mother Nature are alive with an inner spiritual reality, as many of us believe, then we must take into account options which bring us beyond objective, mundane reality. Perhaps these cannot be defended in a court of rationality, but they can be experienced. If they exist, it is our duty to attempt to find and experience them, rather than to deny their existence. The latter is the easy way out. Anybody can set up a rational system based upon an ideology; not everybody has the intention and strength to explore and make friends with the hidden, irrational side of Nature.

Ben Charles Harris, a pharmacist in Connecticut, wrote a book about herbalism based on the doctrine of signatures. *The Compleat Herbal* (1972) defends the merit of this approach. He writes,

> *If at times the examples of correspondences throughout this work appear far-fetched, let me offer as warrants of the doctrine's usefulness some fifty-five years of living with and experiencing the healing herbs, as well as close to four decades of professional pharmacy and teaching of herbalism.*

Although the doctrine of signatures depends upon a subjective examination of natural phenomena, this should not be seen as a flaw but as a strength. Through study of the natural history, environmental patterns, chemical properties, taste, smell, appearance, etc., a person can learn to see similarities between plants and people. Through experience, the interior eye is trained and certainty in knowledge and practice is increased. Although we start in a place of weakness and vulnerability to delusion, we are enabled through experience to arrive at a place of wisdom.

This contrasts with the current approach in science and medicine, which discounts all subjective phenomena, in favor of objective fact, scientific trials, and consensus opinion. There is no instruction to develop therapeutic intuition or receive advice from dreamtime. Healthcare providers rely upon machines but patients are not machines, so this method can never reach out to and comprehend the true wellsprings of healing and disease.

The doctrine of signatures operates through at least two different subjective faculties, the intuition and the imagination. Intuition helps us see patterns in the world. We see several unrelated factors, but suddenly they fit together and make sense. Because of this experience of having things fit correctly, the intuition is satisfying, giving us a sense of perspective, context, and meaning. The intuitive approach is relatively acceptable to modern people because it fits in with rational thinking. The one faculty gathers information, the other fits it in place.

As an example of an intuitive approach to understanding an herb, let us take Angelica. It grows in damp, shady soil, but has warming, drying properties which help it remove damp and cold from the system. The environment where it grows is a signature which makes sense to the intuition and is not too far removed from the rational approach.

The second way that the doctrine of signatures works is through the imagination, the ability to see images. Angelica is notable for the long hollow tube of the stalk. This pictures or resembles the tubes of the body. Hence, Angelica is a remedy for the bronchial tubes. It is also a signature for the blood vessels (especially as the stalks are a bit red or purple), and indeed, Angelica removes stagnant blood and warms and stimulates the circulation. Finally, a magical element is hinted here, because the tube of the Angelica stalk was long used in Eurasian shamanism as a "magician's staff," to help facilitate the shamanic journey. The tube represents a passageway, from one world to the next.

The American Indians take this imaginative use of signatures a step further. If the plant suggests a certain animal, or it attracts certain animals, then an affinity to this beast and the medicine it represents is thought to reside in the plant. My friend Karyn Sanders, a native herbalist in Oakland, calls this the "spirit signature." To continue with our example, Angelica has a brown, furry, resinous root, so it is considered a Bear Medicine.

We can easily see how the imaginative approach to the doctrine of signatures leads us into a territory which is not acceptable to the rational mind. The idea that the landscape is full of cartoonlike images that point out medicinal affinities is preposterous to most modern people. It so often leads us directly into magical thinking, as we have seen with Angelica. Who knows where this will end, says the rationalist?

The poet William Blake valued the imagination deeply as the means by which it was possible to receive new understanding and to judge what was spiritually true and what was fantasy. He pointed out that if one follows the way of the imagination long enough to gain experience, one will learn how to trust it as a faculty of perception and a way of life. He differentiated between images which arise spontaneously in the mind, and those which arise out of remembered images. Spontaneous images relate to our inspirations and new spiritual gifts, the others reflect the known world. He also pointed out that one can learn to tell the difference between images which are generated within oneself, based upon doubt or self-will (these he called "fantasies") and those that come from beyond us ("vision"). He showed that the imagination is not just a source of random images, but the faculty of seership itself.

This leads us back into dreamtime. If we develop not only the intuitive, but even the more risky imaginative approach, we will return to that magical source of life and inspiration, the world of dream. The doctrine of signatures, with its appeal to both imagination and intuition, stands at the boundary line of dreamtime and the rational world. By its nature it will tantalize, tease, and dissatisfy the rational mind. Harris says we can either believe that signatures are a sign from God or Mother Nature, telling us what a plant is good for, or we can use them as a memory device.

Through the doctrine of signatures we can begin to see the interconnections between different parts of Nature. At first, these connections will seem remote and hard to believe—or perhaps magical. With time they will begin to make sense and our use of these faculties will become a matter of confidence and wisdom. Eventually we get to participate directly in that magical fairy realm.

Because of its subjective nature, the doctrine of signatures has been discarded by modern rationalists as a survival from a more naive or primitive culture. To look for hidden similarities between different things smacks of "magical thinking." Perhaps the time will come when mere objective thought will be considered primitive and naive.

Signatures can come to us through all of our senses—sight, sound, taste, smell and touch. Harris defined and described different categories into which signatures fall in *The Compleat Herbal*. Here are some of the things we can observe about a plant, pointing to its essence and use.

Habitat. The environmental niche occupied by a plant reflects stresses and conditions which it has had to adapt to, and these often correspond to conditions in the organism. Plants which grow in wet situations often relate to organ systems which handle dampness in the body, such as the lymphatics and kidneys. They correspond to diseases produced by an excess of dampness—respiratory problems, mucus, lymphatic stagnation, swollen glands, kidney and bladder problems, intermittent fever and rheumatic complaints (*rheuma* = dampness in Greek). Here we think of Horsetail (low, wet sands/kidneys), Eryngo (salty, sandy seashores/kidneys), Gravel Root (swamps/kidneys), Swamp Milkweed (swamps/kidneys), Hydrangea (sides of streams/kidneys), Boneset (wet soils/joints and fever), Willow (low ground/joints and fever), Meadowsweet (low ground/rheumatic pains, intermittent fever), Northern White Cedar (cedar swamps and margins of lakes/lymphatics), Labrador Tea (cedar swamps and margins of lakes/lymphatics), various Knotweeds (low ground/kidneys), Sweet Flag (swamps/mucus, lungs and joints), Angelica (damp, shady, cool valleys/damp, cold rheumatic and respiratory conditions). It is interesting to note that sandy, gravely soils are also a signature for kidney remedies (Horsetail, Eryngo, Gravel Root, Gromwell, False Gromwell, Uva ursi, etc.) The old authors believed that plants which broke into the rocks with their root systems and clove them apart were suited to "breaking stones" in the kidneys. Such plants were called "saxifrages." Sassafras, Saxifrage, and Juniper are lined up here, though the best gravel remedy I am acquainted with is Gravel Root, which actually precipitates gravel around its roots. Plants growing in the open sunlight are often warming, drying and cheering (Calendula, Lemon Balm, St. John's Wort, and Rosemary).

Some distinctive environments yield distinctive properties.

Plantain grows on compacted soil from which it is hard to draw nutrients; it is the "herbal drawing agent."

Color. The colors seen in the flowers, leaves, stalks, and roots of plants are often very significant. Purple, indigo, lavender, and purple-red usually indicate low-grade, septic, toxic heat and fever. When the stalk is red or purple-red we often have a plant which will pull out toxic heat, detoxify the interior, perhaps working through the portal vein and often on the liver: Dandelion, Burdock, Gravel Root, Plantain, Wild Indigo, Echinacea. As the color tends towards a pure red, there may be a relationship to the blood and heart: Blood Root (congestion of blood to the head, migraine, menstrual problems), red-stemmed Melilot (congestion of blood), Red Clover (mildly thins the blood), St. John's Wort (nutritive, blood building), Raspberry (nutritive), Hawthorn berry (heart), Cayenne Pepper (heart). Passing on to orange and yellow we have a signature for the bile, liver, and digestive tract (spleen, lymphatics, stomach, liver, gallbladder, and intestines): Goldenseal, Barberry Root, St. John's Wort, Chamomile. Brilliant blue is one of the most reliable of the color signatures. It almost always indicates an antispasmodic: Lobelia, Skullcap, Blue Vervain, Chamomile (the oil is blue), Blue Cohosh, Wood Betony. White saps usually represent a consciousness-diminishing property: Opium, Wild Lettuce. The white marbled leaves of Milk Thistle were taken as a signature of galactagogue properties. White can also represent the bones: Boneset (white flowers), Solomon's Seal (white rhizomes), Comfrey (white roots under the black covering), Black Cohosh (the same). Black does not often appear in plants, but represents necrosis. Wild Indigo has beautiful green leaves and pods, which on ripening or injury, turn completely black. This plant was used for necrosis, gangrene, typhoid, putrid deterioration.

Form. This is where we have the most fun. The appearance of the plant is often cartoonlike in the way it represents the utility of an herb. Often these signatures are so strange as to defy judgment, yet they work. Thorny nuts and pods represent mental tension, obsessive thought, and mental illness (Thornapple, Horse Chestnut, Wild Cucumber). Sweet Leaf *(Monarda fistulosa)* has a crownlike ring of petals around the compound flower head, representing mental restfulness. Eyebright has a figure like an eye on the flower. Thornapple looks like an ear and middle ear tube; it is a remedy for ear infections with obsessive thought. Self Heal looks like a throat and is, of course, a remedy for tonsillitis. Star Anise looks like the sinuses radiating outward from the the root of the nose and clears sinus congestion, especially of the maxillaries. Pulsatilla has a yellow flower and is for yellow mucoid discharges. Elder has hollow, tubular stalks and opens tubes, blood vessels, blood stagnation, pores of the skin, fever, detoxification, the intestines, etc. Angelica also has hollow, tubular stalks and acts in a similar manner. Both of these plants are used for shamanic journeying, because the tube represents a passage to another world. Sweet Leaf has tubular flowers and is one of the greatest diaphoretics. Lacy leaves and umbel flowers represent aeration of the lungs and bloodstream: Elder, Sumach, Fennel, Dill, Angelica, White Pine. Large leaves stand for surface area and gas exchanges or breathing, hence the lungs and skin: Burdock, Elecampane, Comfrey, Mullein. Hairy, hirsute leaves stand for the hairs of the skin and the villa of the mucosa, and usually for respiratory and digestive remedies: Comfrey, Mullein. Thick, mucilaginous leaves and parts represent mucus. Knobby swellings indicate glands—see especially the incredible nodules on the roots of Red Root or the nodular roots of Figwort. Right angles represent the gallbladder and joints (Werewolf Root, Solomon's Seal, Agrimony, Celandine). Knobbiness can also picture swollen, rheumatic joints: Mustard, Devil's Claw (looks like a knarled hand) and Leatherwood *(Dirca palustre)*. This shrub has prominently swollen joints with, as some people have suggested, the face of a wolf etched on them. Homeopathic provings hint that Leatherwood may be useful for rheumatoid arthritis and lupus. A number of plants look like bones, knuckles, vertebrae, and joints, especially Solomon's Seal, Horsetail, Boneset, Comfrey. Hands and arthritic pain are pictured by Marijuana; hands and the workplace by Cinquefoil. Lady's Slipper has roots shaped like testicles, hence is an old aphrodisiac and a modern nerve tonic. The flower looks like a slipper; it is a medicine for edema where the shoe does not fit right.

Texture. Hairy or hirsute leaves and stems are a signature for the hair of the head (Agrimony) or the body hair or hairs of the mucosa (Comfrey, Mullein, Lungwort, Coltsfoot). Mullein is definitely the remedy for harsh coughs which have worn down the villa of the lungs. Leaves that are thick from the content of mucilage (Slippery Elm, Coltsfoot) are good lung and mucosa remedies. The oily leaves of many mints, especially Sweet Leaf and Lemon Balm, signify soothing, balsamic properties.

Taste. This is a very significant property and gave rise to several important classification schemes which will be mentioned in the next chapter. The action of herbs upon the palate and mouth is not adequately described by the word "taste." There are at least three major reactions. First, the five flavors, then the temperature (in the Greek method this includes hot, cold, damp, and dry), and finally the impression made on the nerves (diffusive, tingly, or heavy, dull). Thus, I speak of these three elements of "taste" (flavor, temperature and impression).

Aroma, scent. The smell of a plant conjures up different feelings and physical reactions in people, all of which have psychological and medical significance. These scents are often based on the presence of volatile oils and resins which have proven medicinal virtues, so we are not just talking about something purely subjective, but substances which have long histories of use in medicine and commerce. Many of the mints are blessed with high contents of volatile oils, and these usually determine most of their medicinal power. The warm, rich, drying aroma of Rosemary has a salutary, cleansing, sharpening quality to it. This plant was long used to fumigate rooms, but it also awakens an old system, running off edema due to cardio-renal failure in a harmonious, safe manner. Spearmint, Chamomile, Wild Bergamot, Lavender, Thyme, Pine, and many other plants possess properties directly related to volatile oils. The presence of resins often indicates a respiratory action. As herbalist Michael Tierra explains it, the resins penetrate into the respiratory tract, attach themselves to the mucus, loosen it up and bring it to the surface. Here we think of Pine, Propolis, Poplar bud, Gumweed and others.

Sound. Not many plants have distinctive sounds. However, the sound of wind blowing through the tall White Pine has a peculiar relaxing effect, which this plant carries into its medicinal action. Pine is soothing and strengthening to the nerves, at the same time it is an expectorant and antiseptic (it brings up viscid, green, saplike mucus), and a powerful drawing agent (think of the power it takes to draw that sap up the tall trunk).

Times. The period during which plants bloom, and perhaps when they leaf out and the seasons they thrive in, often correspond to the timing of symptoms. For instance, Blood Root flowers slowly unfold from morning to noon, then slowly fold back up again (used for migraines, worse from morning to noon, better from noon to night and relieved by lying in the dark). Pulsatilla blooms early in the spring, and has mental suggestibility "like an April day," according to homeopath William Boericke (1927).

Jonathan Carver (1766), a British officer travelling in the interior of North America, recorded a signature which suggests that the Indians also used time as a signature. He mentions the widespread use of Rattle Snake Plantain by the Indians as an antidote for snakebite. "It is to be remarkèd that during those months in which the bite of these creatures is most venomous, that this remedy for it is in its greatest perfection, and most luxuriant in its growth."

"Spirit Signatures." Bear, Wolf and Turtle Medicines have already been mentioned above. One of the most important in this category are the Snake Medicines. These plants are used for snakebite and toxic poisoning. Because of the necessity of using good snakebite medicines on the frontier, and also because the Europeans had a tradition of using plants which resembled snakes (Bistort, Plantain) for snakebite, this nomenclature was adopted by the pioneers. Snake Medicines known to the Indians and the pioneers include Plantain or Snakeweed, Black Cohosh or Black Snake Root, Virginia Snake Root, Senega Snake Root, Rattle Snake Master, Echinaea, Rattle Snake Plantain, Button Snake Root, and Corn Snake Root.

The way to work with signatures is through patience, waiting for them to "click in" and make sense. There is a big difference between reading about a signature and "feeling the tumblers click." They do not come to one in a rational flow of insight, but scattered over many months and years, during which time one is observing people, plants, and nature. Sometimes our knowledge is more rational, sometimes less so.

It is difficult to organize signatures into an overall scheme—believe me, I have tried. In the European tradition, I believe the best work in this direction was done by William Coles in *Adam in Eden* (1657). He matches the plants to the human frame, part by part. This follows an ancient tradition. The idea that the human body is a representation of the world around it, a microcosm of the macrocosm, is intimately associated with the doctrine of signatures.

The Wisdom of Nature

If we struggle with the uncertainties of imagination and intuition, after some time we may begin to feel that there is indeed a hidden logic with

Mother Nature. Images, similars, signs, correspondences, and coincidences infer a different way to look at the world; they give rise to a different kind of knowledge.

Paracelsus, the wandering Swiss doctor, surgeon, and mystic of the early sixteenth century, worked out an entire system of knowledge and vocabulary based on the experience of Nature as a living, intelligent being. The name he gave to this was *naturgewissenshaften,* meaning "Wisdom of Nature," or *natura sophia* in Latin.

Paracelsus used the expression *lumen naturae,* or "the light of Nature," to describe a different way of perceiving the world that was based on the innate intelligence in Mother Nature. He made clear that this light had always been available to housewives, woodsmen, folk-doctors, herb-pickers, sages and all sorts of people living close to Nature, close to the experience of life. It was not available only to philosophers. As Paracelsus demonstrated in his own rough, wandering, persecuted life, it was associated with direct experience, not abstractions and ivory towers.

Out of his experiences of this other way of perceiving, Paracelsus developed a system of medicine with its own peculiar terminology. The following are the more essential themes of the system, as described in the works of Paracelsus and related writers.

The philosopher's stone. The old alchemists continually emphasized that all wisdom began with the dirt under one's feet. The primal substance from which they worked was called the *lapis philosophorum,* or philosopher's stone. It was hidden and rejected, and yet common and found everywhere. There is no doubt that mere dirt was in fact the starting place for their chemical studies, but they also used the expression as a metaphor. What is the mere dirt under our feet, the starting place for all knowledge, which is common but ignored? It is experience. People constantly ignore their experiences!

The alchemists maintained that true knowledge could only grow out of direct personal experience, not out of theory, book knowledge, or consensus opinion. This kind of knowledge is alone wisdom or *sophia,* and thus the philosopher (lover of wisdom) is not an abstractionist, but a practical observer and experiencer of life.

The vital force. Within nature there is a hidden, invisible animating force which is, however, visible in its effects. Living beings are intrinsically different from inanimate ones. The laws by which they operate are innately different. Each organism has its own separate blob of energy assigned to it from the greater storehouse of Mother Nature. The life force is molded into configurations or signatures, activated by similarity, and traced through correspondence. It maintains the viability, integrity, and health of the organism.

The vital force has both a substancelike quality to it, which Paracelsus called the *mumia,* and an intelligent, spiritlike side, which he called the *archeus,* or arch governing principle. The homeopath James Tyler Kent pointed out that it was more effective to refer to the life force as a substance, since we tend to visualize substances as more real than "energies."

The doctrine of signatures. As we have seen, each plant is a personification of pattern, of vitality brought together into a configuration. As such, there are certain patterns in the plant—the way it grows, where it grows, and what it is like to our senses—which reveal its medicinal properties. Each is a *signatum* or sign which shows what the medicine is for and how it is to be used.

The law of similars. Signatures work by virtue of the similarity between a disease, organ, or people, and a plant. Thus, the idea that "like treats like," or the law of similars, is implicit in the doctrine of signatures. This is the original way in which similars were observed and used.

About 1790, a German doctor, Samuel Hahnemann, introduced the "pathogenetic" interpretation of the law of similars, namely that the medicinal agent causes the same symptoms that it cures. This became the basis of homeopathy, which was thus based on a pharmacological principle, rather than a spiritual or philosophical experience.

Hahnemann and many of his followers considered the law of similars to be a universal healing principle, and there is good evidence that this is true—that it operates on every level whether it be spiritual, psychological, or physical.

The doctrine of correspondence. The word "correspondence" has been traditionally used to describe the special relationship between two things which are similar according to their hidden essential nature. If they reflect the same or similar essence they are said to be "in correspondence" or "correspondents." Working in this vein, we see that all the things in creation—plants, diseases, and the human organism—are in correspondence with each other in different ways.

The eighteenth century Swedish mystic and seer, Emmanuel

Swedenborg, contrasted correspondences with representatives, which resembled one another but did not have the same essence. Correspondences, as he showed, operate between the spiritual, psychological, and physical planes of existence.

The microcosm and the macrocosm. Because all elements, functions, and organ systems within an individual are in correspondence to elements in the outside world, the individual is a microcosm, a small world, reflecting the construction and properties of the greater world, the macrocosm. Paracelsus taught that true healing treatment resulted from linking the cure in the macrocosm (say, Celandine) to the diseased organ in the microcosm (say, the gallbladder).

The archetypal human. Since the individual is a reflection of the macrocosm, it can be said that the entire universe is laid out as an enormous human being. This is called the *anthropos* or "Grand Man."

Some authorities describe the archetypal human being as God. The ancient Hermetic writings state, "the Heavenly God is an Immortal Man, the earthly man is a mortal god." Paracelsus, like many of his contemporaries, viewed the *anthropos* as the archetype of humanity, Adam, which had fallen at the beginning of the creation.

The soul of the world. The totality of the life force existing behind the outward shell of the material world constitutes an entity called the *anima mundi,* or soul of the world. It could also be called the all-life. In this soul we are all connected, all related, as the American Indians say.

These are the concepts that come into play when we build an herbal approach based upon the doctrine of signatures. They are somewhat different from those used to build an approach based on dreamtime, and certainly different from those predicated by modern science. They are, however, akin to the type of thought which lies behind the construction of archetypal classification systems—the subject of our next chapter.

Half of the sea becomes earth,
half the flash of lightning.

HERAKLEITOS THE DARK

Elements, Temperaments, and Constitutions

The Hippocratic movement was contemporary with the appearance of Socrates, Plato, and Aristotle, about 400 B.C.E. Like the philosophical tradition, it represented the emergence of intuitive and rational modes of thought out of the old mystery schools and temples. We have already seen how the basic method of Hippocratic medicine developed out of the ancient quest for a healing vision or dream. There were other strands of tradition in the Hippocratic corpus as well. One was the emphasis on temperaments or constitutions.

The doctrine of signatures places the emphasis on pattern, but it does not organize patterns into an overall classification scheme. Instead, signatures remain like dreams, a tumble of different messages without order. One of the most characteristic ingredients of ancient and traditional medicine is the use of a set of basic patterns, "elements", or constitutions. We have the four elements of Greek and Western philosophy, the four directions of American Indian medicine, the five phases of Traditional Chinese Medicine, and the three doshas of Ayurveda. Similar systems are found in Africa and Polynesia, so we can speak of this as a universal component of traditional medicine.

These primal organizational themes give us a fixed set of patterns to work with in classifying disease, organs, and medicines. However, they have a much deeper meaning as well. The psychiatrist C. G. Jung, working with the Western tradition of four elements, pointed out the inner satisfaction and holism which the fourfold symbol or *quarternio* carries for the psyche. The mandala or cross represents the primary psychologi-

33

cal functions which he catalogued: rational thinking, intuition, emotive feeling, and physical sensation. Thus, it is a symbol of wholeness, unity, and integration.

There is also deep psychological and spiritual significance in the other plans used in traditional medicine. The fivefold system used in China can be arranged as a five-pointed star. This is also an ancient symbol. It does not represent wholeness, but change and transformation. The threefold classification is likewise of great significance. Three often represents two opposite qualities and the relationship or reconciliation between them. Finally, we have the two opposites of *yin* and *yang,* or water and fire, or *mercurius* and *sulphur,* which represent basic polarity.

These primal classification schemes relate to basic functions within the body-psyche continuum, and are therefore important in bringing about healing, although they are not used in conventional medical practice. Such symbols strike us at a deep level as intuitively real, though they may not be real in a strictly materialistic or rational sense. That is not their prime function. They are a part of the mythopoetic universe which is essential to our wholeness.

The American Indians deeply value the idea of the four directions of the medicine wheel. Each of the four directions represents a department of life, a psychological function. This is one area where the Indian and the European approaches dovetail rather nicely. In fact, the colors of the four directions are identical to the colors of the four temperaments (red, yellow, white, and black).

The Four Humors

It is likely that the doctrine of the humors is based on a mythological construct native to the Greek mystery schools, reflecting ancient shamanic thought rather than the result of strict medical observation. The humors represent more of a psychological truth than a physical reality. The way in which they are used in Greek medicine, however, is simply empirical. During the healing crisis which results from fasting there is a discharge of the humors that are in excess. Afterwards the system is brought back into balance. Health represents a balancing or "tempering" of these humors, but exact balance is never possible, therefore, there are four basic "temperaments" or tendencies in people.

The sanguine temperament. These people possess an excess of red bile or blood, therefore they are robust, excessive in following their impulses, joyful, but lacking in restraints and tending towards hemorrhage by way of carelessness, injuries, aneurisms, or internal bleeding. The principal organ is the heart.

The choleric or bilious temperament. These people possess a surfeit of yellow bile or choler. They tend to be willful, angry, and frustrated, and tend towards jaundice, liver, and digestive problems. The principal organ is the liver.

The phlegmatic temperament. This person is full of mucus, or white bile, and is therefore dreamy, sentimental, subtle in moods, and tends towards sleepiness, diminution of consciousness, lethargy, respiratory problems, and mucus discharges. The principal organ is the lungs.

The melancholic temperament. The black bile (or melancholia) is the most dangerous of the four humors. It is not an actual secretion of the body, but a metaphor for toxic waste products and stagnant, necrotic tendencies in the organism. It is seen in a blackish complexion to the skin or discharges. The corresponding mentality is melancholy (which literally means "black biliousness") and the diseases tend towards inactivity and death of the tissues. The principal organ is the spleen.

The Hippocratic authors also wrote about the healthy or unhealthy effects of climates, geography, and waters, the nature of cycles and timing of disease, the use of simple surgical techniques, and a few basic herbal medicines. They taught the use of purging, vomiting, sweating, and bloodletting in an effort to remove excess humors. It was the last technique which came to be unduly emphasized in the declining era of humoral medicine during the Age of Enlightenment.

The Hippocratic system was based on empirical observation, a basic rational technique of healing through fasting, and a rational organization of knowledge, even if it sometimes depended on intuitive or mythic concepts such as the four humors. It was rightly recognized as the seedbed of rational medicine, even after the original methods had been discarded, forgotten, and misunderstood by the medicine which grew up around its foundation.

The Four Qualities

The ancient Greeks debated about the nature of primal matter, arguing in favor of two, three, four, or five primary elements or constituents.

Herakleitos the Dark gave an especially vivid definition, cited at the head of the chapter. Eventually, the preponderance of opinion came to rest upon four essential elements: earth, air, fire, and water. These have come down to us through mythological and astrological teachings and are still a part of our cultural heritage, though not relevant to the modern scientific thinker.

While some of the ancients were interested in the nature of the absolute particles comprising matter—coining the word "atom" as a result—others were more interested in the patterns which underlay their world. This was the approach taken by Aristotle. He reasoned—or intuited, really—that all phenomena in the world could be divided into four basic categories, or "qualities": hot, cold, moist, and dry. Plants, animals, people, stones, and diseases could all be classified in this manner.

Aristotle's students were satisfied with his overarching definition of qualties and moved to apply them in the world. One of them, Theophrastus, attempted to classify as much of the known natural world as he could. He wrote what is essentially the first book of botany, in which he attempts to classify different qualities in plants and other natural substances according to the four qualities.

Over the succeeding centuries, physicians began to classify medical phenomena and herbs in this fashion. In the second century C.E., Galen of Pergamum organized these efforts into a comprehensive medical system. He taught that the four qualities could be further subdivided into four degrees. Thus, a person, condition, or medicine could be "hot in the first degree and dry in the second." Herbal medicines were then matched to organic problems on the basis that "contraries cure contraries" (hot to cold). If the organism was slightly too warm, this condition was counteracted by the use of slightly cooling vegetables or herbs. Thus, the use of green salads was introduced to counteract the heating effects of the summer—a practice still with us today in Western cuisine. The physician had to be careful to match the relative degree of temperature, in order not to suppress or disturb the innate temperature of the organism. Thus, a cold sedative like Opium was not used to treat overheating in the summer time, but mental raving or pain.

A very important point to be made is that the four degrees do not refer primarily to a gradation of hot to cold, as in degrees of temperature on a thermometer, but refer to the actions of the plants.

Plants hot in the first degree act as warming diaphoretics to remove chill and fever. Plants hot in the second degree act more deeply. Not only are they diaphoretic but they cut through humors and mucus. Those hot in the third degree not only promote perspiration and cut tough humors, but act on toxic heat conditions, where there is evidence of sepsis, toxemia, putrefaction, and deterioration. Medicines hot in the fourth degree plunge to a level of surfeit, where the quality damages or suppresses the system. These agents are utilized in small doses to raise blisters and irritate the repressed system into activity.

Cool or cold medicines also act through four degrees from a superficial level to a deep one. On the most gentle level (the first degree), they are used as food (i.e., salads) to cool during summer heat. On a deeper level (second and third degree) they cool fever in the internal organs, especially the stomach, liver, and intestines. These are especially the remedies which "cool the choler" or the heat of the liver. Some of them are also used to cool inflammation on the surface, as seen in boils and skin eruptions. They also can sedate the mind and calm the spirits. Finally, herbs in the fourth degree of cold dull the mind and senses.

Plants damp in the first degree calm the cough and bring up mucus from the lungs. (Most of these are what would be called mucilages, or slimy medicines that coat and lubricate tissue). Those that are increasingly damp nourish the blood and spirits. Some of them are mildly purgative. In excessive doses they dull the functions of the body.

Plants dry in the first degree help restore the tone to the tissues. These are generally what we would call "astringents" today. In large doses they start to cause withering and wasting.

This system is further developed by the combinations of hot and cold with damp and dry. In all, there are about a dozen basic categories for classifying herbal actions.

Here are some examples of medicinal herbs classified according to the traditional Galenic method:

Hot in the first degree. *Basil, Chamomile, Lemon Peel.*
Hot and dry in the second degree. *Caraway, Cardamon, Catnip, Chicory, Dill, Fennel, Frankincense, Lady's Mantle, Marjoram, Myrrh, Peppermint, Sweet Leaf, White Hoarhound.*
Hot and moist in the second degree. *Red Clover, Balsam Fir, Grape Vine, Olive Oil.*
Hot and dry in the third degree. *Clove, Ginger, Hyssop, Lobelia,*

Mugwort, Pennyroyal, Rue, Spikenard, Thyme, Wormwood.
Hot and moist in the third degree. *Garlic, Fenugreek.*
Hot and dry in the fourth degree. *Cayenne, Celandine, Mustard Seed, Nettles, Prickly Ash.*
Hot and moist in the fourth degree. *Onion.*
Cold and moist in the first degree. *Eyebright, Garden Lettuce, Mallow, Raspberry, Violet.*
Cold and dry in the first degree. *Cabbage, Lemon Juice, fresh Olives.*
Cold and moist in the second degree. *Borage, Comfrey, Cucumber, Linseed, Mango, Melilot, Pumpkin, Purslane, Sesame Seed, Water Lily, Watermelon.*
Cold and dry in the second degree. *Plantain, Radish, Rose, Sumach.*
Cold and dry in the third degree. *Hops, Juniper Berry, Marijuana, Sheep Sorrel.*
Cold in the fourth degree. *Poison Hemlock, Opium, Wild Lettuce.*

Greek physicians and philosophers of the generations following Hippocrates and Aristotle worked out an arrangement by which the humors and the qualities were seen to integrate with one another. They classified the yellow bile as hot and dry, the red bile or blood as hot and damp, the white bile or phlegm as cold and damp, the black bile or melancholia as cold and dry. These relationships could be shown in a beautiful mandala which expresses an underlying harmony.

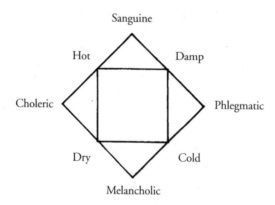

The Four Elements

The ancient Greeks debated on the kind and number of primal constituents in the world. Some speculated that there were one, two, or three elements, while others subscribed to the "atom" theory. Empedocles suggested that there were four elements: earth, air, fire, and water. Plato adopted this idea and his student, Aristotle, modified them into the four "qualities" of hot, cold, dry, and damp. This model reflects an everyday experience of Nature. Even in modern terms, the four element theory is not entirely without merit: the four elements correspond to the modern chemical concept of three "phase of matter" (solid, liquid, gas), plus the combustible state (fire). However, the four elements also have a deep psychological and mythological basis. They corrrespond with the "four winds" and directions which seem to encompass the known world, and four elemental beasts or beings are often found in archetypal and mythological literature, representing the totality of forces in the world.

During the Roman era the Greek philosophical tradition came into collision with another indigenous but very different Mediterranean culture, the Judeo-Christian. Here again, there were four basic archetypes. The late Hebrew prophets such as Daniel and Ezekiel reported the vision of four beasts before the throne of God: the lion, bull, eagle, and human. These creatures reflect the astrological culture of Babylonia in which the late prophets came to maturity. These are the symbols associated with the four "fixed" signs of the zodiac: Taurus, Leo, Scorpio and Aquarius. Later, when Christian literature appeared, these four symbols were used to represent the four Gospels. The picture of the Creator surrounded by the four beasts, the four gospel writers surrounding Christ, and ultimately of Christ crucified on the fourfold Cross, appealed to the sensibilities to the Graeco-Roman mind, steeped as they were in the idea that the material world was built on a fourfold edifice.

There was also an undercurrent of thought which supported the addition of a fifth element. This is commonly called the *quinta essentia* or "fifth essence" in the Western tradition. The fifth element represented a semi-material, spiritual agency which operated on and through the four material elements to bring about change. It also represented the higher, spiritual nature which transcended the physical world. To what extent these ideas were related to the ancient Indian concepts is unclear, but the Vedic or Hindu seers also maintained a system of four material elements and a fifth spiritual element, the *akasa*.

The four-element theory remained unchallenged until the appearance of Paracelsus and his system of three primal alchemical substances. Paracelsus did not deny the existence of the four elements, but he reduced their importance. He saw the world as composed of primal substances which were bound together by the life force, but which were separated into inanimate pieces after the death of the body. These primal substances were driven out into the open by the action of fire. As he explains, "that which burns is *sulphur,* that which goes up in the smoke or vaporizes is *mercurius,* and that which remains in the ash is *salt.*" These had their closest material analogues in oil, distilled spirits, and ash, salts, or precipitates.

The Paracelsian view differed from the Greek four element theory in that it was based upon a chemical way of looking at the world. The Greek tradition was more interested in the philosophical harmony and psychological wholeness inferred by looking at the creation as it was, without breaking it down into invisible particles. Chemistry did not develop any further than simple cooking, where one saw the four elements change. People had not yet observed the derivation of hidden elements out of the break-down, decomposition, or destruction of the world into invisible components.

The Paracelsian paradigm represented the beginning of a chemical worldview, a move away from a holism based on looking at Mother Nature as she presented herself, towards an emphasis on chemical reduction to finer parts. Paracelsus rightly saw that his system was intrinsically different from the four element theory. In the years after his death, the Paracelsian tripartite system and the four element theory battled it out for supremacy, until the whole idea of primal elements seemed to become a delusion for intelligent thinkers and chemists. At the same time, the first of the modern chemical elements began to be discovered. As a result, the earlier paradigms were abandoned. It was not appreciated that they were mythopoetically relevant and even chemically accurate for people working with cruder tools.

One of the curses of the Western system of science as it developed was a disregard for the achievements of past generations, as if people were innately deluded or less knowledgable because they were not privy to current knowledge. This is an absurd chauvinism, discounting the hard-wrought results of experience in favor of current theories and consensus opinion.

By contrast, Traditional Chinese Medicine absorbed opposing systems to build an edifice based on more subtle ideas. The American Indians, in placing value on the "ancestors," or those who have gone before, also would not countenance such a lack of respect towards other generations, times, and world views.

The Four Psychological Functions

C. G. Jung worked out a psychological model which resembled the four-element theory of the Western tradition. He identified four different psychological types, functions, or ways of looking at the world which were implicit or suggested in the four elements. As evidence of the mythological basis of these psychological patterns, Jung turned to alchemy. This may have been more intellectually acceptable than astrology or tarot, but the closest analogue to Jung's thought appears in these systems, where the four elements are treated as psychological entities. Thus, after Jung's work was published and digested, it was assimilated back into these metaphysical systems.

The principle difference between the traditional approaches in astrology, tarot, and the American Indian medicine wheel, is that each element or direction is looked upon as an entire department of life, with psychological, physical, and social references. Jung instead saw four psychological functions or ways of looking at and adapting to the world.

Jung named the four functions intuition, thinking, feeling, and sensation. (We are, of course, dealing with the English terms used in translation, which are not as expressive as the original German.) Everybody has all four functions, but there is a tendency to favor one. The intuitive person tends to look for connections, patterns, and relationships between different objects and people. He or she tends to see how a pattern will work itself out in human society, in individual psychology, or even in the physical organism. The thinking person looks for what makes sense according to deductive reasoning and rational thought. The pattern does not matter as much as the logic behind the process. The feeling person does not care whether the experience makes sense or fits a pattern, but what it feels like emotionally. (Unfortunately, English is a little ill-prepared for these concepts. "Feeling" is used to describe emotional experiences, physical sensations, and intuitive "hunches.") Sensation people are somewhat more difficult to recognize or define. They do not look for the pattern, the logic, or the feeling, but learn from the sensation of what they are doing. These people are the ones who have to learn from experience. Theirs is a hands-on knowledge, a physical feeling of "what it felt like," which helps them to proceed from one experience to the next. They have a hard time trying to explain why they did something or what somebody else should do; they would rather just show you how to do it. And if they have not had the experience, they will not attempt to explain it. The four functions match the four elements: intuition (fire), thinking (air), feeling (water), and sensation (earth). Jung laid out the four functions on a cross, as follows:

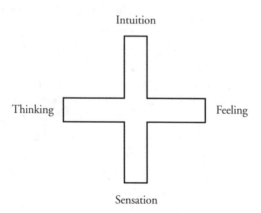

Jung found that each person tended to have a dominant function, a secondary function that he or she was fairly good at using to supplement the first, a third function that could support the others, and an "inferior function" that was difficult to grapple with or use with ease. This function was the Achilles' heel of the psyche. On the cross, the inferior was always the one opposite the dominant function. The two supporting functions were on either side.

In addition to these four functions, Jung identified a fifth which he called the "transcendent function." He placed this in the center of the cross, or *quarternio*, like the quintessence. This function was not immediately available to ordinary consciousness, but through special development or critical experiences, it could be brought to bear on solving the issues of life. This function tended to look above and go beyond ordinary functioning with the four regular faculties of the psyche. These, after all, tended toward domination and inferiority. The "transcendent function" was so named because it jumped above these prejudices and brought in new solutions for the soul. Jung identified this function with the "active imagination," or the imaginative faculty actively used.

Jung wrote extensively on alchemical symbolism, attempting to show how the four psychological functions were suggested in the mythopoetic universe of the past. It is ironic that he utilized the alchemical tradition, which is largely dualistic or tripartite, rather than ancient philosophy. In his works on the subject Jung attempted to show that the three substances of Paracelsus were actually derived from the four elements. This is simply not true. Had Jung known more about the American Indian concept of the four directions, his mythological argument would have been enriched from this direction as well. The "medicine wheel" also represents four departments of life and the totality of a whole life.

The Five Phases

The ancient Chinese philosophers and doctors seemed to have first worked with a model based on *yin* and *yang*. Another school appeared which saw the world in terms of five elements, or phases of transition, really. These two schools fought it out for a while, but succeeding generations just took what was good from both, and integrated them into a single system. To this day, Chinese medicine has a fluidity and adaptability which shows evidence of this open-minded, synthesizing approach to knowledge.

The Chinese have five basic elements, instead of four. Essentially they have put the "fifth essence" found in the Western and Ayurvedic tradition on an equal footing with the other four. These five elements are wood or wind, fire, earth, metal, and water. The fifth element of the Chinese system is wood or wind, since wood is organic and changing, while wind brings in movement and change. Metal corresponds to the Western element of air, which is sometimes associated with metal (as in the tarot deck.)

By adding the fifth element, the Chinese set up a system which is geared towards showing change and transformation. This is appropriate, since the "fifth essence" is the one responsible for change in both traditions. Because of the emphasis on change, many people feel that the five elements of China ought to be represented as five "phases," or states of change. This word is beneficial in separating the two different systems.

When the Chinese put the five elements into the shape of a mandala, they put earth in the middle. The Chinese sages evidently felt that earth was the element that served as the foundation upon which the other elements rested. In ancient China the rich land in the center of the country supported the rest of the kingdom. In Chinese medicine, the earth element is associated with the digestive and assimilative functions (stomach and spleen) which occupy the center of the body, more or less. There is also the point that the spleen "stores the thoughts" or images, and thus serves as a sort of switchboard for mental functioning.

All of these associations, but especially the last, show that the ancient Chinese sages were thinking of the connection between the earth and the Underworld. To place the earth element in the center, as is done in China, is equally as good as placing the quintessence in the center, as is done in Ayurveda and the West. It is as if one system placed Nature in the center, where the other places Spirit.

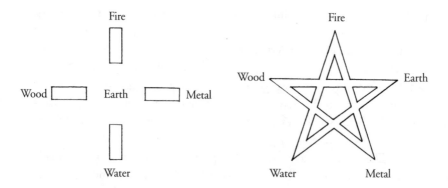

One of the most important applications of the five phase system for herbal medicine is in the area of tastes. The five phases are associated with the five basic flavors received by the human tongue: bitter (fire), sweet (earth), pungent or acrid (metal), salty (water), and sour (wind). Although the flavors fit the elements neatly, they function very pragmatically, as guides for knowledge about herbal properties. The bitter flavor in large doses stimulates heat and activity; in small amounts it sedates heat. The sour flavor is puckering and affects the tone of the tissues, adjusting the tension, which is related to the liver and gallbladder. It also helps sedate fire. The sweet flavor in moderate doses is nourishing, building blood, *chi,* and tissue. It acts particularly on the stomach and spleen, or digestion and assimilation. In excess, these organ systems are destroyed. The pungent or acrid flavor is what we usually associated with culinary herbs (Oregano, Thyme, Curry, Cumin, etc.). It acts directly on the respiratory tract to stimulate function and raise mucus. It also removes gas from the stomach and digestive tract and breaks up congealed, carbonized blood—which helps the respiration. Its action is aerating.

A perusal of Chinese herbal materia medica shows that the uses of herbs usually reflect their flavor and temperature very closely. Sometimes properties related to the doctrine of signatures are also evident.

It is interesting to compare the Eastern and Western methods of incorporating taste into herbal analysis. The Chinese emphasized the five flavors, while the Greeks emphasized four temperatures. Still later, Samuel Thomson, one of the founders of frontier American herbalism, placed the emphasis on the impression the herb made on the nervous system.

If we place all of these approaches to "taste" together, we have a rather comprehensive way of analyzing plant properties: flavor, temperature, and impression. Since there is no word which accurately includes all of these experiences of the tongue, I have called them "taste." Throughout the text I will refer to these analytical methods of understanding properties.

Yin and Yang

The simple beauty of the yin/yang system is based on the observation that everything has two sides. The word yin designates the shady side of a mountain; the word yang represents the sunny side. By extension, yin came to mean all things dark, cool, damp, hidden, withdrawn, interior, feminine, while yang represented all things light, warm, dry, exteriorized, visible, masculine. Chinese philosophers extended these ideas towards the philosophical horizon. "Heaven and Earth" were seen as the primal forces of the world we live within. Chinese doctors extended the yin/yang theory in a pragmatic way, in order to describe simple medical phenomena.

Thus, beginning students of Traditional Chinese Medicine learn the "eight parameters," or eight fairly obvious categories of disease expression: hot and cold, excess and deficiency, interior and exterior, and yin and yang (which encompass the others). The yin substance in the body is visualized as a fluid which lingers in the interior, sedates the system, and tends to cause heat by deficiency and cold by excess or stagnation. Yang is visualized as a fire which causes activity and heat, tends towards the surface which it protects, and causes heat by excess and cold by deficiency. However, there is the "yin within the yang," and vice versa. The primal fire of the body moves the waters while the primal waters sedate the fire. The primal yin and yang of the body reside in the kidneys, which are thus the origins of fire and water and the gate of life and death. The kidney yin is the primal water of the body which lubricates and cools, the kidney yang is the primal fire which activates and warms, not unlike the renal and adrenal functions associated with the kidneys in modern scientific medicine. Thus, ultimately, yin and yang become quite material and substance-like, and cannot be viewed as mere philosophical abstractions.

Galenic Humors and Paracelsian Essences

For Paracelsus, the plant, the person, and the disease had an innate personality. For Galen and his followers there was merely a relative excess of hot, cold, damp, or dry, without any primal personality. It is no wonder that Paracelsus was treated as a medical heretic. In the centuries following his appearance, doctors and herbalists tried to work out a compromise between the two systems. Thus, the seventeenth century herbalist Nicholas Culpeper differentiated between the "physical" or "manifest" properties of the plant, and their "hidden" or "specific" properties. The latter were often called the *arcana* in the literature of this time, meaning something hidden or secret.

Culpeper noted that using the "physical" properties of a plant—hot to cold—did not get to the core of the problem, but only palliated. He warned, in fact, that such cures based on "antipathy" (opposition) would weaken the system by working against it in a forceful manner. On the other hand, the "hidden" properties of the plant would radically cure. They acted in a "sympathetic" manner (by similarity). The essence of the problem would be addressed by the essence of the plant.

When we are dealing with the subject from a modern energetic standpoint, however, I do not believe that the Galenic and Paracelsian views are so incompatible after all. Many of the Galenic remedies work by affinity to the problem, rather than simply by balancing humors or artifically changing the "temperature." Angelica grows in cold, damp ground along flowing streams, but is warming and drying in temperature and moves cold and damp out of the system. Is the essence of this plant cold and damp or warm and dry? In reality, all of these aspects reflect the essential nature of Angelica and the conditions to which it is remedial.

What is important to distill from all of this is the value of the essence. My friend Fred Siciliano, O.M.D., of Ventura, Ca., coined the phrase "the law of the essence," to take this into account. Although it is possible to palliate or even suppress conditions by the use of medicinal plants, generally they are rather mild, and their action often really does reflect the essence within, rather than humoral balancing or philosophical scheme. This will be demonstrated throughout the pages of this book.

Constitutions and Homeopathy

The battle between the followers of Galen and the Paracelsians can be seen as a precursor to the fight between allopathy and homeopathy. About two and a half centuries after Paracelsus died in 1541, Samuel Hahnemann sought to practice medicine based upon a single, universal principle, the "law of similars." This is the basis of homeopathy, meaning the cure is like *(homoion)* the disease *(pathos)*. Although his ideas differed in many respects from those of Paracelsus, there were also many similarities.

Hahnemann taught that it was impossible to know the hidden, internal workings of the organism. The life force manifests itself through symptoms, and these are the only true signs of the disease which our senses can perceive. The homeopath sets out to find the similarity between the symptoms produced by the disease and those produced by the medicine. This is the essence of Hahnemannian homeopathy pure and simple; there is no place for constitutions, patterns, and essences.

Some of Hahnemann's writings suggest that he was sometimes looking in the direction of the medical essence. For instance, in his early writings he used the word "specific" to designate the exact remedy homeopathic to a condition. Later he discarded this is favor of "similar," showing that he was more interested in the similarity of the remedy to the disease, than in its innate character. Occasionally, Hahnemann noted characteristic symptoms that led to a certain medicine or allowed simple generalizations linking remedies to common problems, but he did not encourage people to look for patterns in the symptoms. This would have opposed the general tenor of his teachings. His successors, however, were eventually driven in this direction.

If we look at homeopathic textbooks written through most of the nineteenth century, we find a fairly exclusive emphasis on symptoms. Towards the end of the century, however, we find more and more interest among Hahnemann's followers in grouping symptoms into patterns, temperaments, and constitutions. There is even some attention to the doctrine of signatures. However, the revolutionary change in homeopathy which brought constitutions into the picture came towards the end of the nineteenth-century through the work of James Tyler Kent.

Kent was a brilliant and original thinker with a strong personality. In his *Lectures on Materia Medica* (1905) he was able to bring the picture, the personality of the individual needing the remedy, so vividly before the reader that his students began to think in terms of constitutions or types fitting the different remedies. Although Kent did not actually introduce the idea himself, his students made the leap based on his descriptions. From this time foreword homeopathy has seen more and more emphasis on the constitution. Finally, at the present time, "constitutional prescribing" is the norm, and the symptomatic approach of Hahnemann is not as commonly used.

Nor Wonder, if by fire
Of sooty coal the empiric alchemist can
Turn, or hold it possible to turn,
Metals of Drossiest ore to perfect gold,
As from the mine.

MILTON

Alchemy and Chemistry

As we have already seen, the move from the four elements of Greek tradition to the three primal substances of Paracelsian alchemy represented a paradigm shift towards a chemical world view, in which the familiar bodies of every day life were broken down into primal constituents which had been hidden in the interior. This heralded the appearance of the alchemical, and then the chemical world view.

In time, chemistry superseded alchemy and the latter came to be associated with fantasy and confusion. However, when the basic concepts of alchemy are understood, the system does make sense and it provides a unique concept for understanding substances and their properties. The alchemical view is valid, but our Western cultural bias in favor of present verses past knowledge has caused us to lose the thread of alchemical thought, just as the thread of Hippocratic medicine has been lost.

Since alchemy is a "primitive" system of chemistry based on the idea that there is a spiritual essence in the substance, it will be helpful to discuss it here. That is part of the vision of plant properties communicated in this book. We will find both physical conditions and medicinal plants which are better described by alchemical terminology than by any other. Traditional Chinese Medicine relies upon a Taoist alchemical system because it provides some useful vocabulary. We also will learn a great deal from the modern chemical viewpoint which superseded its predecessor.

Alchemy

Alchemy began with simple chemical operations such as cooking, paint and dye manufacturing, glass-making, and metallurgy. The early metallurgists noticed that the ores they were refining could be defined into two categories: the essence, or pure metal, which was malleable and fusible; and the impurities in the ore which separated out. These were named *mercurius* and *sulphur,* because the former metal was malleable and fusible even at room temperature, while the later substance burned and smelled, like an impurity. From Europe to China, Cinnabar (HgS) was held in great esteem, since it contained both these materials.

Generalizing from metallurgical experience, early scientists speculated that there was an essence or mercurius in all living and nonliving material. It was incorruptible, spiritual, refined, the source of genetic types. Heat separated it out from the unrefined ore. In organic materials, heat was used to distill and set aside this essence. All substances isolated by distillation over heat, such as alcohol, were thought to contain the essence or "spirit" of a thing—hence our word "spirits" for liquor. All substances were also thought to contain the combustible material as well. This burned off and could not be reclaimed. It was likened to the life force, which burns and is consumed.

At a later date, the concept of a third substance evolved. This was called *salt.* It was considered to be analogous not only to the physical body, but to the spiritual body which would resurrect after the death of the physical vehicle. The last judgment was viewed as an inescapable fire, from which the purified spiritual body would arise. From ancient time, salt had been used as a metaphor for character. Jesus says, "have salt," meaning spiritual strength, character, staying power. We still say a person with character is "a salty dog."

The doctrine of three primal psychological components is as old as the earliest surviving literature, and as current as the work of Freud. The descriptions, the angles on these elements change somewhat, according to the perspective taken by the viewer, but essentially we have a higher, spiritual self, a conscious, everyday self, and a subconscious, instinctive self. The three selves are an element of shamanic tradition as well as psychology, as shown by Max Freedom Long in *The Secret Science Behind Miracles* (1948).

Far from being a labyrinth of confusing ideas, either on the psychological or the chemical level, it turns out that alchemy is actually a simple, practical approach to both. If all one had to work with was a primitive fire and a few pots, the model is sufficient. However, alchemy is distinguished from chemistry in that the primal substances are given spiritual, as well as physical correspondences.

The Chinese entertain a similar concept of "three precious substances." The first substance is the *jing*, or essence, which is also considered to be analogous to mercury and purified metals in general. The second is the *chi*, or energy, also associated with sulphur. The third is the *shen*, meaning "spirit" or "mind."

The English word "spirit" is quite poorly defined. Generally, it means something vaporous and insubstantial. This meaning is related to the *mercurius*. However, it also means someone with a lot of character, vision, or staying power, like a "spirited horse" or an athlete who's "got a lot of spirit." The German word *gheist* represents this second meaning. We can see that these represent two different ways of viewing spirit.

In Chinese philosophy the third element is not viewed as a spirit in a vaporous sense, but can in fact also be viewed as a body. There is an ancient expression in the literature referring to the Shen: "In Heaven Shen is image, on Earth it is body."

East or West, the three substances are basically the same. There is the essence, the energy, and the body. Each substance represents both a spiritual and a material factor. That is the nature of alchemy. For quick reference, we can draw up the following chart:

Mercurius / Jing. This is the primal essence from which all configurations or genetic types arise. It corresponds most closely to the genetic/hormonal materials which guide the development, maturation, and propagation of the individual type or species. The bones or skeletal frame are the most dense expression of the essence, since they appear like a blueprint and their maturation is regulated by hormonal unfoldment. When the mercurius is deranged, there are birth defects, incomplete maturation, and destruction of the pattern of the individual type. Often, the bones are malformed.

The essence corresponds to the "spirit," in the sense of something more subtle than the physical. In alchemy, the mercurius is isolated by distillation or evaporation and condensation. It is, however, not actually spiritualizing in a psychological sense, because the essence favors the propagation of the type, rather than the development of personal, individualized experience.

Sulphur/Chi. This is the primal energy which lies at the root of all activity. The chi is often thought of as the life force. However, sulphur or chi is more broadly equivalent to the idea of "potential energy" in chemistry. Any movement or activity connotes the presence of energy; that is sulphur or chi. The life force is only one kind of chi.

On the level of the organism, the chi corresponds to all energy processes, including metabolic processes and that mystery which we call the life force. In alchemy, it corresponds to that which is combustible. Each of us has a blob of energy which is with us from birth to death. When it is all burnt up, we die. The sulphur or chi corresponds to the life force.

In the psychological sphere, sulphur corresponds to the conscious being which is experiencing being alive. This includes not just the conscious self, but the entire psyche or soul which is experiencing life in the body. The soul does not yearn for spiritual experience per se, but for the psychological. Thus, although chi is thought of as a spiritualizing principle, it is in fact, neutral energy brought to consciousness and simply interested in experiencing being conscious per se.

When the chi is operating smoothly, the fire of life burns strongly, there is evenness in the flow of metabolic and life events, and waste products are burned up and removed. When it is deranged, the fire burns impurely, there are metabolic waste products and a vitiated, frustrated, angry psychological life.

Salt/Shen. The third is the principle of embodiment, so that there is an abiding place for the mercurius or archetype and the sulphur or psyche. Salt corresponds to body in a physical sense, but also ironically in a spiritual sense, for it is out of the experience of being in a body or separate unit that experience arises and this becomes "spirit" or character.

The alchemists looked upon salt as the precipitate which remained after the destruction of the body by fire, and in the Christian West they looked upon it as the essential spiritual experiences which remained and arose when the fire of life had been consumed.

In terms of health, salt is associated with solids in the body, but also with the control of water, which is dependent on the electrolyte salts. If the salt is functioning in a healthy way, the person will feel grounded, the tissues will be watered and fed, the waste salts and waters will be excreted, and there will be a perfect balance of solids and fluids in the organism. If the salts fall out of solution, there will be deposits of tartar around the body, resulting in arthritis, gout, kidney disease, and, as these salts pass through the kidneys, diabetes and kidney failure.

The Chinese labeled the three substances as "precious" because they are the foundation of life, and when they are squandered, life is wasted.

During the seventeenth century, emerging scientists began to fall away from the established alchemical models. There was an increasing awareness of the existence and nature of ultimate substances such as phosphorus, gold, iron, sodium, sulfur, etc. The old model was not sufficient to describe these "elements." Unfortunately, rather than preserve the old models which had their utility from a certain perspective, there was a tendency to ridicule them as old-fashioned and deluded. They were a part of a reality in which spirit and body were fused, where mercury meant a specific metal, a class of substances, and a spiritual entity. This was not the way the emerging rational mind wanted to look upon things. Thus, alchemy began to pass into history, and with it, a mythopoetic vision of life and the world.

As I showed in *Seven Herbs, Plants as Teachers,* the seven principal stories of the book of Genesis are mythopoetic descriptions of the struggles and lessons of spiritual life. The story of Noah is the one that refers to the testing of the integrity of the psyche. It features the principal elements of the alchemical approach: the vessel within which the work of remaking takes place, the totality of animals representing the libido or psychic energies ("the Antediluvians are Our Energies," as William Blake said), the three levels of the vessel representing the three psychological components, the top one of which is open towards the heavens, and the four couples (Noah, his three sons and their four wives) representing the four directions. There is also the appearance of the rainbow, or what the alchemists called the "peacock's tail," representing the completion of the work. The threefold and fourfold maps are not incompatible, as Paracelsus saw them, but complimentary. The same could be said of the work of Freud and Jung, dwelling as each did on the three- and fourfold psychological motifs.

Chemistry

In 1663 Robert Boyle published *The Skeptical Chymist,* in which he pro-posed that the three Paracelsian substances were not actually a valid model for chemical work. He backed up his assertions with reference to practical laboratory work, and of course he was entirely right in one sense. The chasm between alchemy and chemistry had opened up.

The seventeenth and eighteenth centuries saw the development of knowledge about simple aspects of inorganic chemistry. In the early decades of the nineteenth century, chemists first began to realize that organic bodies had a different kind of chemistry. This gave rise to the field of organic chemistry.

Through much of the nineteenth century it was still only possible to isolate broad categories of organic substances, such as mucilages, bit-ters, volatile oils, alkaloids, and glycosides. During this period, conven-tional doctors started to classify plant medicines according to these cate-gories. They learned that mucilages had a certain set of uses, bitters another, etc. This was a quite practical classification scheme, following rather naturally in Nature's tracks. It is still used in European medicine and in the more modern approaches to herbal medicine in America.

Bitters. A wide variety of chemicals have a bitter taste and these function together as a class, regardless of their structure. Bitters have been shown to stimulate secretion of digestive juices and hepatic elimi-nation, thus they act strongly on the entire apparatus of digestion. In addition, they irritate tissues and this causes activity. In large doses they cause irritation to the point of fever, in smaller doses they have a stimu-lant effect. At the turn of the century it was commonly believed that bit-ters were a necessary element of the diet. Bitters can easily be detected by their taste.

Tannins. Originally isolated from Oak Bark and used as an astrin-gent to tan hides, the tannins are used (in considerably smaller doses) as astringents to bind and tone tissues, especially the mucosa of the diges-tive tract, the uterus, and the skin. They increase tissue tone, regulating permeability and reducing excess discharges, as in diarrhea and bleeding. In addition to Oak Bark, astringents such as Wild Geranium, Bistort, Agrimony, Lady's Mantle, and Raspberry Leaf contain tannins.

Volatile oils. This class of substances is composed of oils which eas-ily evaporate or volatilize. They are found in strongly scented plants, especially in the flowers. The mints are especially endowed with volatile oils, but many other plants contain them as well, including Garlic, Pine, Cedar, and Cloves, for example.

Volatile oils are often very beautiful in aroma, and many of them are extracted and used in the production of perfume. They are highly permeable, moving through all the membranes of the body and even through the placenta into the fetus. As medicinal substances they are highly reactive, and even a small amount has a strong influence.

These oils have a wide range of important medicinal actions. They are antiseptic, and have therefore been used for hygienic as well as medical actions. Most of them are soothing and anti-inflammatory, making excellent applications for wounds and burns (St. John's Wort, Lemon Balm, Lavender, Sweet Leaf). They can act deeply throughout the nervous system, soothing and relaxing like Chamomile and St. John's Wort, or stimulating like Lavender and Peppermint. As we know from smelling a flower, volatile oils can stimulate feelings and they act deeply on the nervous system, senses, and mind. Some of them, like Lemon Balm and St. John's Wort are used for depression. Sweet Leaf seems to act on the senses themselves. Some volatile oils are irritating (Mustard oil) or numbing (menthol and camphor). The primary areas impacted by volatile oils are the skin, nervous system, mucosa, and the respiratory, digestive, and urinary tracts.

Because they are highly volatile, they are easily dissipated by heating, drying, or preparation, and care needs to be taken in their application. They also combine with each other easily, so that mixing plants together in a preparation can create new volatile oils not found in the original ingredients. Some plants even pick up scents from around them, altering their taste and smell—Sweet Leaf is especially notable. It can taste like a nearby asphalt road.

Resins. These substances are often produced by plants and trees for protection against fungal infection or injury. They are strongly antiseptic and also stimulate local white blood cell production. Descending down the air passages readily, like volatile oils they have an additional soothing and expectorant influence. They also operate on the mucosa of the digestive and urinary tracts. *Grindelia*, Pine, Spruce, Poplar bud, Propolis (a bee secretion collected from tree buds), and Myrrh contain medicinal resins.

Carbohydrates. Plants which are high in carbohydrates, including sugars, are often used as food sources. When these nutritive substances occur in combination with medicinal substances, they can be especially nourishing to certain body systems and tissues. Thus, Chinese herbalism has long recognized sweet herbs as tonic. Some of the common Western herbs containing nutritive sugars and carbohydrates are Raspberry Leaf, Red Clover, Alfalfa, Burdock Root, Dandelion Root, and Solomon's Seal. Carbohydrates combine with other chemicals to form gums and mucilage, a very important class of substances in herbal medicine.

Mucilage. These complex carbohydrates have a filmy, coating, lubricating quality so that in the body they produce an effect similar to mucus, coating and soothing raw, exposed, irritated, dried membranes. Their action directly relaxes the mucosa of the digestive tract, stimulating a reflex action that runs through the spinal nerves to related areas, such as the respiratory and urinary tracts. Thus they coat, soothe, lubricate, and cool the mucus membranes of these tracts when the normal secretion of the body is down. Comfrey, Slippery Elm, and Marshmallow are the most prominent mucilages or demulcents. Plantain, Coltsfoot, and Solomon's Seal are also mucilaginous.

Salts and Minerals. Some plants, like Alfalfa, Horsetail, Lungwort, and Nettles are high in minerals, which make them beneficial as nutritive, mineralizing agents. Some of them contain valuable salts which not only nourish, but enhance the electrolyte activities of the body, thus furthering cellular nutrition.

Saponins. Substances that bond with both oil and water are called saponins, or soaps. They have medicinal properties, especially in the stimulation of expectoration, as seen in Senega Snake Root. However, they also serve as building-blocks or chemical precursors for steroids, cortisone, and hormones. Some, like Wild Yam, serve as sources of chemicals for the body to use in building its own chemicals. Others, such as Goldenrod, Chickweed, and Figwort contain anti-inflammatory properties.

Alkaloids. These nitrogen-rich compounds have a powerful effect on the mind and body, acting as hallucinogens, poisons, and medicines. Strangely, they do not seem to serve any known function in the Plant Kingdom; so that we are left to speculate that they are gifts from Mother Nature to be used in an appropriate fashion. The Nightshades (including Tomatoes, Belladonna and Cayenne) are one clan rich in alkaloids.

Phenolic Compounds. A large selection of important plant constituents are based on the phenolic compound, and like the acids (see below), they vary much in nature and application, making this a less significant grouping, from the standpoint of pattern. However, very famous botanical substances belong to this group, including salicylic acid (Willow, Meadowsweet, Lady's Mantle, Poplar, etc.), the original source of aspirin, eugenol, and thymol.

Flavonoids. These are a class of phenols which are very widespread in the plant world, and fairly important in medicinal terms. They have a number of applications, but the most prominent is an action on the vascular system, which includes decreasing capillary fragility and permeability, lowering blood pressure, and relieving hypertension. Some of them also have diuretic, antispasmodic, anti-inflammatory, antiseptic, and antitumor properties. Simon Mills (1993) writes, "They act as a stabilizing and calming factor in the peripheral circulation, and with additional anti-inflammatory and diuretic properties, their influence is likely to be well rounded." Plants in this category include Rue and other members of the citrus family, Elder, Yarrow, and Hawthorn.

Cardiac Glycosides. Closely related to the saponins which also have cardiac activity, these have the ability to strengthen and regulate the beat of the heart without increasing the amount of oxygen needed by the cardiac muscles. Thus they increase the efficiency and steadiness of the failing heart. Included here is Foxglove, the source of the famous cardiac drug digitalis, Lily of the Valley, and Squill.

Coumarins. The smell of newly mown hay and the vanilla-like flavor detected in some members of the clover family, including Melilot, Alfalfa, and Red Clover, indicate the presence of coumarins, which are a natural blood-thinning, anticoagulant factor. Coumarins are used in conventional medicine to thin the blood.

Acids. Weak organic acids are found throughout the botanical kingdom, but they usually do not exist in a free form. Citric acid, formic acid (the sting in Nettles), and valeric acid (Valerian and Hops) are examples. However, there are many kinds of acids, with significantly different medical properties, so that this constituent does not make a natural grouping with which to classify plant actions.

Anthraquinones. These bitter tasting compounds stimulate the peristalsis of the large intestine, removing constipation. Some of the more active laxatives and cathartics contain anthraquinones, including

Rhubarb, Yellow Dock Root, Senna, Buckthorn, Cascara Sagrada, and Aloe. They often cause gripping and need to be given with carminatives like Ginger.

When the different constituents in a plant are understood as operating together in a supplementary or synergistic fashion, it is often possible to see the "logic" behind the diverse properties of a plant. We thus detect a pattern or personality by which we can use the plant in a specific, individualized fashion. Authors and teachers who understand how these constituents work together can relate the properties of a plant in a way that is fully holistic because the pattern is inferred in the sum total of parts.

Unfortunately, the tendency in conventional science and medicine is towards a fragmentation of the plant into ultimate constituents, without a sense of how they work together, so that no sense of pattern or individuality is seen in the plant, drug, disease, or person. From this perspective, herbs are sources of chemicals only, not useful repositories of knowledge and medicine.

Modern medicine and science has never proved that herbs do not work, they simply have ignored them. The fad of the hour is to break down substances, not into patterns, but into piles of unrelated constituents. Herbs are not ultimate discrete substances and therefore do not fit this paradigm. They are inconvenient.

There are many different ways of understanding how herbs work. If we have an open mind, we can see the crossovers, the benefits, in a number of these approaches. The job of the true physician is not to push an ideology, but to meet the sick person on his or her ground, without judgment, then to reach for a healing solution, wherever that solution may lead, and finally to get out of the way and let nature cure. Sickness is something which has outsmarted the little bit of nature within us, so it is very intelligent. If we hope to contend with it, we have to be humble. It is well to recall the first aphorism of Hippocrates: "Life is short, the art takes a long time to study, observation is faulty, experience difficult to obtain."

Now, ere the sun advance his burning eye
The day to cheer and night's dank dew to dry,
I must up-fill this osier cage of ours
With baleful weeds and precious-juiced flowers.

SHAKESPEARE

Using Medicinal Plants

The medicine plants described in *The Book of Herbal Wisdom* personify various principles, doctrines, experiences, and patterns which are of significance when we follow an approach based on the Wisdom of Nature. Each medicine is a healing agent and a repository of wisdom. I have selected plants which are widely regarded in the tradition, which have been most useful in my practice, or which are particularly important as teaching aides. The selection is somewhat limited. The intention is to present enough herbs, enough teaching aides, to get a good look at how medicine plants operate and how the human organism works from this vantage point.

When herbs are used according to their essence they operate in a manner which is subtle. It does not take much to influence the body or the mind if we have the right medicinal substance. The approach is homeopathic. In small doses herbs stimulate the self-healing ability of the body.

In my own practice, I use plant medicines in small doses (one to three drops of the tincture). This is all that is needed when we are trying to help the body help itself. With this dosage I have seen radical changes occur in a short time, major cures accomplished, as well as the occasional "aggravation" common to homeopathic remedies. This is a very effective way to treat objective physical and subjective psychological problems. Anyone who thinks larger dosages of herbal medicines are necessarily more powerful is incorrect.

If possible, pick and prepare your own herbs. There will be no substitute for the knowledge you will gain from immediate experience of the herbs in the field. There is also no better way to check in with the spirit of the medicinal plants and to start on a respectful path with them. The Indian people traditionally ask permission before picking a plant; sometimes the plants will tell people where is a better place to collect. Some people talk or sing to plants. But at the least feel comfortable with them; then they can slip into our consciousness.

I like to make tinctures from herbs, preserving them in alcohol. The method I follow is quite simple compared to the basic alchemical technique or the official standards in the various formularies and pharmacopoeias published earlier in this century. Like many herbalists, I pack the fresh herb in alcohol, store it for a week to three months, and pour it off through cheese cloth. Occasionally, the dried plant material is preferred (Elder and Walnut bark). This approach is similar to the methods developed by Dr. Robert Cooper, an English homeopath, and Dr. Edward Bach, of flower essence fame, both of whom worked with the subtle properties of plants.

Dr. Cooper would bottle an entire plant in "spirits" at the height of blooming. He called this an "arborivital" remedy and used single drop doses at widely separated intervals. There was a case of hopeless cancer cured by him with a single drop of Star of Bethlehem. Dr. Bach prepared his remedies from the flowers, placed in a glass bowl in the sunshine, until they wilted, then bottled in brandy. He then used small doses (four drops, four times a day). He was a close personal friend of Cooper's son, Dr. LeHunt Cooper, who also used the arborivital remedies, and it is likely that these methods are related.

Dr. Bach felt that the essence was heightened in the flower. American Indian tradition would not agree with this. Following the example of the bear, Indian practitioners consider the root and the bark to be the more powerful parts of the plant. They also look for the part of the plant that looks like the organ or disease.

Generally, plants are chopped up and placed in alcohol to soak for a certain period—three days to three months. This is called "maceration." During the preparation period, store the macerating herb in the dark, unless it is one that likes sunshine—Calendula or St. John's Wort, for example. It is best to have the bottle filled to the top with alcohol so that there is little air to cause oxidation of the preparation. Or, alternatively, cover the top of the liquid with plastic wrap. After an adequate length of time, pour off the liquid, squeezing out the maceration. The "marque" or remnant of the plant left behind ought to be treated with respect. Place it at the base or in a crook of a tree especially set aside for this, or add it to the compost pile.

Homeopathic pharmacy begins with a tincture of the plant which, according to the directions laid down by Hahnemann, is usually made by macerating the fresh plant parts in grain alcohol. This is called the mother tincture (ø), since it is from this that the homeopathic attenuations are derived. These are made by a process of dilution and succussion (shaking). There are several different scales used in this process. On the decimal or "D" or "x" scale, one drop of the original mother tincture is diluted in nine drops of alcohol. This is shaken a fixed number of times. We then have the first dilution, or "1x." If we take a drop of the 1x, in nine drops of alcohol and shake it, we have a "2x." This process is repeated to give the 3x, 6x, 12x, 30x, etc. These are called "potencies," meaning that although they are diluted, they are "potentized" by the shaking and dilution. The other popular scale is the centesimal, abbreviated with a "c." These potencies are made by placing one drop of the mother tincture in ninety-nine parts of alcohol to yield the "1c," then the 3c, 6c, 12c, 30c, 200c, etc. At higher potencies the abbreviations change: 1000c becomes 1m, 10,000c becomes 10m. There are several other scales and abbreviations I have not used in this book.

The quality of the alcohol used will affect the quality of the tincture produced. Dr. Bach recommended brandy, and I must agree from experience that this produces a tastier and better quality preparation in most cases. Most herbalists use vodka. It is important to avoid grain alcohol, cheap brandies, or any other kind of alcohol that is composed by the addition of odds and ends at the distillery. This results in an agent which is essentially a compound. A spectrum chromatograph of good quality brandy will be completely different, compared to a cheap brandy made from the leftovers at a distillery. The first has very nice, definite lines of demarcation, the second produces a chaotic jumble.

Different alcohols have different medicinal influences. Grape alcohol stimulates the circulation, and I do think it helps the remedy get into the body quickly. I specifically recommend E & J's White Brandy. The cheapest kind of vodka should be used, because federal law dictates that all vodka be made the same way.

Medicine plants are not just material bodies to be hurled about at diseases in large and increasing doses, because we guess we have the right remedy! That is not a respectful way to work with plants. (I have often noticed that Indians do not trust non-Indian herbal practitioners, often because of practices just like this.) Nor are medicine plants far-off archetypes or essences removed from our everyday world. After many years of experience working with herbs, I can say that they are power itself. I have seen them change and save lives. The trail they blazed is engraved upon the bodies and souls of my friends and family and myself.

Needless to say, I have had my share of failures in the medical arena as well as successes. We can never be smug or overconfident about healing. Anyone can coverup or rearrange symptoms, or dash around with big doses of herbs used according to the latest scientific or popular fad, but cure is a mystery which comes to us from the hidden vortex of God and Mother Nature. We do not own it; it comes to us as a dispensation from beyond.

The nature of disease is to force us to go beyond where we are stuck. Sometimes that means way beyond this life into the next world altogether. More often, it means a change during the unfolding adventure of life. Change is a deep and profound action which is essentially spiritual in nature. That is why healing, and the herbs that help to heal belong to Divine Providence and should be treated with respect.

Leaves of Light

Under the leaves and the leaves of light
I met with virgins seven.

OLD ENGLISH CAROL

And there were whispering voices in all the leaves,
which seemed to converse with the internal principles
of the breast in their own occult tongue.

THOMAS LAKE HARRIS

The texture of the branches was so even—the
leaves so thick and in that conspiring order—it
was not a wood but a building. I conceived it
indeed to be the Temple of Nature,
where she had joined discipline to her doctrine.

THOMAS VAUGHAN

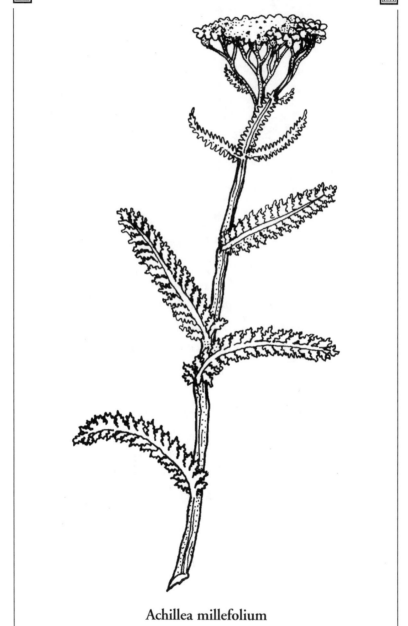

Achillea millefolium

Yarrow

Achillea millefolium

Yarrow

Yarrow is a familiar wildflower found in open fields and waste places throughout the northern hemisphere. It has a long history of use in the herbal traditions of Europe, Asia, and North America.

There is some controversy about the botanical origin of Yarrow. One suggestion is that the Old World species, *Achillea millefolium*, travelled across to the New World, where it met with an almost identical native species, *A. lanulosa*. These two plants are essentially identical and can only be separated by examination of the chromosomes. The former is a haploid mutation, having a double set of chromosomes. However, haploid mutations must also occur among the native plants as well. As far as the herbalist is concerned, there are no essential differences between these two plants and they have long been gathered indiscriminately.

In the spring, the soft, lacy, delicately cut leaves rise like plumes from the ground. They curl over in such a way as to suggest the tail of a squirrel. The Anishinabe or Ojibwe name for the plant is "Squirrel Tail." As the stalks rise, the leaves shrivel. The flower tops are flattened off like a table top or mesa. It is a member of the Asteraceae (or Sunflower) family, so the "flower" is actually a collection of many little flowers together (an inflorescence). They are usually bone-white, though occasionally one finds a clump that is tinged pink, faint brown, or light purple.

Yarrow is widely used in folk medicine. It has found a niche in the imagination of practically every culture endowed with a supply. There are many magical and ceremonial uses as well. Divining sticks are made from the stalks in China. Ornamental varieties are grown in gardens. Finally, it is a powerful medicine plant.

In traditional practice, Yarrow is usually regarded as an important remedy for hemorrhage and fever. It is also used as a "bitter tonic" to stimulate the digestion. The application as a wound remedy is prehistoric. The name *Achillea* comes from Achilles, the great warrior. Homer gives a vivid account of the use of Yarrow. The arrow shaft is cut away, the dried blood is washed out with warm water, then yarrow root is sifted into the wound.

Roman centurions knew this plant under the name *Herba militaris.* In later times it was called "Soldier's Woundwort" and "Carpenter's Weed." The Teton Dakota name for the plant, *tao-pi pezu'ta,* means "medicine for the wounded." Yarrow was used as late as the American Civil War.

According to the doctrine of signatures, the lacy leaves of Yarrow are said to resemble the teeth of a saw. This is stretching things a bit. The leaves feel as gentle as feathers between the fingers. I could think of many leaves which look more like saw-teeth than these—Cinquefoil, Agrimony, and Spearmint for example. The name *millefolium* means "thousand-leaved," as if each finely cut piece were a separate leaf. However, the lacy "teeth" are actually the ribs and veins of a single leaf which has been cut back through evolution.

Several parts of the plant are used in herbal medicine. The young leaves in the spring are full of healing juice. The second crop coming on in the fall is also beneficial. As the stalk shoots up, the leaves die back to inconsequential, lackluster vestiges. The stalks and mature leaves should be avoided. The flower tops picked from plants growing on rough, gravelly soil, produce a poignant, sharp preparation. This is what I like the best.

Yarrow is only slightly known in homeopathy—which calls it "Millefolium." It received a modest proving in the nineteenth century which justified the traditional uses, but an understanding of its genius and applications did not develop, so that it is seldom utilized in homeopathic practice at the present time.

Cuts to the Bone, Cuts to the Blood

I was first taught about this medicine some years ago by herbalist Victor Rangel when we were both working at Present Moment Herbs in Minneapolis. "Yarrow is the remedy for cuts to the bone, and cuts to the third level of the blood," he said. I asked him what that meant. "I dunno," he replied. I guess he was playing the part of an unconscious trance medium for the plant. After thinking about this for some time, Victor cut his finger to the bone. He tried Goldenseal to staunch the bleeding, but it didn't help. Then he put on some Yarrow. The bleeding stopped immediately and the wound healed without complication.

Victor and I speculated about the meaning of "the third level of the blood." We thought it might refer to an idea in traditional Chinese medicine. According to the theory of "hot induced fever," heat penetrates the four levels, from the *wei chi* (surface defensive energy) to the *ying chi* (internal nutritive energy) to the blood and finally to the primal fluids of the body. The symptoms of heat entering the blood level are high fever, skin that is hot to the touch, skin eruptions of a purple or black color, disturbed mind or delirium, a deep red tongue body, and a deficient, rapid pulse. Heat entering the blood can cause the blood to become agitated and spill out of the vessels, resulting in nosebleed, coughing of blood, and blood in the stool. This is called "reckless marauding of the blood."

The symptoms of fever calling for Yarrow are indeed rather similar to this. It is suited to conditions where the mind is sometimes dimmed or restless, the tongue is red, dry in the center but moister towards the edges, and the pulse is rapid, nonresistant and full. It is sometimes used for skin eruptions caused by fever clearing poisons from the blood. Yarrow is especially called for when hemorrhage results from fever.

Achillea has a long history of use in folk medicine as a fever-remedy. After more than a dozen case histories, I can offer a picture of the characteristic patient, though I am afraid we are still somewhat poor in peculiar or keynote symptoms. When Yarrow is required, there is a suffused, reddish complexion showing congestion of blood, the pulse is usually full, nonresistant and rapid, and the tongue red (usually dry on the inside, wetter on the sides.)

An interpretation of these symptoms will help the reader to understand the peculiar genius of *Achillea*. The fullness in the pulse gives the impression that the blood mass has been infected. The full, rapid pulse is seen in Traditional Chinese Medicine as an indication of heat invading the body and calls for pungent, bitter, cold herbs to expel heat. Yarrow is just such an herb. According to Chinese medicine, heat entering the blood causes it to become "reckless," resulting in hemorrhage. Yarrow is for hemorrhage with resulting fever, or fever which results in hemorrhage.

I mentioned the idea of "the third level of the blood" to my friend Halsey Brandt, an herbalist in Bisbee, Arizona. "I know what that means," he said, without batting an eyelash. He gave a different interpretation which is just as valid. "The capillaries are the first level of the blood, the arterioles are the second, and the arteries are the third." This is an excellent idea, because Yarrow is suited to deep cuts which penetrate to the arteries, resulting in profuse hemorrhage of bright red blood. The idea also applies to fevers. The Yarrow fever cuts deeply, past the superficial level of defense, penetrating to the deep vasculature. Yarrow churns up the blood deep in the interior, bringing heat to the surface.

The old herbalists noted that Yarrow both caused and cured bleeding. John Gerard (1597) said that was sometimes called "Nosebleed," since a good sniff could cause bleeding from the nose. Maude Grieve (1931) comments, "It seems to act either way." This is a clear demonstration of the homeopathic law of cure: what an agent causes, it will cure. However, there is another important lesson here. Like a number of good blood medicines, Yarrow both stops hemorrhage and breaks up congealed blood.

The concept of "cuts to the bone, and cuts to the third level of the blood" also ties in with the doctrine of signatures. One year I was teaching a class in Oregon. One of the students, Malcolm Gardner, was an experienced botanist. He was dissatisfied with my meager rendition of signatures for this plant and suggested another. The lacy "leaves" are actually a single leaf which has been cut back to the rib or vein through evolutionary processes. The plant itself is literally cut to the bone and the artery.

Yarrow is particularly good for blood blisters or bruises associated with bleeding. Here it should be compared with Arnica. This homeopathic and herbal remedy is suited to bruises without bleeding, since it irritates exposed capillaries, causing them to bleed. This causes a black-and-blue mark around the cut—another example of something causing what it cures. Yarrow has more affinity to cuts and bruises of violent origin; it is "the wounded warrior remedy." Arnica, on the other hand, is suited to bruises, strains, sprains, and overexertion.

One of my students, Pam, became a real expert in the use of Yarrow as an antihemorrhagic and wound medicine. The first time she had an opportunity to use it occurred on a family outing at the cabin up north. She was taking a leisurely sauna. When she got out, one of her friends notified her that her twelve-year-old son had a severe cut on the lip. He fell off a swing and it hit him on the return. He had developed a huge blood blister on the outside of the lip. There was slight bleeding on the inside. "I was picking Yarrow that morning," Pam noted. "So why not use it?" She applied a Yarrow poultice and the swelling went down while she was watching. Her son could hardly believe it. "He looked at me and I looked at him. Could it work that fast?" She had to apply it an hour later, when the swelling started up again. That was all that was needed. When her son woke up the next day, he had no discolored skin or swelling, no black eyes, and only a little mark at the lip.

A more dramatic case was supplied by Pam's husband. He was out cutting wood with a chainsaw when a birch sapling snapped back and smashed him in the nose with such force that it knocked him to the ground, where he lay unconscious for a few seconds. He awoke to find blood gushing from his nose in all directions. Fortunately, the chainsaw had not injured him. He knew enough to put on Yarrow compresses and the next day there was only a small mark. He got back home the next day. "See anything different about my nose?" he asked Pam casually. She started to lift her finger to his nose. "Don't even think of touching it," he said. "It doesn't look bad, but it hurts."

Another student was a little less fortunate and gave himself a nasty cut with a chainsaw. It was three and a half inches long, extending down to the shin bone, the width of a chainsaw blade. He was too freaked out to look at it for the first ten minutes and went on working. By that time the margins of the cut were swollen and purple and his pants were soaked with blood. He walked to the edge of the woods, picked some Yarrow leaves, chewed them thoroughly and placed them on the cut. Every few minutes he changed the dressing. The bleeding stopped, the swelling disappeared, and the pain went away—all within fifteen minutes! He was astonished. The next day the lips of the wound were joined together. I saw it the following day and it looked like a little cut. A month later there was a red mark but no scar.

Yarrow seems to actually help the arteries suck up blood that has flowed out through a torn vessel into the tissues. The importance of this should be considered in something like an acute brain aneurism. The brain tissue is destroyed by the blood flooding out from the ruptured vessel. In some cases, the leakage is slower, but death is usually sudden.

One of my students called me for advice. A friend of hers had just been taken to the hospital unconscious from an aneurism in the brain. "I knew that if he was conscious, he would have wanted me to give him herbs," she said. She went down to the hospital, pretended to be a member of the family, and starting dripping Yarrow, Wood Betony, and Dr. Bach's Rescue Remedy onto his lips. She told the man's children to continue after she left. Although the doctors were not expecting him to regain consciousness, he woke up after a week. After several months of medical therapy he regained most of his previous functions. Two years later he has problems with his short term memory.

This same student also saved the thumb of a man who caught it in a log-splitter and the thumb of another woman who got hers caught in a meat grinder at a butcher shop. In both cases she gave Yarrow and St. John's Wort.

Although Yarrow is not widely advertised as an important wound-wort by the herbal products industry, I have talked with a great number of practicing herbalists and found that many of them have had remark-able healing experiences with this plant.

In addition to stopping bleeding caused by trauma, Yarrow is also suited to fevers which cause bleeding. According to traditional Chinese medicine, heat enters the blood and causes it to get agitated, so that it can overflow from the vessels. This is called "reckless heat marauding." I have few experiences with this malady, so I will refer to another writer for some dramatic case histories.

Dr. E. B. Nash (1905) was one of the few homeopaths who used Yarrow, but it is noteworthy that he learned about it from a lay herbal-ist—his grandmother. "When a young man I was troubled for a long time with frequent attacks of profuse epistaxis," he writes. "Dr. T. L. Brown prescribed for me several times, but without success. I became weak from loss of blood. Finally my old grandmother told me to chew yarrow root, and showed me the plant growing in my father's yard. I did so and was quickly cured." Later he put this knowledge to work in his own practice. "While on my vacation at Blue Mountain Lake, in the Adirondacks, I met a man there in the last stage of consumption. He had his medicine from his doctor in New York with him. He was spitting daily large quantities of blood, with severe cough, and his Secale was not able to control it in the least." (*Secale* or ergot was used as a vasoconstrictor in late-nineteenth-century allopathy.) The man implored Nash for help. "Doctor, can you do anything to stop this bleeding?" Nash didn't want a terminal case like this on his hands and he was on vacation anyway, so he gave some simple advice while blowing off his acquaintance. "I stooped down...pulled up a little root of yarrow growing at our feet, handed it to him and told him to chew it. He looked surprised, but did so, liked the taste of it and kept on chewing. It stopped his bleeding and soothed his cough so much that he dug up a basket of yarrow and took it home with him. That controlled the bleeding. He went to Florida for the winter, but died the next spring." Yarrow did not cure tuberculosis, but palliated the symptoms.

The cutting quality of Yarrow extends to the nonmaterial level as well. Richard Katz and Patricia Kaminski of the Flower Essence Society (FES) cite Yarrow and Pink Yarrow as flowers for psychic protection. Almost every line of flower essences contains Yarrow, so it is a highly thought of remedy in this tradition. FES also recommends "Yarrow Special Formula" for use in problems caused by radiation. This flower essence is made in a carrier of sea salt water. Flower Essence practitioner Yolanda LaCombe of Los Angeles says, "It has a beneficial effect not only on nuclear radiation but also from radiation therapy or electromagnetic smog." She cites one case where a fourteen-year-old girl was environmentally ill and highly sensitive to electromagnetic energy. She had to stay home and was taught by a tutor. Very gradually, the Yarrow Special Formula was introduced. Eventually she was able to attend school half time. Yarrow is also used to heal burns. It is excellent for radiation burns and deeply penetrating burns.

American Indian practitioners have used Yarrow to revive people from a coma. This makes a great deal of sense, since a good sniff of the flowers make a sharp impression on the senses. Yarrow both dulls pain and heightens consciousness. In a similar manner, it causes bleeding, stops bleeding, and breaks up stagnant, coagulated blood. Such opposite traits are common in herbal medicine.

A Deep Fever Medicine

In addition to its properties as a woundwort, Yarrow is suited to many acute febrile conditions. It has a bitter and pungent flavor, a cold, dry temperature and a sharp, biting impression. Gerard called it "meanly cold." These properties indicate a plant which is suited to sudden, violent invasion of "external pernicious influences," to use the Chinese phrase. It contains volatile oils and bitter principles which stimulate the mucosa of the respiratory tract. Yarrow has long been used in traditional herbalism for acute conditions such as cold, fever, flu, and bronchitis.

Richard Hool (1922), a Lancashire herbalist, is one of the few writers who left a detailed description of the specific indications calling for *Achillea* in fever. The symptoms, he says, include a hot, dry, and constricted skin. There is arterial excitement resulting in restlessness, wakefulness, and delirium. He says Yarrow causes the skin to become soft, moist, and flexible while making the mind calm and rational and inclining to sleep. He combined one part each of Angelica and Yarrow as an all-purpose fever remedy.

I would like to add a few additional indications from personal experience. The pulse is highly characteristic. It is usually full, rapid and nonresistant. The quickness indicates heat, the fullness reflects the infection of the blood mass, and the nonresistance shows that the heat is overwhelming the defensive perimeter and "having its way" with the system. The tongue is red, drier towards the center, wetter towards the outside and seldom coated. This shows that heat is attacking the fluids in the interior of the body and driving them off through the exterior. The face is often flushed, as if the patient had been out in the wind. This is common to the sanguine or bloody temperament, and to remedies for "heat in the blood," such as Wild Indigo, Echinacea, Safflower, and Arnica. It results from congestion of the capillaries of the cheeks and face. Often, the Yarrow personality has a ruddy, robust, sanguine complexion even in health.

In my practice, Yarrow has proven to be as valuable as Aconite and Belladonna, the two well-known homeopathic remedies for fever. The characteristic symptoms for these remedies are distinctive. The Aconite personality has a rapid, bounding pulse that feels like the back of a deer jumping over a fence, indicating that the blood wants to force its way out of the vein. This was the classical indication for bloodletting in ancient and medieval medicine. The Arab physicians described this as the "gazelling pulse." The use of Aconite by homeopaths, and later by allopaths was credited as one of the practices that brought a close to the era of bloodletting. The Belladonna personality has a throbbing pulse and arteries, the characteristic "strawberry tongue" with inflamed big red points, often showing through a thin coating, eyes dilated, sensitive to light, with moaning and delirium. These remedies should be compared with Sweet Leaf *(Monarda fistulosa)* and Elderberry *(Sambucus* sp.) to provide a wide selection of fever remedies. The former is characterized by damp, clammy skin, with heat in the interior. The latter has dry, red skin on the cheeks, but also some evidence of stagnant blood—a blue, perhaps swollen aspect over the bridge of the nose and mottled red and pale skin in the forearms, calves, and other parts of the body.

Here are a few experiences from my own practice showing how yarrow works. A thirty-one-year-old man had been relapsing into febrile conditions for most of the winter. He was a robust fellow who worked at a gym. Face slightly red, pulse full and rapid, tongue red. A few cups of Yarrow tea removed the condition promptly.

I was asked to make a house call to visit a quadriplegic who was subject to recurrent bladder infections. Recently he started to pass a large amount of blood in his urine. His family and attendants were worried that he was about to die. The complexion was flushed, sweaty, and hot, with an expression of torment and anger. Pulse full, tense, and slightly rapid. I was intimidated by the concerns of the family, so I hesitated and gave two remedies instead of one. My intuition favored Yarrow for the heat and hemorrhage, but I also gave Agrimony for the torture and as an astringent hemostatic with an affinity to the kidneys. Our friend took a few drops of each tincture every few hours. The next day he passed a clot of blood, the bleeding stopped, the heat and sweating went away, and the expression became comfortable. I suspect it was the Yarrow that had the principal influence here.

As I became better acquainted with Yarrow I was able to observe more specific symptoms. A student in one of my classes caught the prevalent flu in the first months of 1992. She was a thirty-nine-year-old woman, robust, active, sanguine in appearance and temperament when in health. The pulse was rapid and hard, muscles painful and achy, fever up to 103 degrees. The only remedy that I know of with this particular pulse is Barberry Root *(Berberis vulgaris),* which is a remedy for intense heat. I gave her the homeopathic 6x potency and within a minute she was more relaxed and comfortable. Now the pulse was rapid and full. I could predict what was going to happen. She would need *Berberis* to remove the harshness of the initial attack of influenza, but the fever would descend into the blood, then it would burn out the blood resulting in red cell die-off. She would need *Berberis vulgaris, Achillea,* and finally homeopathic Ferrum phosphate (for anemia with fever). This was exactly the way the condition transpired; she was back to work on the third day.

This woman had a dream which contributes further to our knowledge of Yarrow. After she took the tincture in the afternoon she fell into a deep sleep (remember Hool's comment about Yarrow bringing on sleep). She dreamed she was trying to turn off a camping cook stove that was burning out of control. She struggled and finally succeeded. She woke up breaking out into a sweat and the fever was relieved.

A "Bitter Tonic" for the Digestion

Yarrow has a strong affinity for the digestive tract. As a hemostatic, it stirs up stagnant circulation in the portal vein draining the intestines. This cleans out the tract "from the bottom layer up," since it opens the drain and allows decongestion through the bloodstream. Yarrow may also be a catalyst to digestion. Biodynamic gardeners report that a leaf of Yarrow put into a compost pile will catalyze the fermentation and get the compost digesting faster. As a "bitter tonic," it tones the mucosa of the tract, increasing cellular activity and secretion.

Richard Hool considered Yarrow to be one of the most important remedies for the digestive tract. "No remedy which I am acquainted is more to be depended upon in chronic affections of the mucus surfaces of the internal organs. Its value in this respect is peculiarly apparent in chronic dysentery, diarrhea, and other diseases of the bowels. When false membranous formations have occurred in the small intestines, produced by the gradual exudation of plastic lymph, Yarrow may be relied upon for their removal."

William LeSassier, of New York City, one of our most experienced contemporary practitioners, ranks Yarrow highly as one of the most important digestive medicines. He uses it for diverticulitis and colitis. It is especially indicated, he says, when there is a crack down the center of the tongue which opens up to display a "chaining" effect (little lines crossing back and forth.) It looks like a little red feather running down the center of the tongue—think of the feathery leaves of Yarrow. "This configuration indicates that heat is burning down to the blood level," says William. It commonly occurs in the middle of the tongue and downwards, indicating irritation of the mucosa of the digestive tract, possibly even bleeding.

I have several case histories that demonstrate this use. A forty-five-year-old stone mason had been diagnosed with diverticulitis. The doctors informed him that he would have to have a colostomy. This was hard for a big workingman to take. When I saw him, he had a mild fever, indicated by the rapid, full, nonresistant pulse, sweat on the brow, and reddish tongue, dry in the middle. (I didn't know William at the time, or I would have looked for the red chaining.) Yarrow tincture, a few drops three times a day, completely cured the condition in a few weeks. His condition is still better, five years later.

A twenty-six-year-old woman had been diagnosed with colitis while she was still a teenager. She was married and had a child. Periodically, she had bleeding from the colon, only temporarily abated by medical drugs. She had a somewhat rapid, full, non-resistant pulse and a red tongue. Yarrow put the condition in remission for two years. "Nothing has ever helped me like this before," she said with real gratitude and a bit of wonder in her voice.

Culpeper considered Yarrow nearly a specific for bleeding hemorrhoids. Hool considered Burr Marigold *(Bidens)* to be a better specific for this problem, followed by Yarrow.

Achillea is sometimes listed as a remedy in adult onset diabetes. It does not have a direct effect on the Beta cells which secrete insulin. It probably helps by cleaning up "background noise" bothering the pancreas. Yarrow thins the blood and decongests the portal circulation which drains the abdominal viscera, as well as the arterial supply in the area. This probably removes stagnation and inflammation affecting the pancreas.

I saw one case where a woman came down with diabetes, high

blood pressure, insomnia, and repeated small strokes, all at the same time. The doctors saw no connection between these symptoms. The pulse felt like blobby oatmeal passing under the fingers, indicating a very stagnant blood supply. She had a red, robust complexion. I tried Sassafras to thin the blood, but the pulse stayed the same, so I tried Yarrow. The congestion started to dissipate. I have not heard back from this woman, so I cannot claim a cure, but this is the kind of case that would call for Yarrow. I have seen this pattern twice more since then. A man in his fifties dropped by on a social call. He had the same pattern. Diabetes set in with high blood pressure and a single damaging stroke. "Did insomnia start at the same time?" I asked. "Why, yes, as a matter of fact." I informed him I didn't want to take on a case like this without some remuneration. He said, "Well, I'm not sure I believe in alternative medicine." He was a nice fellow; I hope he doesn't have another debilitating stroke.

By thinning and decongesting the blood, Yarrow has an influence on the cardiovascular system. The blood pressure is sometimes lowered, the blood thinned, the peripheral vessels decongested. This takes a burden off the heart. The famous French herbalist Maurice Messegue says that Yarrow is "antispasmodic, soothing to the heart and circulation and particularly to be recommended for people subject to angina and pain in the thorax."

In a similar fashion, Yarrow acts on the liver. The organ is an intensely vascular structure, receiving the portal circulation coming off the intestines, as well as a large amount of red blood from the hepatic artery. The liver even fashions a supportive structure from veins. Thus, Yarrow has the capacity to benefit the liver, though the influence is less direct. By increasing the health of the liver, Yarrow would have an additional benefit back on the intestinal tract. It is, as a result, considered a "blood purifier," and Maurice Messegue recommends it for herpes and acne.

An Important Woman's Medicine

Many years ago a woman came into the herb store and sat down by the stove for a talk. She recounted how she had missed her period for three months that summer. She knew she was not pregnant. One day she was walking in a field on the north shore of Lake Superior. She sat down and in a few minutes noticed that her period had started. She looked around and saw she was seated in a clump of Yarrow. For many years I just remembered this story as an odd fact; eventually I saw how it fit into the profile of this medicine plant. Eventually I also learned that some of the most potent Yarrow grows on the hardscrabble soils along the Superior shoreline.

Because Yarrow has such a strong affinity to the blood and bleeding, it is an important remedy in female complaints. It works both ways, to staunch excessive bleeding and to break up stagnant blood. In addition, it tones the mucus membranes of the female tract and reins in heat and restlessness associated with hormonal episodes. Yarrow is a menstrual regulator of great worth. Although it does not have a special affinity to women (unlike Black Cohosh, Blue Cohosh, Squawvine, Pulsatilla, Lady's Mantle, and other herbal agents), it is so useful here because of the affinity to the blood.

In both American Indian and Traditional Chinese Medicine, we have the concept of stagnant blood, or adhesions of blood, remaining after injuries or due to poor circulation, becoming an encumbrance on the system and a source of disease. In both traditions many gynecological problems are traced to retention of blood in the female tract. The idea is that blood, which needs to be thrown off at every period, is retained, causing adhesions of stagnant blood which produce hard, immobile masses giving rise to sharp, fixed pains. Uterine fibroids are considered to be a form of "stagnant blood" in Chinese herbalism. This concept is very effective therapeutically, whatever its merits from a scientific angle.

The most comprehensive account of Yarrow as a female medicine is probably rendered by the late Maria Treben, an Austrian herbalist. She recommended that every woman, from age thirteen to ninety take a cup of Yarrow tea once in a while as a general safeguard. Yarrow will help bring on a suppressed period, will staunch menstrual flooding and will help stir up stagnant blood in the gynecological tract. It is useful for irregular menstruation in young girls, mental restlessness in menopausal women, inflammation of the ovaries, prolapse of the uterus, uterine fibroids, vaginal discharge, and many other conditions. Even women past the time of life can benefit from the herb, she says. Elisabeth Brooke in her fine book, *Herbal Therapy for Women* (1992) gives it a well considered account.

Here is a case history which illustrates the affinities to restlessness caused by hormonal shifts. A thirty-two-year-old woman, seven months pregnant, came to see me when I worked at Crescenterra chiropractic clinic. She was feeling overheated and restless during the last three months of her pregnancy. She was sullen—getting out of an abusive relationship. The pulse was full and rapid, the tongue red, dry in the middle, moist on the sides, the complexion robust. I diluted the *Achillea* to about 1x (one part in ten) because she was pregnant and it is a strong remedy. This cured the condition in three days.

Yarrow is effective as a simple menstrual regulator when there is excessive bleeding. Jessy Diamondstone, an herbalist in Vermont contributed an interesting case. A woman came to her with excessive menstrual bleeding and diarrhea. Tea made from Yarrow promptly cured both problems.

For the cure of uterine fibroids, Treben recommends a sitz bath. About two times a week is sufficient. She recommends that a hundred grams of the whole, cut herb be steeped in cold water all night, brought to a boil in the morning, and poured into the bath. Immerse up to about the diaphragm. I have seen this treatment work so many times—dozens—that I long ago lost count. This is also a good way to remove varicose veins, if there are blue veins and reddish skin on the legs. This approach works best for women with the typical indications calling for Yarrow—a red, sanguine complexion, full, rapid, nonresistant pulse, red and blue coloration on the arms and legs, red hemorrhagic menstruation and so on. The other herbs I have seen cure uterine fibroids are Shepherd's Purse and Trillium. The former has a more heavy, clotted, dark menstrual flow, blue, swollen veins without red color, and a greater tendency to prolapse. The muscles are more likely to be involved when Shepherd's Purse is indicated. Trillium is an active little thing with red hemorrhagic tendencies and specific symptoms established in homeopathy.

I was consulted by a woman in her late thirties, just after an operation to remove a cyst from each ovary. "They were filled with blood, according to my doctor." Since the operation she had been unhealthy. At the time, I didn't know about Yarrow and stagnant blood or "blood blisters," so I gave Echinacea and Wild Indigo because of the possibility that there was some sort of lingering, septic infection after the surgery. This helped for the time being. A year later she had bronchitis with harassed respiration. Agrimony helped for a few months, but the problem returned. The gynecologist also reported that the cysts were growing again. By this time I understood the properties of Yarrow. The woman had a reddish, sanguine complexion. *Achillea* tincture, a few drops a day, cured the bronchitis and the cysts. "I can't believe that it would cure both things," she exclaimed. Her gynecologist couldn't believe it either.

One of my students liked Yarrow a great deal. She had a lot of blood stagnation in the legs, evidenced by thick blue arteries running through reddish skin. This was coupled with a great deal of extra weight in the hips and legs. She'd taken Yarrow tea internally on the advice of a good herbalist, and this had accomplished a lot, emotionally and physically. However, looking at the blue-red discoloration in the legs, I could not help but think that she needed a stronger dose, so I suggested the sitz bath. She liked it so much that she took two baths and three cups of tea a day. After two and a half days she started to have blood in her urine. I told her to lay off Yarrow for a while and resume it on a more conservative basis. Eventually, she lost ten pounds, her legs became less discolored, the varicosities went down, and both her personality and physique appeared to be in greater harmony. She continued on a more gentle regime with Yarrow for several months.

When Stagnant Blood Turns to Bad Blood

Indian medicine people suggest that the stagnant blood resulting from a bruise can linger in the body to produce what is called "bad blood," which may eventually turn into cancer. In order to prevent this, the treatment of bruises is given special consideration. This is why Sassafras is used in American Indian and folk medicine to "thin the blood" and prevent cancer.

The Chinese have the same concept. Stagnant mucus can precipitate into "soft, moveable tumors," which are generally non-malignant, but stagnant blood, they say, can turn into "hard, immobile tumors," and some of these can be cancerous. The same idea also shows up in the writings of J. Compton Burnett, a turn-of-the-century London homeopath. He described how cancer can set in at a site where there has been a serious blow, even a long time previously. Burnett recommended English Daisy *(Bellis perennis)* as a remedy for bruises to deep lying tissues and organs, and cancers resulting from such injuries. Modern doctors have also noted that cancers set in where there has been a trauma from a blow, bruise, or chaffing years before. They also understand that many cancers prefer to grow in an oxygen-depleted, stagnant, venous blood supply. This gives us a great tip to the treatment of cancer. Herbalists have followed up on this hint, but doctors have not. They do not understand the thinking behind traditional medicine, which attempts to treat general conditions of hot and cold, excess and deficiency, etc., rather than specific pathological lesions and entities.

Yarrow is widely used by American Indians, even at the present day, as a medicine for cancer. I have heard this from Winnebago, Anishinabe (Chippewa) and Dakota people. This usage fits the profile for Yarrow. Many cancer patients show symptoms of infected blood mass, or "heat in the blood" as well as "stagnant blood." Yarrow at least proves palliatives in some cases and may prove curative in others. I have not seen it outright cure cancer, as I have seen with Sheep Sorrel, Red Clover, Poke Root and a few other agents. Yarrow is, however, an excellent herb for countering the side effects of radiation therapy and the hot flashes which result from the use of the cancer drug Tamoxiphin. I have seen it stop these hot flashes three times, yet I have never been able to get Yarrow to work for menopausal hot flashes.

One Sunday afternoon I was standing around in Present Moment Herbs. It was my day off, but I needed to buy some toothpaste. Someone directed a man to see me. He was a nice guy in his late-thirties, who hoped that herbs might help him with a patch of skin cancer. As a matter of fact, herbs can help. The patch was about the size of a half dollar and lay on the side of the head, behind the right eye. The area was red, burning and stinging. In a few spots it was excoriated and raw. He told me he had been burned by a fleck of hot metal which flew up behind his mask when he was working with an acetylene torch. The cancer set in at the site of the burn. The tongue was red, lips red, forehead warm and sweaty. It looked like there was a lot of internal heat in the system. The pulse was fine and rapid. Surgery was scheduled for two weeks. I suggested that he might put on Thuja tincture, cover it up with "Sting-Stop" salve (*Echinacea, Urtica,* and *Ledum*), and take some Yarrow tea.

The logic here was threefold. Thuja is an old homeopathic remedy for skin cancer. It is better suited to skin tags, tumors, moles and what not, so it may not have been applicable here. *Echinacea* is used for cleansing and local lymphatic drainage, heat in the blood and has some anticarcinogenic reputation. *Urtica* is a burn remedy. *Ledum* was not relevant, as it is indicated for cold, blue mottled skin tone. Had I known about Sweet Leaf at the time, I would have recommended that. I thought the Yarrow was the most important of the bunch, because it is for penetrating injury, repairing damage to the blood, and lessening the internal heat.

A few days later I got a phone call. "Is this supposed to cure cancer?" the man asked in an astonished voice. What? I responded. "The pain is gone, the patch is reduced by about half and the raw spots are scabbed over." I was quite surprised. "Well, I don't know," I said. He came in and I took a look at him. The lips were no longer dark red, the tongue was lighter, and he no longer looked hot.

The patch on the skin completely cleared up in a week, but the cancer continued to "boil up" from below, causing new eruptions, and he eventually had the surgery.

Wounded Warrior, Wounded Healer

Chiron was the eldest of the race of centaurs and the teacher of Asclepias, Hercules and Achilles. He taught many different ways to heal, including the use of the hand *(chiro)* and the herb. To Achilles, the great warrior, he imparted knowledge of the healing properties of Yarrow. Ironically, both Chiron and Achilles were killed by being shot in the heel (or back of the hoof, in the case of our centaur friend).

Although Chiron was a wise and noble individual who instructed both men and gods in the healing arts, his descendants, the centaurs, became famous for their riotous behavior. Some of them were once partying outside his cave. When Chiron went out to see what all the noise was about, he was shot in the foot. He suffered great pains which could not be healed. It had been prophecized that Prometheus, who had been chained to a mountain for bringing mankind the gift of fire, could only be freed if an immortal was to die. Chiron volunteered for this assignment and Prometheus was freed.

Yarrow has long been considered a remedy for the wounded warrior, but it is also a remedy for the wounded healer. Different herbalists have emphasized one side or the other. Elisabeth Brooke reminds us of its reputation as a remedy for warrior. Richard Katz and Patricia Kaminski of the Flower Essence Society teach that it is good for people who are too delicate, too susceptible to their environment. These polarities belong together. Herbalist Barbara Park, from Olympia, Washington, put it very well to me one time. "Yarrow is a remedy for the wounded warrior. It's good for professionals—doctors, lawyers, therapists—who jump in to put out the fires, but get hurt. It's also a remedy for the wounded healer."

The Magical Uses of Yarrow

Just as Yarrow is a remedy for cuts and bruises, I believe it also has the capacity to act in a deeper, magical fashion, to prevent the tendency to such discomfitures. A person who works around sharp tools or has a tendency to accidents would do well to put a sprig of Yarrow in the toolbox, or amongst the power tools. This sends a message that accidents are not welcome. One sprig in the spring and one in the fall is a good measure.

A tendency to accidents is a good indication for Yarrow. A woman came to me one time for help with painful menses. She experienced excessive bleeding, cramping, and pain. She remarked, "For a week or two before my period I get clumsy and hurt myself." This was something I'd never heard about before—one of those little secrets of womanhood we men don't always hear about—but apparently a feeling of clumsiness is not unknown as a symptom of pre-menstrual syndrome (PMS.) I gave her Yarrow, but I am afraid I didn't hear back on this case. However, since that time I have used Yarrow with success in similar cases and I often ask about clumsiness before the period.

Preparation and Dosage

The young leaves, which appear in the spring and again in the fall, are acceptable for use. The mature flower tops, found during the summer, are probably the best representative of the plant. At least they are the part I prefer to use. The mature stem is somewhat woody and the mature leaves are shriveled, so they add little to the medicinal properties of a preparation and need not be included. The root has been used, as Homer informs us. The plant is more powerful when it is found growing on sandy, gravelly, stony, and light soils. I have it growing on my farm, but the soil is too rich, so I have to pick it elsewhere. Generally, if the plants grow above three feet high they are too well nourished and should be avoided.

Make an infusion by pouring a cup of boiling water over a tablespoon of Yarrow. The fresh flowers make a nice tincture, somewhat sweeter than the leaves, but still finely sharp and focused. Even the dried flowers make a decent tincture. Set the flower tops in brandy for at least a week and pour off. My standard dose is one to three drops. Most people use much more.

A few simple formulas using Yarrow might be mentioned. I seldom employ combinations, but I do not discourage others from doing so. A standard old fever remedy is one part each of Yarrow flower tops, Elderberry flowers, and Spearmint. This can be improved by the substitution of Sweet Leaf *(Monarda fistulosa)* for Spearmint, a vastly superior article in fever. This is a nice combination because Yarrow churns up and thins the hot blood congested in the depths, Elderberry decongests and starts the blood flowing through the vessels towards the outlets while bringing heat to the surface and adjusting the pores, and Sweat Leaf draws out heat, tones the pores, and cools the interior. For fever and influenza, Richard Hool preferred Angelica and Yarrow. I have not tried this remedy; it may be better suited to the climate of Great Britain. Boneset or Blessed Thistle could be added to this formula. Another traditional combination for tension and restlessness, even for essential hypertension, is Yarrow flower tops and Linden flowers. To prevent coronary thrombosis, the *British Herbal Pharmacopoeia* suggests a combination of Nettles, Melilot, and Yarrow.

Analogous Medicines

Yarrow is similar to the other great bruise remedies used in homeopathy and Chinese medicine, Arnica and Safflower. All of these plants have the characteristic blue and red swollen bruise, the red showing that inflammation is active and the wound is recent. Sassafras (the favorite Eastern American Indian remedy for bruises) is better suited to a black and blue contusion. Vegetable charcoal is an old folk-remedy for bruising introduced into homeopathy (under the name *Carbo vegetabilis*) as a medicine for stagnant circulation. The complexion here is usually blue and yellow, showing stagnation, and fitting this remedy better to old bruises. Elderberry *(Sambucus* sp.) has blue and swollen tissue, which occurs more readily in association with sprains in the wrists and ankles. Poison Hemlock *(Conium maculatum)* is used in homeopathy (small doses) as a remedy for the pitch black bruises one sees in old people. As a fever remedy, Yarrow has few good analogues, though it is similar to Safflower.

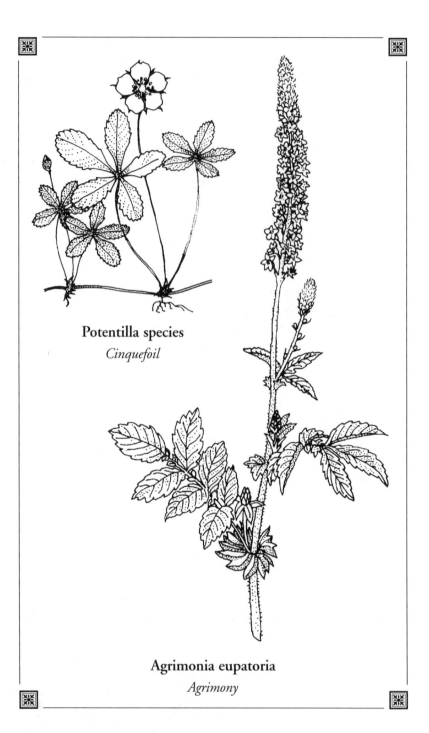

Potentilla species

Cinquefoil

Agrimonia eupatoria

Agrimony

Agrimonia eupatoria

Agrimony

This small woodland herb is a member of the Rose family. *Agrimonia eupatoria* is the officinal species in Western herbalism. It is native to Europe, but there are representatives of the genus in North America and Asia. As a matter of fact, I prefer the variety found in my neighborhood, *Agrimonia gryposepala*. All members of the family I am acquainted with can be used interchangeably. In fact, the closely allied Cinquefoils (*Potentilla* sp.) can also be used in their place.

Agrimony occupies a small niche in the herbal pharmacopoeia of Europe, China, and Indian America. Earlier this century it was brought to attention by Dr. Edward Bach, of flower essence fame. It also occupies an obscure position in the homeopathic pharmacopoeia. Over the years I have used it so frequently, with so much success, that I now include it among the top three or four most important medicines in my practice.

Ironically, from a position of greater familiarity with traditional literature, I now realize that the old herbalists used Cinquefoil or Tormentil *(Potentilla recta, P. tormentilla)* where I would use Agrimony. These two clans, both in the Rose family, have nearly identical properties. This late realization presented me with a dilemma. Should I give an account of Cinquefoil, in order to include the more extensive historical material, or Agrimony, to reflect my personal experience?

In the end, I decided to give an account of Agrimony, with references to Cinquefoil mixed in. Although this is a bit complicated, I believe that the remedies are similar enough that it does not do a great deal of harm to our study. We learn, indeed, from a comparison of source material.

The principal difference in the use of these plants seems to be the association of Cinquefoil with magic. Because the leaves look like a hand, Cinquefoil was used to protect people against meddling, interference, and witchcraft. This gave Cinquefoil a higher profile, and I believe it was for this reason that it was more often used as a healing herb. Cinquefoil is widely used in European, American folk, and Indian tradition.

Having said this, however, I have to say that if there is one plant I know from over a decade of clinical experience to have had an effect which is magical—that is, it will change the environment around the person using it—Agrimony is the one. This remedy also prevents meddling and interference.

Since Cinquefoil seems to have about the same medicinal properties as Agrimony—both are excellent for tension, mental, or physical—it is hard to tell where to draw the line between them.

Historical Uses

The Roman physician Dioscorides (70 A.C.E.) renders a brief description of Agrimony. He says that it is used to cure cuts, assuage inflammation, subdue dysentery, and remove cramps. He gives a more extensive account of Cinquefoil, which was clearly a popular remedy in his era: the root is "of much use" he says. Dioscorides calls it *Pentaphyllum*, or "Five Leaf." This name has the same meaning as the Latin, *Cinquafolium*. The plant Dioscorides describes has been identified as *Potentilla recta,* though it is not likely that the Greeks and Romans recognized much difference between various representatives of the genus.

Dioscorides says Cinquefoil is used to assuage toothaches and clear up rotten ulcers in the mouth. It also stops the flux of the belly or dysentery, acts on "griefs of the liver, & the lungs," swellings and hardnesses, edema, suppuration, growths on the fingers (here the doctrine of signatures has had an influence), condylomata, and skin eruptions. He adds that people use it to cure ague (alternating chills and fever) by giving four leaves for a quartan ague (recurrent after a four week cycle), three for a tertian (three week cycle), and one for a quotidian (one week cycle).

Note how Dioscorides says "people use it" in this magical way, not that he himself does. This is rather typical of Dioscorides: he does not revel in magical uses and seldom speaks of them from personal experience, but he does not ignore them. He evidently felt they may be of importance and did not pass judgment upon them.

The English translator, John Goodyear (1665), rather enthusiastically adds to this account. From him we get a good sample of the magical ideas which surround Cinquefoil. He uses the name *Pentadactylon,* meaning "Five Fingers." This is generally the more common name used by writers interested in the magical properties. He writes:

> *If any bear Pentadactylon about his body, he remains without any grief,*
> *& it helps ye eyes, ye Strumas [swollen glands], ye hardened Tonsillae,*
> *ye Vua and ye griefs under ye tongue, & ye joints, & ye griefs of ye*
> *nerves & ye teeth, & ye Psora got by pernicious famine, drawing down*
> *ye menstrua of ye afterbirths; but being poured on the hands it is excel-*
> *lent good against fears & enchantments, therefore take ye herb when*
> *ye moon increaseth, ye sun arising.*

Agrimony labored in relative obscurity compared to Cinquefoil, but by the time of the Renaissance, it had worked its way up to the level where it enjoyed a modest popularity, especially in Germany. The English herbalists, dependent on the German literature, began to give it some space in their herbals as well. John Gerard (1597) gives a short account. Rather colorfully, he relates that "Egrimony is good for them that have naughty livers, and for such as pisse bloud upon the diseases of the kidnies." Culpeper renders a more comprehensive account. Agrimony taken internally "openeth and cleanseth the liver," benefits the bowels and stops dysentery, helps "them that have foul, troubled, or bloody water," causing "them to make water clear and speedily," and removes intermittent fever. Externally, it "draweth forth thorns," heals old sores and ulcers, and helps "strengthen members that be out of joint."

Gerard and Culpeper describe Cinquefoil and Tormentil under separate headings. These accounts build somewhat upon Dioscorides and the traditional authorities. The one unique point comes up in Culpeper's account of Cinquefoil, where he speaks of his extensive experience using this plant for the ague. "You shall very seldom miss the cure of an ague, be it what ague soever, in three fits, as I have often proved to the admiration both of myself and others," he writes. "Let no man despise it because it is plain and easy, the ways of God are all such." He repeats the information about four leaves, three leaves, and so on, then complains: "A hundred to one if it be not Dioscorides [who said this]; for he is full of whimsies."

This is rather unfair. Dioscorides was merely reporting a common usage which probably led to Culpeper's familiarity with the plant. It was not his style to disparage folkpractice, though he never claims that such magical beliefs are proven. This is, I must say, a truly scientific attitude, well in advance of the prejudice of our own age, when ridicule is heaped on anything which cannot be proven according to some narrow line of rational enquiry.

Culpeper goes on to give the real secret to his success with Cinquefoil. "The truth is…if Jupiter were strong, and the Moon applying to him, or his good aspect at the gathering, I never knew it miss the desired effect."

By the early nineteenth century, Agrimonia had dropped into relative obscurity in England and North America. It was still widely used in Germany, and it was probably through German immigrants that Agrimony entered back into use in the United States. Indeed, in that curious little souvenir of early pioneer history, *The Indian Doctor's Dispensary, Being Father Smith's Advice Respecting Diseases and Their Cure* (1812), Peter Smith indicates just such a source. "An old man of my acquaintance, after a spell of the gravel, which nearly took his life, was for several months unable to retain his urine, but it dript from him continually. He was at last advised by Dr. George Foulk, a German, to drink agrimony: this being the only medicine he used." He was "a well man in a few days." Smith is known to have been read by the "eclectic fathers," and they were the ones who introduced Agrimony back into practice.

It was Dr. John Scudder, the great light of eclecticism, who established the first reliable characteristic symptom upon which Agrimonia could be prescribed ("pointing pains in the kidneys"). By the early twentieth century the properties of Agrimony were well known to the eclectics. Despite this tradition, Agrimony was never widely used by the lay herbalists of North America. Indeed, it was little used by the American Indians.

There is scant mention of Agrimony in anthropological literature relating to Native Americans. I have only met one Indian who knew how to use it as a medicine. "Yes, I was shown that plant when I was a boy," remarked Mark Olson, a member of the Mille Lacs Lake band of the Anishinabe. "The Indians don't use it anymore, they use acetominephin or Tylenol instead." Evidently it had been used for pain.

Cinquefoil also fared somewhat indifferently in the United States. It was used as a charm by some. As a remedy, however, Cinquefoil fell into relative oblivion. We do not find either it or Tormentil in the herbal literature of the nineteenth century. Dr. Edward Shook (1947) seems to have single-handedly revived the use of Tormentil in American herbalism, and Dr. John Christopher (1976) follows and develops on his work.

The homeopathic authors hardly noticed either of these plants, but William Boericke (1927) gave a short entry for *Agrimonia eupatoria* and it became an official medicine in the U.S. homeopathic pharmacopoeia. He recommends it for bronchial discharge, menstrual difficulties, urinary tract infections, and kidney pain. These are probably clinical symptoms picked up from eclectic sources: *Agrimonia* never received a homeopathic proving. I have noted several symptoms generated by the remedy during my use of it, so that we now have a few pathogenetic indications.

The great boost in our knowledge of Agrimony came through the work of Dr. Edward Bach. It was one of his thirty-eight remedies. He developed a psychological profile for the remedy. It turns out that there is a perfect correspondence between the physical symptoms found in eclectic literature, the mental indications in the work of Bach, and the signatures seen in the plant. Agrimonia provides another excellent illustration of the doctrine of correspondence, showing how the psychological and physical properties converge to paint the same picture. It is the great remedy for tension on any level.

The "Caught in a Bind" Remedy

Agrimony is about as tense a plant as you will ever see in our American woodlands. The leaves are sharp-edged, the seedpods are a kind of cocklebur, and throughout, the plant is covered with stiff hairs standing on end. Those of us who find our cartoon characters in the wilderness like to say that it looks like a cat sticking its paw into an electric socket, with the hair standing on end.

I used this image in my classes for several years before I had confirmation of its accuracy. Eventually, I had a case which incarnated the picture. The patient was a twelve-year-old female cat who had been diagnosed by biopsy, two years previously, with cancer of the liver.

89

Through tender loving care and the ministrations of a holistic vet, she had survived in relative comfort. In May 1990, I was called by her owner. In the last several weeks she had started to look sick, withdrawn from the company of other cats and people, moved with obvious discomfort and refused to eat. When I arrived I could not help but notice that she looked like the cartoon cat with its paw in the electric socket. The hair almost seemed to bristle with tension. I had to give Agrimony. The Bach flower remedy (stock tincture) was used a few drops, three times a day. There was immediate improvement. The cat was her ordinary self in five days. Six months later she needed a few doses of homeopathic *Lycopodium* for symptoms of kidney stress, so the problem with the liver had evidently receded. Three years later she remains well. I said to the owner, "Well, I guess it's O.K. if she had cancer, as long as she dies of old age."

The characteristic mental state of the *Agrimonia* patient revolves around tension, frustration, anger, and inner torment. The person feels "caught in a bind," as if he or she is in the wrong place at the wrong time, unable to do the right thing, go with the flow, or be a good person. Often the problem revolves around the work situation. The person is in the wrong job for his or her interests and talents, or working for a frustrating employer or supervisor. This mental tension builds to such proportions that the patient feels tortured. Instead of manifesting this tension outwardly, what is so highly typical of the *Agrimonia* patient is the effort to hide his true feelings behind a facade. He pretends to be cheerful, good natured, humorous—but it is all a facade. Dr. Bach pointed out the mental symptom which I find most characteristic: the patient is more cheerful than seems appropriate. I like to say the person is "torturedly cheerful." No peace, restless, always doing things, busy, trying to prove he or she can do it right, be good, etc. There is desire to live on the dangerous side of things, for drugs and alcohol to suppress his anguish. An alcoholic family background is not uncommon. Flower Essence practitioner Yolanda LaCombe says, "One hallmark of a full blown constitutional Agrimony type is to deal with tension by driving waaay too fast. Then they go back into their life situation with a smile."

Here is a case which illustrates the mental state very well. She was a patient at the chiropractic clinic where I used to work, a thirty-eight-year-old woman, seven months and a week into her second pregnancy. She came down with a respiratory infection, accompanied by mental restlessness and insomnia. Pale and anemic. Hasn't been able to sleep for four nights. Close to tears. "I'd kill for sleep," she said. "My job is to sleep, but I can't make it happen." (Caught in a bind; occupational terminology.) Craves drugs to put her to sleep, the last two nights. "I'd let somebody shoot me, knock me over the head, if I could sleep." (All of this was highly atypical for this woman.) What is the problem? "I'm suffering from anxiety," she reflected. "In terms of calendar. I only have a few weeks left to see people, get things done, before the baby comes, then it will be too late." The respiratory symptoms included the following: one nostril plugged, the other one drips, changes back and forth; paroxysmal sneezing; eyelids red, eyes watering, feels close to tears; no appetite; a slight, hollow cough; breathing restricted, holds the exhalation back. I do not know if the other symptoms are characteristic of Agrimony, but this breathing pattern is typical. *Agrimonia eupatoria* tincture, five drops, three times a day. Mental relaxation was immediate, she slept well that night, respiratory symptoms cleared up in three days.

I had a case where *Agrimonia* produced mental tension. The patient was an eight-year-old-boy suffering from "hyperactivity." I had some success with homeopathic Carbo vegetabilis and the mother wanted more reaction. I felt somewhat "caught in a bind" and gave *Agrimonia eupatoria* 12x, as my next best guess. It caused him to manifest new and atypical behavior problems. He became boisterous, uncooperative, "acting out" a lot at school. He sometimes talked in an artificially loud voice. These symptoms disappeared when the remedy was discontinued. Thus, they may be considered "pathogenetic," or artificially produced by the remedy.

If we analyze Agrimony according to its taste, we do not come across such powerful indications as we do from the doctrine of signatures. The flavor of a good quality leaf of *Agrimonia gryposepala* is faintly sweet and sour, about neutral in temperature, with a moderately astringent impression. It is reminiscent of its cousin, Raspberry leaf. The European genus, *Agrimonia eupatoria,* is also faintly sweet with an astringent impression. Agrimony leaf contains some tannins and a volatile oil. These properties have won it a reputation as an astringent tonic, much like Raspberry, which mildly astringes and builds up the tone of the intestinal and urinary tracts.

In conventional herbalism, Agrimony is not used to release tension, but to improve the tension, the tone, on the tissues. And yet, if we look deeper at these indications, we will see the relationship. Herbalist

David Hoffman points out that Agrimony is especially good for bed-wetting in children who are having anxiety about toilet training. Is that a condition of relaxation of the tissues of the urinary tract or is it a state of tension? As we so often see in our herbal studies, a single plant unites opposite properties together under one roof.

"Constricted Liver Chi"

Whenever we have a mental state where there is anger, frustration, and fighting against the flow or a lack of confidence in the natural progression of events, the liver will usually be involved. These mental conditions correspond with the old idea of the "choleric" or liver personality, in Greek and Chinese medicine. There are also correlations with physical changes in the liver and its related structures in the organism.

The liver receives toxin-ladden blood coming up from the intestines through the portal vein. This would easily kill hepatic cells, if it were not for the life-giving, antidotal supply of arterial blood coming down through the hepatic artery. This balances the portal blood supply at all times. If it does not, liver cells will either be killed by the influx of too much venous blood, or the excess of arterial blood will not allow complete processing of the dirty blood. The autonomic nervous system, through the solar plexus, controls the tension of the hepatic artery (and the arterial system as a whole). It relaxes the arteries after a meal, allowing the arterial blood to flow into the liver. Thus, the liver is able to maintain its environment by balancing the inflow of arterial blood with the influx of venous blood. We can appreciate how the inability to relax, both physically and mentally, was seen to indicate a liver pathology in ancient medicine.

The element of hepatic functioning corresponds with the sphere of influence of the remedy *Agrimonia*. It is called for in cases where the mind and circulation is tense, resulting in the appearance of sharp, shooting pains in different parts of the body. In severe cases, there is damage to the liver cells, resulting in cirrhosis. *Agrimonia* is an old remedy for cirrhosis, as well as alcohol and drug abuse.

It was Scudder (1870) who set the use of *Agrimonia* on a path to certain use as an agent with specific, individualized indications. He noted the "pointing pains" in the lumbar region as a characteristic symptom. His concept of its role in renal affections will be taken up shortly.

Scudder also gives interesting indications for the location of the pain in the liver. "Sometimes the pain will seem to involve the lower portion of the liver." (Perhaps this occurs because the lower part of the liver is more strongly bathed by the toxic-laden blood from the portal vein.)

Agrimony is also associated with the gallbladder, which is naturally paired with the liver. It is a remedy for tensions and constriction in the gallbladder which can interfere with liver functioning, or can result from liver tension. Agrimony is also good for migraines, or what the Chinese call "gallbladder headaches," where the pain travels up the gallbladder meridian from the hepatic area, over the shoulder blades, through the neck and into the head. I have had several positive experiences using *Agrimonia* for migraine, but it is not a major remedy compared to *Chelidonium* or *Iris*.

Although *Agrimonia* seems to have a direct influence on the liver, it also has an influence throughout the body. The Agrimony patient often suffers from problems because of tension in other parts of the organism. Consequently, pain in the liver area is not the most common or typical symptom seen in the Agrimonia person. One of the areas most strongly affected is the sexual-urinary tract.

Constriction and the Kidneys

Constriction in the circulation can become centered on the kidneys. In his early writings, Scudder says that "pain, simulating colic, pointing in the lumbar regions, or uterine pain associated with lumbar uneasiness" is the "strongest indication for agrimonia." In his last writings Scudder was even more positive about the relationship of *Agrimonia* to the kidneys. "Given a pain in the region of the kidneys, and I always think of agrimonia as the remedy." He had seen "wonderful results" from it in long-standing cases where all other remedies failed. "I have found other uses for it, but this has been so prominent that I always associate the medicine and the position of the pain." Nephralgia is one of the severest kinds of pain; notice Scudder's choice of words. "It is a torture that might be borne for an hour or a day; but continued night and day for a fortnight or a month, the sufferer may well pray for relief or death." The urinary problems with which this pain is associated are diverse. "I have seen cases where the urinary deposit felt like pounded glass; cases with muco-pus in large amount; cases where the triple phosphate would make the lower third of the urine turbid as if with albumin; cases where not more than an ounce or two of turbid, dark-colored urine would be passed in the day; and still cases where the normal amount of clear urine of specific gravity 1020 would be passed."

A subsequent eclectic, Finley Ellingwood (1919) gives more descriptive detail of the kidney pains. "Deep soreness or tenderness over the kidneys. Tenderness that seems to be due to irritability in the structure of the kidney. Sharp cutting, deep-seated pain, with general distress in the lumbar region. Pain extending from the lumbar region through to the umbilicus. Inflammation of the kidneys, or bladder, with foul-smelling urine, containing a sediment when passed, accompanied with discoloration, and dirty appearance of the skin. Renal congestion, general irritation of the urinary organs."

Agrimonia is an old remedy for relief of pain from the passage of gallstones and kidneystones. This symptom may be considered pathogenetic. In 1990 a man requested Agrimony flower essence after I had described it in class. The next day he passed a gallstone. I have several case histories which demonstrate the usefulness of *Agrimonia* in kidney-stone and gallstone colic. In 1989 I saw a woman who was complaining of an extremely sharp pain in the right hypochondrium. The complexion was the strained, gray-yellow look which is indicative of *Agrimonia*. The tongue was purple-red, a possible indication for gallstone colic. The pulse was tense. She did not seek a medical diagnosis. Agrimony flower essence eased the pain right away and the stones passed away in less than twenty-four hours.

Tension Harassing Respiration

The constriction characteristic of Agrimony can affect the lungs as well. One often hears the evidence calling for *Agrimonia*. A person holds their breath, letting it out as if it were under pressure—like steam from a teapot. This symptom need not be associated with respiratory complaints. Agrimony people often hold the breath due to pain somewhere else in the body. Horses so often do this that it has a name, "cribbing," and is sometimes considered a serious problem. It is a natural way to get a release of endorphins—natural painkillers—from the brain.

In some people, the tension directly affects the lungs and the constricted breathing is directly associated with respiratory problems. Both

Scudder and Bach used *Agrimonia* in bronchial troubles, including asthma. Dr. Bach gives a case history. "A lady of about forty had suffered from asthma from childhood, and had spent about four months each winter in bed. She had had an enormous number of injections of adrenaline and had been given every type of asthma treatment without effect. She was, like many cases of asthma, whooping cough, and other chest complaints, tortured by her disease. She was first seen in December, 1930, and by the end of January 1931, Agrimony had completely removed the disease. There was a slight return in the winter of 1931 which was easily controlled, the patient not having to go to bed. Since then there has been no trace whatever of the disease."

Here is an excellent case history from my own notes. A forty-one-year-old man was brought in to see me by a friend. He was suffering from "allergy induced asthma and respiratory problems" and used a ventilator constantly. He had a harassing, gagging, tormenting cough, much fluid in the lungs, mucus expectoration, sneezing, nasal congestion, dripping and irritation, watery eyes, and gasping for breath from time to time. He appeared to be tortured, but commented with a laugh, "This is nothing." The symptoms were chronic, but worse in the winter and from changing weather, cats, animals, pollen, dust and mold, smoke, but not tobacco. The tongue was red along the sides with a thin, dry, yellow coating all over the middle, torn off or ulcerated in one spot. Pulse slippery and wiry. I gave him *Agrimonia gryposepala* tincture, three drops as needed, to relieve the torment. Four months latter I ran into him at a party and asked him how the asthma was. He thought for a moment. "Oh yeah, it completely cured it and I stopped taking it." The symptoms came back after a while, so he started using the ventilator. He was going to go back to the Agrimony.

Here's a respiratory case where the condition was probably associated with liver damage from hepatitis. The patient was a pleasant, cheerful, seventy-one year-old woman. She had chronic sinusitis. This cleared up promptly under Kali bichromicum and Kali muriaticum, two good homeopathic remedies for that kind of problem. However, she still had mucus in the bronchial tract. The tongue had a long dry, reddish patch down the middle, surrounded by a yellowish coating; the sides were clear. The shape of the red patch reminded me of the eliptoid ulceration typical of *Agrimonia,* except that it was not ulcerated and it was much larger. The tongue had been in a similar condition when I gave the Kali salts, but more swollen. Her pulse was wiry. I was immediately drawn to the liver as the source of the problem. The woman then mentioned that she caught hepatitis twenty-five years previously. Current symptoms: clearing of the throat, "comes again and again," accumulation of mucus in the lungs, epigastric pain, gums sore and tender, pain in the kidney region. *Agrimonia* tincture, three drops per dose, one to three times a day, as necessary. Two hours after the first dose she experienced pain and soreness "under the breasts...in the lungs and liver." Chills and sweating the next day. The second day she woke with fever, pain in both hypochondria, sore and achy all over, couldn't lie on her right side. "Had to lay on the left for relief." Reduced her to one dose per day. The aggravation subsided after five days. Afterwards she had only occasional problems with bronchial or sinus infection.

Intestines and Skin

Our fun little tension can also extend to the abdominal viscera. This results in a similar way, in ulceration, enteritis, colitis, and bleeding from the bowels. The mucus membranes are affected up to the mouth. Ellingwood gives the indication, "Ulcerative stomatitis, with foul smelling breath." Sometimes the tongue displays oval, lengthwise ulcerations.

Agrimonia has an ancient reputation, both in Western and Chinese medicine, as a remedy for ulceration and bleeding from the intestines and the "lower extremities." It definitely has an action on the skin as well as the mucosa. Toxic intestines are sometimes associated with skin conditions.

The following case illustrates the relationship of this remedy to ulcerations on "the lower extremities." A nurse in her mid-thirties had taken a prescription drug, some months previously, for cystitis. She had an allergic reaction, her heart stopped, and she was rushed to the hospital. Since this time she had been experiencing swelling and burning of the right labia of the vagina. We tried *Apis* (homeopathic honeybee) internally and herbal Nettles externally, but the condition continued to deteriorate. Finally, ulcers started to appear. They were cultured and showed the presence of "rare, difficult-to-treat strains of staph." She decided to take antibiotics, but this only accelerated the condition. By now she was taking drugs for the pain. The ulcers were excoriating away the tissue in small patches, so as to amount almost to a fissuring process. Nothing the doctors did helped her, and in desperation she came back to me. When she arrived she was constricting her breathing from tension caused by the pain, letting her breath out almost like a current of steam from a teapot. More out of sympathy than a need for information, I asked if it "really hurt." "Oh, it doesn't feel so bad," she explained with a smile, as she held her breath. I gave the Bach flower essence and had her put a compress of the bulk herb on the ulcers. The pain subsided within twenty-four hours, she took only one more dose of demerol, the ulceration was gone in seventy-two hours. The remedy also affected her mental state. The morning after taking the remedy she woke up knowing she had to terminate her job—which she promptly did. She felt like it wasn't the right thing for her.

I had another patient in whom *Agrimonia* caused the reappearance of ulcerations on the "lower extremities," so the symptom may be considered pathogenetic. A thirty-three-year-old woman had been given "hundreds" of cortisone injections for chronic nephritis over the past decade. She came to my house one Sunday afternoon, in a rather desperate state. One dose of *Apis* 30x completely stopped the nephritis. However, the damage done by the cortisone apparently had not healed. Two years later she had tension caused by her work situation. I recommended Agrimony—she had the Bach flower essence kit. This produced a tremendous detoxification and release of tension. The next day she woke up feeling like she had a hangover "from a really big binge." Her eyes were dull and glazed over. She continued to take the flower essence. The second day she began to feel itching on the buttocks which rapidly developed into deeply etched, burning ulcerations, situated exactly where she had the cortisone shots years before. At least a dozen of these appeared and disappeared over the next five days. Afterwards she was mentally and physically much better. She too, quit her job.

Dr. Bach supplies us with a case history which demonstrates the use of Agrimony to cure just such welts on the skin. "A boy of ten years had had periodic attacks of urticaria on the back, neck and chest for two years. He was a cheerful lad who made light of his trouble, although the discomfort and irritation during an attack kept him awake at night and impaired his general health. His temperament indicated the remedy

Agrimony, which was given as a medicine and lotion, and within a few days the condition had cleared up." A slight relapse, two months later was quickly cured by the same remedy. He had no recurrence for five years.

Agrimony is also beneficial for acne, according to Yolanda LaCombe. Frequently, the flower essence will produce acne as a detoxification and sometimes it will cure it. "I have heard of Agrimony being used successfully for skin conditions which create a masking effect," she continues. She cites various kinds of lupus and sarcoma.

Tension and the Female System

According to Chinese medicine, the liver "holds in the blood" and has an influence over the release and timing of the menses. We can see why this would be the case, from our discussion of arterial tension and hepatic function. *Agrimonia* has an influence in this sphere as well.

In one case recently, a thirty-eight-year-old woman came to see me for high blood pressure and infertility. She had two boys but wanted a girl. With both pregnancies she suffered from toxemia. She was not ovulating so the doctors put her on fertility drugs, but nothing happened except that they caused very large benign cysts on the ovaries. She had her thyroid removed some time ago as there was a large benign tumor on that organ. The high blood pressure sometimes shot up to as high as 200/150. She suffered from alopecia and skin rashes, especially "pimply stuff" on the lower face, and a reddish complexion caused by "blood vessels going up to the skin." She was under stress from remodeling her house and dealing with contractors. By this time I knew that Agrimony (or Cinquefoil) was almost specific for alopecia and toxemia, and often curative for high blood pressure. She took Agrimony tincture, three drops, three times a day, but she called me after ten days to report that she had been ovulating every three days and was exhausted! We cut it back to once a day and she asked me a few days later if she could continue to take it if she was pregnant! It brought down the high blood pressure and she did get pregnant. (Yes, Agrimony is safe during pregnancy.)

This case illustrates a profound action on ovulation and fertility. As we shall see, Agrimony and Cinquefoil have powerful influences on toxemia and delivery as well. And, not surprisingly, there is a major impact on menstruation as well.

The eclectics developed the use of *Agrimonia* extensively in women's complaints. Ellingwood writes that it is "useful in a form of dysuria which affects women and girls, especially those who are suffering from some form of dysmenorrhea; or those in which there is difficulty in having a normal menstrual function established, this function being accompanied with much pain and general distressing symptoms. With this there is often an irritable condition of the bladder. At the same time there may be hysterical symptoms, which result from uterine or ovarian congestion, which on its part, may be increased by the urinary irritation."

A hair stylist in Wisconsin had been suffering from severe, horrific menstrual pains for her entire adult life. By telephone I suggested Prickly Ash, which grew on her farm. This helped only a little. A year later, at the end of the first day of a weekend class, she commented, "I told my church group to pray that I didn't get my period during the class—it's so debilitating." I said, "No, it would be better if they prayed for you to get the period during the class, so that we could see the nature of it, then get the right remedy." The next morning, she was sitting in a rocking chair, bundled up in blankets, trying not to complain about her menstrual pain. Every once in a while she would hold her breath from the spasm. Agrimony made her condition much better for the rest of the day and slowly brought the whole condition under control over the next year. "Agrimony tries to hold back the pain and not complain," I noted to the class. "But Chamomilla sighs and tries to attract attention and lets you know she is in pain."

Years ago, I helped a forty-year-old woman who was suffering from severe menstrual bleeding. She had a slightly yellow, pinched complexion that indicated hepatic tension, a wiry pulse, and two or three longitudinal ulcers on the tongue. She was under great pressure. Her marriage of fifteen years and two children had just broken up. Her father had been an alcoholic. For several months she had prolonged periods with profuse bleeding, the blood turning black and coagulated. From loss of blood she developed anemia. Her doctor recommended a DNC. "Don't fool around," she said. "This is a serious problem." (More pressure, I thought to myself.) From the look of the tongue I presumed there were ulcerations in the uterus, and speculated to myself that the DNC might cause further trouble. We didn't need to find out, fortunately. The Agrimony flower essence cured all symptoms. The menses were normal in three months. She also took an iron supplement to build up the blood. At the time, I did not realize that Agrimony was traditionally used to treat anemia. It operates indirectly, by improving tone in the alimentary structures and therefore digestion and assimilation.

I have already mentioned a case where Agrimony cleared up tension arising during pregnancy. It is my belief that Agrimony helps prevent birthing problems. Over the years I have noticed that many people who need Agrimony had problems when they were born or when they gave birth. One problem I suspect Agrimony would help is "keeping the cord from wrapping around the neck of the baby." (The Indians have remedies for that condition.) Having a cord around your neck while trying to descend the birth canal is an awfully serious illustration of being "caught in a bind." I have no proof of this belief, but I offer Agrimony as a possible solution to an age-old problem. Cinquefoil, which imitates the hand of an able midwife, may also turn the baby.

The wife of a friend down in Indiana suffered from a serious chronic illness. The disease began after "shunning" by her church, then a serious infection of postpartum toxemia which went into sixteen years of suffering, including rash and edema, which came and went. An herbalist eased the symptoms with Cinquefoil.

I had a very surprising opportunity to verify all these indications. The following case not only illustrates the use of Cinquefoil as a remedy in two serious physical conditions, but sets the stage for its use as a magical agent, which will be mentioned further on in our little discussion.

Magic or "good medicine" is sometimes simply a matter of the proper timing of events, while poor timing can be the source of "bad luck" or "bad medicine." Someone might say it is "the spirit" acting through our lives. I wouldn't object to that sentiment. However, I would add a further idea: plants can influence this element of timing. They participate in the life of the spirit just as we do. We should not be so chauvinistic as to believe that we are the only ones on this planet who enjoy that life. Whether we find the right healing remedy or not may be a matter of timing, or being open to the spirit, or believing in the possibility of healing from an unorthodox source, or believing that miracles can happen. Plants, just like any of us, would like to participate in the occurrence of a miracle.

One day I went out to lunch at the little cafe in the small town near where I live. After a while I noticed a woman across the aisle who looked exactly like someone I had known five years before. I couldn't imagine what that woman would be doing sitting in that particular small town diner in the middle of nowhere. The last I knew, she lived in an exclusive suburb on the other side of the metro area. I tried to catch her eye, but she didn't look up. After a while one of the town paramedics came over—a friend of mine—and started talking. I had never run into him there either. After a minute the woman across the aisle joined in. "I thought that was you, Matt, but I couldn't tell until I recognized your voice." The paramedic left and we visited.

"Jean" and her husband were now living near me. She had been sick about a year, but didn't have time to take care of herself "until today," when she got in the car and started driving over to my farm. Halfway there, she decided she'd better call ahead, so she came into the little cafe to call. I wasn't home, so she sat down to have some lunch. "You better come out and see me," I said.

Jean had been suffering from a slight edema of the legs, with some varicosities (probably unrelated) and some reddish sores. When she described how the swelling came and went, I thought of the case I had heard about were Cinquefoil was used. I started to tell her about it. When I mentioned toxemia she burst out, "Toxemia! That's what they told me I had in a dream a month ago!" "They" used the word eclampsia. She didn't know what that meant and looked it up. "It means toxemia following pregnancy." Since she hadn't had any children for twenty-five years, she didn't think it made sense and forgot the dream until that moment.

Well, we certainly were going to use Cinquefoil! We talked for a while and I kept thinking I should mention that the primary use the Indians make of Cinquefoil was to fight witchcraft. I thought that would be a bit much for her, so I decided not to say anything. As I was pouring off the tincture she said, "One last thing: do you think this could have anything to do with witchcraft?"

Jean explained that she and her husband had been members of a huge Lutheran church. She opposed some action the board took in fundraising; they turned against her and a campaign of shunning and behind-the-back talking began which finally forced them to sell their home of fifteen years. She felt the entire episode to be something akin to witchcraft.

My friends lived in a cozy little suburb. Underneath that surface there were strong fixed thought forms of conformity and convention. If someone was different, these might generate unacknowledged emotions of hatred and fear. One or two spiteful or fearful people who don't want their comfortable boat rocked focused this energy. The people involved in doing this probably weren't even aware that they were causing a deep, serious, negative influence on other people. This is the stuff of real "witchcraft," not little old ladies with warts on their noses and brooms in their hands.

Perhaps my friends never truly fit into that suburban setting and the experience ultimately served to loosen them and send them on their way to a more appropriate place to live. The body, however, remembers the trauma, and needs help unlocking the experience that remains impressed upon it. Until this is released, a "residue of the curse" remains.

My friend took the Cinquefoil and slept almost nonstop for three days. On the fourth she broke out into a rash of "blood blisters" from head to foot. "Oh, yeah," she said. "I forgot to mention that. I've had those things for years." After that, the edema and spots disappeared completely.

I believe that Agrimony would probably have worked in this case just as well, but I had learned to use Cinquefoil from the case history mentioned above, so that was the remedy I pulled out of the cupboard.

Several months later I found a call on my machine from Jean, filling me in on details she hadn't revealed at the time. (Remember, Agrimony has the outward facade.) "I think the reason I went to see you was because I had glaucoma and the doctor said I was going blind." (Oh, that's pertinent!) "Well, I went to the optometrist again recently and he was shocked. The damage to the optic nerve was entirely gone, as well as the blind spot." She wanted me to know the whole story before she moved to Arizona. Also, "I want you to know: **miracles do happen!**"

The "Bad Hair Day" Remedy

The image of the cat with its hair standing on end seems to have a literal application for Agrimony. The following three cases, remarkably similar in some details, occurred within two days. They taught me much about Agrimony.

The first was a woman, aged thirty, who was outwardly jovial but very tense within. She had a clowning personality, and in fact she was struggling to make a living as a professional clown. Hands and feet always felt cold, sometimes numb. Dizzy when bending over or standing up, sees stars. "Acts hyper, but feels hypo." Hair does not grow, is weak, breaks, so she has to dye. It was a bright, artificial yellow. "I have to bleach it because it is so thin and spindly," she explained. "It grows out to about four inches and that's it. The bleaching makes it thicken up some." Eyes and skin itch. Ringing in the ears. Eating causes bloating. Anemia and eating disorders in the past. Hands feel ice cold. Pulse changes in intensity, "comes and goes," from moment to moment. Tongue has fine red points towards the tip. Feet cold, "so cold I can't sleep." Dysfunctional, alcoholic family, sexually abused by her father, physically abused by her brother. Drinks alcohol to excess "about once a month." Constantly flustered, hard time breathing, tension in breathing. Worries a lot. Heart hurts, "pains when I need to catch my breath." Holds her breath once and a while, as we talk. *Agrimonia eupatoria* 12x immediately restored warmth to the hands. "This is the first time in my life that my hands and feet have ever been warm." Warmth persisted for a week.

This client showed the Agrimony personality through and through. Not only did she get better from the remedy—as I heard through a friend—but she stiffed me for the fee. In over ten years practice, I never had anyone who got a profound healing baldly refuse the customary payment. Her attitude was so exaggeratedly abusive that I couldn't do anything but laugh. That was money worth losing. Anybody who treats the world as she does will not last very long. The cure would undo itself soon enough. Besides, I soon counted myself rich by what I learned from her about the hair.

The very next person booked at the clinic was a thirty-seven-year-old woman. She arrived with an entry complaint of "terrible circulation." She was worried about her heart, though the doctors had found nothing wrong. She gets cold easily, hands and feet cold. Used to do a lot of street drugs. Probably has a toxic liver. Nails breaking off, hair breaks, she has it dyed. "I always have to do something with my hair," she commented. It seemed to be more of a psychological impulse. I was certainly thinking of the previous person as she spoke. Pulse wiry, low, hard, cordlike.

Tongue darkish in the middle. Sun produces prickly sensation on skin of face. Pain in the left ovarian region, scanty periods. Urine difficult to hold in, runs, drips. Constipated, but very gaseous. Cold in wrists, elbows and ankles. *Agrimonia eupatoria* 12x restored the heat to the hands, feet, and joints, removed the constipation, contained the urine, and promoted a general sense of well-being.

The next day my friend at the front desk in the clinic called in sick, but decided to come in to see me. She complained of poisoning from incomplete combustion due to the gas heater in her living room. Nausea, headache, feels like crying, feels anxious, suspicious, of insidious influences, a little scared, angry. Throbbing pain in the liver, right side of body sore. Sore throat. "Yuck feeling" in the mouth, tastes very bad, breath feels "yuck." Tongue feels swollen, pasty, looks atonic. Flulike feeling, body ache. Hands limp and clammy. Eyes look lusterless. Hair is "strange," she says, ends dry and thinning out, doesn't have good body, feels "disconnected from the rest of me," want to "do something to it." Wants to be held and rocked, cry, scream at somebody. Mad at old boy friend, wants to rip down curtains, she's so mad at him. Nausea "up and down." How could I have given her anything but Agrimony after the two previous cases? I wouldn't have thought of the remedy, but *Agrimonia eupatoria* 30x totally cured the whole train of symptoms. She was visibly relaxed after one dose, completely cured in 6 hours.

The peculiar relationship to hair pointed out in these cases bore fruit a few months later. A twenty-nine-year-old man was diagnosed with alopecia. There were spots on his scalp and beard denuded of hair. No other strong physical symptoms, and the only marked indications of any kind were mental tension due to job stress. I gave *Agrimonia* 12x, thinking to at least help the stress. Almost immediately the hair started to grow back. His barber was amazed and he was quite pleased. He also received the benefit I had expected in the area of tension. About two weeks after receiving the remedy he said, "I realize that my supervisor has poor abilities in handling employees, and that the problems I am having are due to her, not myself."

Later, the hair stylist from Wisconsin explained to me that bleach makes the hair thicken up, but damages it in the long run. Each hair has a nerve attached to it, and she speculated that Agrimony may act on these peripheral nerves.

Chills, Influenza, and Intermittent Fever

Another condition associated with constriction of the liver chi in Traditional Chinese Medicine is intermittent fever (chills alternating with fever). The old Western doctors also associated "ague" (intermittent fever and chills) with "biliousness" and "liver problems." Our folk-medical theory says that when chill enters the body it causes a constriction in the fibers and the general flow of things, including the circulation and the equalization of hot and cold. This particularly impacts the liver, which is responsible for the proper "flowing and spreading of chi." This chill or constriction is called "wind invasion" in Chinese herbalism. It causes a kind of "constricted liver chi" in which intermittent fever symptoms are associated with biliousness and indigestion. The gallbladder nerve reflexes may be "pinched," bile is excreted at the wrong time, resulting in indigestion, a bitter taste, diarrhea and constipation, and so forth.

The old Western physicians credited *Agrimonia* as a remedy for intermittent fever. Culpeper says, "A draught of the decoction, taken warm before the fit, first relieves, and in time removes, the tertian or quartan ague."

In three cases I have seen *Agrimonia* produce fever, chilliness and perspiration as an aggravation, so these symptoms may be considered pathogenetic. As we learn from homeopathy, the symptoms a remedy generates (pathogenesis) will also be cured by that remedy.

One of my neighbors selected Agrimony for himself while reading my manuscripts. He had antibodies to three kinds of hepatitis, an extensive history of drug abuse, and is still an alcoholic. One drop made him so sick, he felt like he had influenza for three days. He tried it again, months later, with the same result. Some livers are best left alone.

We have already seen that Cinquefoil was used by Culpeper to cure intermittent fevers with great success. We do not know if it would still work as well, in a different climate and population, but I have one excellent case that cured up quickly under its influence.

One of my long-term students called with a serious flulike condition that was making her miserable. She had already tried the remedies I would have used. Marie was a polarity therapist in her mid-forties. She was suffering from chill alternating with fever, with incomplete sweating at night. This was accompanied by body aches so extreme that the hips were actually dislocated and had to be adjusted by a chiropractor. The stomach felt "very bad," it takes a day to digest a small meal. She was exhausted and tired, the condition has been hanging on for ten days. She told me the tongue was covered with a thick white coating with a crack down the middle. (White indicates a cool condition.) She had a dream the previous night about being an engineer, "trying to build too many buildings." The occupational element reminded me of Agrimony. However, I gave her Cinquefoil *(Potentilla erecta)* because she works with her hands. Relief was immediate and a complete cure followed within a few days.

In Chinese medicine "wind," or constriction, is considered to be a major causative agent in rheumatism, because it tightens the joints and this can result in deposits of material and inflammatory complications. Thus, we should not be surprised that Agrimony also shows up as a rheumatic remedy.

Dr. Bach gave a case history which is pertinent here. "A man of thirty-five had severe rheumatism for five weeks. When first seen almost every joint in the body was affected with swelling and tenderness, he was in great pain, rolling about in his torture, anxious as to what was going to happen. The patient was very ill and looked as though he would not be able to stand much more. *Agrimony* was given hourly for twenty hours when there was marked improvement, pain and swelling had all gone except for one shoulder joint, the patient was calmer and less worried. *Agrimony* was continued for another six hours when the patient slept for four hours. On waking all pain had gone."

Pain, Wounds, and Burns

Any plant which has an association with pain relief is likely to be a vulnerary, or woundwort. *Agrimonia* has been classified in this category for centuries. It has been used for cuts with bleeding and joint injuries. Remember Culpeper's statement that it strengthens the joints. I have used *Agrimonia* several times to cure severe pain associated with muscular/skeletal injuries. The indication was the tormented look and the inability for any other remedy to cure. However, the really powerful vulnerary action of this plant is seen in its action on burns.

I first learned about this from personal experience. While out mowing in the field I put my left palm on the manifold of the brush-mower. In an instant I started back in pain, with the smell of burnt flesh in my nostrils. Huge blisters arose on the skin. I dragged myself over to some Sweet Leaf growing in the field, chewed up the flowers and put some on my hand. I writhed in agony for about an hour and a half, holding my breath as one often does with a burn. I put on St. John's Wort in addition, but the pain was terrible. In a paroxysm of torment, a little picture of some Cinquefoil I had been looking at the day before popped into my mind. That's odd, I thought. I put some Cinquefoil tincture on my hand and sure enough, the pain subsided. It was bearable from that point on.

A curious thing happened the moment I put the Cinquefoil on my hand. I felt a deep relaxation and pain relief emanating from the base of the palm, where the nerves of the five fingers come together. It really felt as if Cinquefoil had an affinity for the hand.

I reflected on my experience and remembered that holding the breath to stop pain is a characteristic symptom for Agrimony. I wondered if this herb—so similar to Cinquefoil—would also be a cure for burn pain. A year later I burned one of my finger tips on the wood stove. A blister raised up immediately. I thought this would be a perfect opportunity to try Agrimony, but I put on Cinquefoil first, "just to make sure." I was going to put on the Agrimony next, but the pain went away and never came back, so I lost that opportunity.

It remained for my friend Susan to prove the worth of Agrimony as a burn medicine. One evening I was over at her house. We were going to have spaghetti for dinner. As she took the pot off the stove, it caught on the burner and boiling water poured all over her hand. I quickly thought about what I had on hand. Agrimony was out in the car. A few drops relieved the pain quickly. She took one more dose that night and everything turned out fine. Since that time I have used Agrimony and Cinquefoil for burn pain and healing.

Magical Uses

More often than any other remedy I am familiar with, Agrimony changes the environment around people who are taking it. This usually has to do with the work environment. People quit jobs that weren't right for them, they get laid off or shifted to a new position, their boss changes the job description, co-workers quit, abusive employers and business partners are left behind, or things just sort of happen where they were stuck before.

Agrimony fulfills the description of a magical remedy as described in the introduction. It does not transform people on a profound level, like Werewolf Root; it changes the outward situation. However, if we turn to the literature for an explanation, we find that it is not Agrimony, but Cinquefoil that has the magical pedigree. This usage goes far back into European and American Indian tradition.

There is an old maxim in folk lore: "What five fingers can bring, Five Fingers can remove" (see Joseph Meyer, *The Herbalist,* p. 229). What this means is that the "hand of the witch" tries to cast the spell, but the Five Finger Grass stops the spell. The plant is hung over the bed of the infant, the lintel of the door, over the window, or in the car, to prevent "interference," disturbance or even theft.

The sensible reader may laugh, but I have seen Cinquefoil and Agrimony remove people from difficult situations so many times that I consider them to be rather reliable for this purpose. I frequently recommend one or the other and almost as frequently see "good results." I've provided a few case histories (one of which is given in the chapter on Sweet Leaf.) It is too bad if people can't believe in a little good "magic."

Five Finger Grass tells us about the power that is latent in the hand: how it can be used or abused. In Hebrew, the word for hand *(yud)* also means power. Even in some English constructions this inference is present. It is with the hand that a person manifests a trade, skill, or work and it is also by the hand that a person, conversely, interferes in the work or calling of another. The hand also refers us to the idea of capabilities or skills necessary to competently undertake a job. Thus, Five Finger applies to work, the workplace, the vocational calling a person feels, and the power that is drawn from working in the right field, manifesting one's spiritual calling or gift.

The misuse of the hand involves a turning away from one's spiritual work. The person who feels a true calling to do something does not suffer from the problem of the idle hand, nor does he or she go a step further and turn the hand to uses that are incompatible with that calling. Going further still, that person does not misuse or pervert the power of the hand to wreck havoc upon neighbors, much less seek actively to take the power of others or to tear down the lives of good people who are dedicated to their spiritual vocation. But this is something we do see in the practitioner of the black art.

There is a difference, a gradation, from the lazy hand to the hand of the interfering busybody, to the hand of the thief, to the hand of the black-hearted revenge-seeker, to the hand of the competent manipulator who can destroy other people's lives.

Fortunately, this is not the kind of witchcraft most of us confront on a daily basis in society. Our problems are more often due to petty back-stabbing. Somebody dislikes us at work, in the neighborhood, at school, or at church. They seduce a bunch of their friends and co-workers to think ill of us and that generates a pool of hostility. Sometimes things resolve and sometimes one has to leave the environment. Or the problem may be that an employer is trying to oversee one's work in an inappropriate way, causing tension, anxiety, and ill-will. It is this type of low-level interference which Cinquefoil is most capable of resolving.

This is not just a theory: these plants really do perform magic! Here is an example "case history." A friend of mine, supporting herself and three children mostly on her own income as a technical writer, was faced with a difficult problem at work. Her boss was getting increasingly unrealistic in her demands, wanted her to work at the office rather than at home (a great burden from the child-care angle and completely unnecessary, except to provide excessive supervision), and was generally becoming obnoxious and bossy. I could hardly think, on the other hand, of a more balanced, nonegotistical, talented person than my friend. Another person was assigned my friend's job and it appeared that her work was at an end. While at this impasse, my friend and her boss ran into each other at the hairdresser (shades of Agrimony?) and the employer started yelling at her in public. Finally, my friend got her to agree to a private meeting at the office the following week. It looked pretty grim.

I heard what happened and I rushed over to present my friend with a freshly cut Cinquefoil leaf. "Put it in the room where you write, under the computer or something," I suggested. I thought it might straighten out the vibes at what we were already calling her "old job." That might help her move on to a new one. To help manifest a new job I was thinking of giving her Solomon's Seal, which is better at bringing in something completely new and unforeseen, but I happened not to have any around just then.

Four days later my friend called. "Thanks for the magic," she chimed. At the meeting her employer took her by both hands, apologized, explained how necessary she was to the company, that they could work around her needs, and hoped everything was O.K. My friend and I were both shocked. The change did seem remarkable.

My friend was telling her story to a friend of hers, who saw a similarity to her own condition. "Oh, please, let me have the leaf for a day," she pleaded. There was to be a company meeting, during which the supervisor was going to address the problems involving the employee. My friend lent her the leaf for a day. When the time for the meeting arrived, the supervisor was three quarters of an hour late and so flustered she had to give ground to save face. Everything was nicely resolved. That evening the Cinquefoil leaf was returned to its position underneath the computer.

More information emerged as I became better acquainted with Agrimony. One day, after helping someone with it I heard a little voice in my ear: "I am a Wolf Medicine. You can see this by looking at the terminal leaflet on the stem. It represents the leader of the pack." Those plants, they're so logical!

Preparation and Dosage

Agrimonia eupatoria is difficult to obtain in herbal commerce in North America. When it is possible to get Agrimony, it is often not the officinal European species, but some local American variety. Fortunately, these seem to have about the same properties as the European.

The lower homeopathic potencies of *Agrimonia eupatoria* are available from several homeopathic pharmacies. I have used them with success. The Bach remedies include a flower essence made from *Agrimonia eupatoria,* but I have not found it as reliable as the herbal tincture.

I make my own tincture from the Agrimony growing in my area *(Agrimonia gryposepala).* It has a slightly sweet, rather refined taste. Agrimony should be picked in June or July, before the leaves get tough. Pick the leaflets branching off the side, so that the top—the leader of the pack—remains. Macerate them in good brandy and you will have a fine product with a slightly sweet favor.

Agrimony is almost identical in properties to Cinquefoil and Tormentil. It is also similar to Avens, another cousin in the Rose family, and has some properties in common with Raspberry (intestinal tonic, birthing remedy) and Meadowsweet (pain relief). It is similar in action to some of our best remedies for "liver tension," including *Bupleurum, Chamomilla,* and *Nux vomica.* The anger of *Agrimonia* is usually hidden ("Oh, no, I'm feeling just great"), while that of *Chamomilla* is displayed (loud sigh, "*Notice* how bad *I'm* feeling"), while *Nux vomica* beats you up.

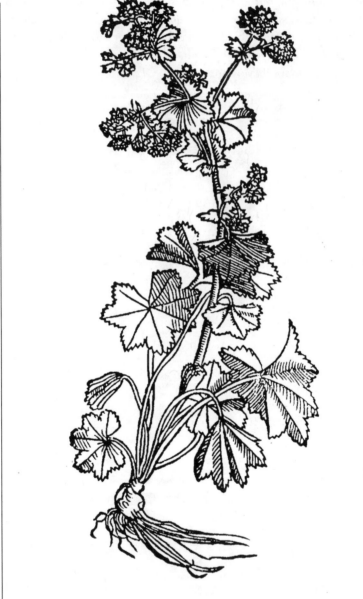

Alchemilla vulgaris

Lady's Mantle

from *Herbarium Imagines Vivae,* published by Christianus Egenolphus, 1535

Alchemilla vulgaris
Lady's Mantle

ady's Mantle is a member of the Rose family native to Europe and Asia, but widely cultivated as an ornamental. The peculiar thing about this plant is that the leaves are "waterproof." Dew and rain bead up on them like little pearls. This, along with the folded aspect, suggests a mantle. Because it was a woman's remedy, it was called *Frauenmantel* in Germany. When the great German herbals were translated into English the name became Lady's Mantle. It was originally associated with the goddess Freya, afterwards with Mary. In France it is more commonly called *Pied de leonis* (Lion's Foot), because of the marked resemblance of the leaves to a lion's paw. Latin writers called it *Alchemilla,* in reference to the alchemists, who placed peculiar value on the dew collected from the leaves. One modern author rather poetically translates this as "the little magical one."

Lady's Mantle inhabits a more northerly range, so it was not included in the materia medica of classical medicine. It seems to have been an important plant to the ancient Germanic peoples, who associated it with the goddess Freya. It remained a sacred herb in Iceland until a late date.

During the middle ages, Lady's Mantle first came to prominence as a wound medicine. It was considered an analogue of the most important vulnerary of the period, Lesser Sanicle. As a result, it was named Greater Sanicle or *Sanicula maioris.* It entered the official pharmacopoeia during the Renaissance, when German authors began to draw on their native traditions. The appearance of the name *Frauenmantel* about 1520 may have changed the way people thought about the plant. From that time onward it developed a reputation as a gynecological remedy, while its use as a vulnerary declined. Today it is principally used as a woman's remedy.

The English Renaissance herbalists gradually took over the German material. Gerard (1597) devotes four lines to the medicinal properties, Culpeper (1654) gives an expanded summary, but William Salmon (1710) provides a two page account in the *Botanologia.* A good contemporary source is *Health through God's Pharmacy,* by the late Austrian herbalist Maria Treben. Another is Elisabeth Brooke's *Herbal Therapy for Women* (1993).

"The Dew of the Philosophers"

The leaves are the part used in medicine. They contain bitters, tannins, and salicin. The taste is moderately bitter and astringent, with a warm undertone. The combined bitter/astringent taste reminds one of the aspirin-like salicin compounds which it contains. This component is often found in plants that grow in wet places or expel water. The leaves are, as we have noted, water-repellent. These properties point to the use of Lady's Mantle to dry up and expel water from the tissues, hence its use in stopping hemorrhage, diarrhea, excessive menstruation, leucorrhea, and infection.

Salmon explains that Lady's Mantle is classified as hot and dry in the second degree. The juice "is not so hot as that of Sanicle, and Therefore more fit for those Wounds which are accompanied with Inflammation." Because it is warm and dry, it mops up "humidities" in wounds, making it a remedy for discharging ulcers and fistulas. He classified it as astringent, drying, cleansing, and strengthening to the tissues. Lady's Mantle has qualities in common with several of its Rosaceae cousins. Raspberry is used as a female tonic during pregnancy, to feed tissues and give them the appropriate tension or tone. It is perfectly suited to these uses, since it is sweet and astringent. Agrimony and Cinquefoil improve pregnancy by removing tension; they are more astringent but sweet enough to provide some tissue-building. Lady's Mantle has also been used as a tonic during pregnancy, like Raspberry, but it strengthens tissues by removing excess dampness and inflammation and is not directly nutritive. Lady's Mantle is better suited to inflammation and tissue weakness and it is not surprising that it is especially recommended to tone tissues *after delivery*. All of these gentle tonics can be used to improve pregnancy and menstrual function.

The pleated appearance of the leaf may look like a mantle or the paw of a large cat, but it has always reminded me of the mesenteric membranes holding the intestines together. I guess my imagination is somewhat medical. This is a signature (or at least a memory device) suggesting the use of Lady's Mantle in astringing, toning, and strengthening the abdominal tissues and structures. It is particularly favored as a medicine to "slim the figure" after child birth.

The fact that dew drops bead up on the leaves is unusual and it is here that we should look to understand the medicinal virtues. Not only does the leaf seem to have a water-resistant property, but it also maintains these droplets for many hours after the dew has burned off other plants. Lady's Mantle may encourage the subtle chemical bonding which makes the surface of a drop of water more cohesive and less capable of evaporation. We can now begin to see why the alchemists found so much of interest in *Alchemilla*. When they looked at Lady's Mantle they saw a plant which was particularly able to generate and preserve one of the most precious substances of all, the *mercurius*.

According to alchemical doctrine, *mercurius* is one of the three primal substances which stand at the foundation of the universe. It corresponds to the essence, the archetypal/genetic/cellular matrix which gives rise to different individuals and species. It gives a person a sense of identity and direction. *Sulphur* stands for the combustible portion, which corresponds to the life force that burns like a candle, from the cradle to the grave. On the psychological level it stands for the soul and psychological passions which animate the life. *Salis* or *salt* corresponds to the body, not just the physical vehicle, but the principle of embodiment on any level—thus with the spiritual body as well as the physical. It stands for the principle of integrity or character.

The *mercurius* was named after the mineral mercury, which maintains itself as a fluidic droplet at room temperature. In the process of purifying ores to yield precious metals, the crude substance is heated to the melting point, so that the molten metal may be separated out. The alchemists concluded that the essence of the metal was brought out by reduction to that state. Since mercury exists as a molten drop at room temperature, it was thought to be particularly close to the essence. In the vegetable kingdom, the *mercurius* or essence was isolated by distillation to produce the vegetable *mercurius.*

It is necessary to understand these associations and think in this manner in order to understand *Alchemilla,* "the little alchemist," because this plant produces the *mercurius* on its leaves. Something within it is distilling the essence and simultaneously helping to preserve it. In a material sense, Lady's Mantle must correspond to processes which encourage cohesion on the surface of the droplet and prevent vaporization, while at the same time (and plants always seem to work in two opposite directions) it must possess the ability to refine and distill fluids into their most subtle expression or "essence."

The process of distillation takes place in the kidneys. The lighter portion of the blood is sucked into the ante-chamber of the kidneys, the glomeruli, by an osmotic pressure maintained by electrolyte salts. The heavier portion, consisting of albumen and sugars—the food in the bloodstream—remains outside the kidney. This pressure continues to pull the fluids and solids down into the inner chamber of the kidneys, the convoluted tubules, where a second process takes place. The convoluted tubules act like little stills and during their stay in them the fluids and solids are graded according to weight. The more refined solids, mostly salts and electrolytes valuable in the chemistry of the body, are allowed to flow back into the bloodstream with some clear, refined fluid, so that they will be available for use again. At the same time, the more turbid sediment is concentrated and eventually flushed away as urine. In this way, the essential renal function of balancing the fluids and solids in the organism is carried on continuously.

The alchemists also acknowledged the difference between the coarse sediments which had to be removed (the *mortuus caput* or "dead head") and the refined salts, which had various uses in inorganic and organic chemistry. These were called the *sal salis,* or "salt of the salts." Reabsorbed back into the circulation, the refined salts acting as electrolytes help bring materials across cell membranes, at the same time maintaining the cohesion of the membrane. Through these electrolytes, the renal function of balancing fluids and solids is carried on throughout the system.

The pulling power of the kidneys not only sucks material out of the bloodstream into the glomeruli, but exerts itself all the way through the urinary tract to its final conclusion and back up into the body at large, so that there is a constant pulling down towards the kidneys. At the same time, the refining, distilling process operating in the inner chamber of the kidneys, the convoluted tubules, not only raises up a refined vapor, so to speak, which ascends back into the bloodstream, but emanates this refining, purifying, cleansing property into the system at large.

The kidneys are, metaphorically, the headwaters of the entire sexual-urinary tract. They are concerned with maintaining the essence or *mercurius,* while at the same time they remove the inessential or waste products. One side of the system is concerned with the manufacture and use of the sexual/hormonal/genetic element or essence, while the other side works to remove the inessential, the waste products.

These relationships are also described in Chinese alchemy and medicine. Here too the essence is likewise represented by mercury, and it is more specifically stated that this genetic/hormonal/archetypal material is "stored in the kidneys." This is the primary function of the kidneys; the secondary function is the maintenance of the waters in the body as a whole.

From these descriptions, we begin to see the physical and medical affinities belonging to *Alchemilla,* the "little alchemist." It has long been used to remove excessive fluids from the tissues, and yet, is not a diuretic. The affinity of the plant is not with the first activity, the pulling of fluids into the kidneys or their release into the ureters for elimination, but with the second activity where the fluids are vaporized and sent back into the blood. If we translate what we see on the leaf of the plant back into the body, we see that Lady's Mantle would help distill the fluids and solids into a purified material which is sent back into the rest of the body. It also helps to maintain the perfect mixture of salts and fluids which strengthens the cohesion of water droplets, and analogously, of cell walls and membranes throughout the body. The refined salts help the transfer of food and fluids across the cell membranes while maintaining their integrity.

Just as Lady's Mantle acts on the yin or feminine element on the microscopic level of the organism, so does it act on the aggregate structures and the whole organism itself. We see how perfect it is that Lady's Mantle should be a woman's medicine. Not only does it help gynecological problems, which are so often connected with fluids, but exerts a psychological or magical influence as well. In the same way in which the subtle, invisible membrane preserving the cohesion and integrity of the droplet is maintained, we can imagine Lady's Mantle making a subtle, invisible membrane around a woman. The influence of the medicine does not stop at the boundary of the person but emanates further out into the world at large, encouraging integrity and cohesion in the people around her.

In its positive expression, Lady's Mantle relates to the woman who maintains a subtle balance, poise, and integrity which emanates into the world at large, so that the people around her are uplifted and improved by her presence. Lady's Mantle is present to help a woman who needs protection, but also self-work and refinement, so that she is lifted out of dangerous circumstances and allowed to exercise her peculiar feminine influence upon the world in a positive way. Perhaps this woman has taken on too big a job and ends up needing protection from the partner she has chosen. The partner may be too disorderly, possibly violent, or at any rate unappreciative of the positive virtues of feminine character.

Let us take a short overview of the renal mechanisms and the remedies which correspond to the various functions. The pulling by which the kidneys bring components of the blood into the antechamber of the renal apparatus is personified by Goldenrod, while the vaporizing element is personified by Lady's Mantle. When the perfect balance of fluids and solids has been achieved, the kidneys are ready to flush themselves. This perfect balance and judgment are personified by Gravel Root.

"An Exquisite Faculty of Speedy Healing"

The use of Lady's Mantle as a wound remedy anticipated its fame as a female remedy. Salmon, writing at the end of the period when Lady's Mantle was used as a woundwort, gives an extensive summary of this tradition.

"In simple green Wounds or Cuts, it has such an exquisite Faculty of Speedy Healing, that it cures it at the first Intention, Consolidating the Lips thereof, without…suffering any Corruption to remain behind." If a wound becomes infected, "it is one of the best of vulneraries, for it digests [corrupted material] if need be, absterges or cleanses, incarnates [new tissue], dries and heals, almost to a Miracle." It is useful for hollow wounds, ulcers, fistulas, and sores. It is most amazing how Lady's Mantle can restore the integrity of torn, ruptured, or separated tissues, as seen in hernias or perforated membranes. It not only supports the cohesion of the cell wall, but of the muscle wall and other such structures, at every level of the body. It is well to remember that Lady's Mantle was used in folk medicine to "restore virginity," i.e., reseal the hymen. This sounds like a folkloric absurdity, but I have no doubt it could restore this membrane, as I have seen it restore others.

One of my students called me up to ask for advice about a friend who had a perforated eardrum. The woman had been struck on the side of her head by her husband, who was abusive—both of them were somewhat hard-living drinkers—puncturing the membrane. After six months, the doctors told her it probably would not repair itself and thought she might suffer a permanent hearing loss. We sent her Lady's Mantle tincture, which she applied externally on the ear and took internally as well. The eardrum sealed up and she left her husband.

Recently a mother brought in her six-year-old son, who suffered two perforated eardrums from an infection which suddenly set in. I gave a mixture of Elder flowers, Violet flowers, and Lady's Mantle. He was on antibiotics and the infection was clearing up. About a month later fever set in with swollen glands around the ears. She brought him into the doctor. The ears were perfectly clear and the membranes were healed over without scar tissue. Perhaps the glands were swollen because they were draining off the ears, or perhaps the herbs had only made a partial cure. I felt, however, that the membrane had probably been influenced by the *Alchemilla*.

Salmon continues his account of Lady's Mantle. "It is an excellent thing also against Bruises, Cuts or Punctures of the Nerves and Tendons; for it suddenly eases the Pain, and alleviates the Inflammation, and thereby induces the Cure." (Remember, it contains salicin.) Lady's Mantle also staunches bleeding, making it "effectual against all sorts of Bleedings both inward and outward," so that it "stops the Over-flowing of the Terms in Women, and cures the Bloody-flux, as also all other Fluxes of the Bowels." And it cures "Bruises by Falls or otherwise, whether inwards or outwards."

Salmon also gives a description of the use of *Alchemilla* to warm and dry the joints, removing pain, gout, and arthritis. For this purpose, he prefers that it be preserved in oil and applied externally. In this form, "it is a famous thing against a cold Gout, and all Pains or Aches proceeding from a cold Cause in any Part of the Body." As a warming and drying remedy it would be effectual against that "cold, wet" complaint, arthritis. "Outwardly applied to the Gout, Sciatica, or other like Pains of the Joints, proceeding from Blows, Over-straining, or the like, it gives Ease, and speedily cures them, adding also Strength to the Part."

"Venus Claims this Herb as Her Own"

As we have seen, Lady's Mantle refines and preserves the fluidic element in the organism, the yin or feminine part, while also acting with a distinct affinity for female organs and problems, and finally as a remedy for women on a more magical or psychological level. Culpeper simply says, "Venus claims this herb as her own." Yet it was not until the time of Salmon, a generation later, that the plant was more fully used as a female medicine. He says it was considered nearly a specific for that most common and quintessential female problem, vaginitis or discharge. "It is a peculiar thing to stop the Whites in Women, being esteemed more powerful for this Purpose than most other things." For this purpose it is injected into the vagina or taken internally. It is also used for excessive menstrual bleeding.

Lady's Mantle also acts upon the uterus, strengthening the muscles and tissues, removing prolapse and excessive dampness and stagnation. It has been used in the last three months of pregnancy as a *partus preparator* and also for the first few months after delivery. As an astringent, nutritive tonic, and drying agent it gets the tissues back in proper form. Salmon explains, "Inwardly also taken, and outwardly applied to Women's Breasts, which are great and over-much flag, it causes them to grow lesser and hard." This use seems to go back to German folk medicine. I know several women who can testify that it does help restore the figure after pregnancy and lactation. This is not just a folkloric joke, but a reliable indication. Furthermore, it is used to promote conception. "Taken by such Women as are Barren, or have a Slipperiness of the Womb, it is said to cause them to Conceive, and to retain the Birth after Conception, for that it dries up the too great Humidity, and stops the Flux of Humors to the Matrix, and so strengthens the Womb." For this purpose Salmon recommended the distilled essence be taken internally for twenty to thirty days, or from a bath in a decoction of the leaves. This "humidity" would correspond to a general condition of dampness and sogginess in the tissues, or what some people today might call chronic yeast infection or candidiasis. In addition, it may have a deeper action, improving the integrity of cell membranes, a fertility problem in older women.

Modern herbalists consider Lady's Mantle to have a gentle balancing and harmonizing influence on the menstrual cycle. It is used for irregular menses in puberty, adulthood, and menopause. Maria Treben recommended combining it with Yarrow to help establish healthy menstruation in young girls. It also relieves menstrual tension and PMS. Elisabeth Brooke recommends giving it as a general remedy whenever a woman is contemplating a hysterectomy, for a variety of reasons. She also says it should be used when there is trauma to the uterus from miscarriage, abortion, use of an IUD, pelvic inflammatory disease, or surgery of any kind. It has a tendency to maintain the feminine organs and psychological security.

By no means is Lady's Mantle exclusively a female medicine. Maria Treben learned from folk healers in Burgenland, Austria, that it strengthens the heart muscle. As a result, she applied it to enhance the muscular tone in general. She used it for muscular atrophy, weakness of the muscles, serious and incurable muscular disorders, multiple sclerosis, poor nutrition, prolapse of the uterus, and hernia. She combined Lady's Mantle with Shepherd's Purse for treatment of prolapse and hernia. I have seen it work several times for hernia. Tis Mal sent some to an old fellow in British Columbia who was suffering from a double abdominal hernia. It completely corrected the condition in less than two months, much to the shock of everybody involved in the case.

Preparation and Dosage

William Salmon gives the most extensive information about the different influences of various kinds of preparations in alcohol, vinegar, water, oil, and salt. As in Chinese medicine, the different methods are seen as changing the direction of the remedy somewhat. It would be too complicated to give all the various preparations under each of our medicaments, so I am selecting *Alchemilla* (which, after all, was the darling of the alchemists) as a remedy to study from the perspective of old-time pharmacy.

Our author recommended the tincture made from wine or vinegar for internal use in complaints of the viscera. "Inwardly taken, [the alcoholic tincture] warms and comforts the Bowels, strengthens the inward Parts, expels Wind, and is an excellent Traumatick, is drying and astringent, and therefore good against all Fluxes of the Bowels, Over-flowing of the Terms, and other Weaknesses of the Generative Parts."

A tincture made from vinegar has the same virtues, but "it opens the more, and removes Obstructions of Stomach, Liver, Spleen, and other Bowels...whereby it effectually stops Vomiting, strengthens the Stomach, and causes a good Appetite and a strong Digestion, but it stops not Fluxes of the Bowels so well as some of the former Preparations." Taken continually all day, so that the amount equals at least four or five tablespoonfuls, "It is a most excellent thing against a virulent Gonorrhea in Men." (Evidently it dries up the discharge.)

The oil of Lady's Mantle, taken internally, eases colic, expels wind, and opens obstructions of the kidneys, ureters and, bladder, expelling gravel, stones, and sand, "cleansing them from any Tartarous Mucilage lodged therein."

Today, Lady's Mantle is commonly used as a tea or tincture. The plant is usually picked early in the summer, before the flowers appear. Since they start to come on by the middle of May, I think this deadline can be extended a little bit. At any rate, they ought to be tender. Prepare an infusion by pouring a cup of boiling water over a tablespoon of the leaves and steep for fifteen minutes. A tincture can be made by macerating the leaves in brandy. Dose of the tincture, one to three drops.

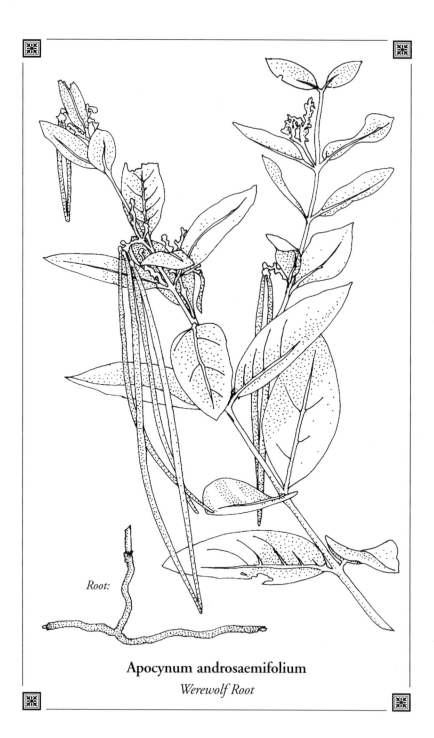

Root:

Apocynum androsaemifolium

Werewolf Root

Apocynum androsaemifolium
Werewolf Root

This plant is commonly called "Spreading Dogbane," but that name will not be used here; I call it Werewolf Root. It is native to dry upland soils throughout much of North America. Like its cousin Milkweed, Werewolf Root has milk-white sap and long seedpods. It rises to about the same height, but is distinguished by the strange way the branches bend away from each other, as if trying to approach a ninety degree angle. The leaves are narrower and smaller than Milkweed, the branches more numerous, and the flowers more dainty and singular, like little pink bells. These are superseded by long, thin pods which hang down together in pairs, so that they look like pincers. The root plunges down about three to twelve inches, splits in two and runs at ninety degree angles north and south, so that it looks like a T square. (According to my friend Halsey Brandt of Bisbee, Arizona, this shape is rarely found in western representatives.) It is a member of the Apocynaceae family, which also includes Periwinkle (*Vinca* sp.) and Indian Hemp *(Apocynum cannabinum.)* Most members of this family are pharmacologically active. Some are toxic, some are medicinal, and some are slightly psychotropic.

This plant is one of the most powerful medicines used by the *m'dewewin* or Grand Medicine Society of the Anishinabe. It is so strongly identified with the *m'dee* that it is commonly called "Medicine Lodge Root" in Anishinabe. Knowledge of its properties is reserved for initiates of the fourth degree, according to anthropologist Huron Smith (1932). Until modern times, this was the final degree and dealt with the initia-

125

tion of the *djahsahkee*. These individuals are described as "tent-shakers" by the older Indians; "shape-changers" would be the "New Age" term. The French missionaries and traders called these men and women *jugleurs* or "jugglers." This old European term refers to a magician who either has occult powers or works by sleight of hand.

The deeper properties of Medicine Lodge Root could hardly be communicated by the Indian medicine men to the rabble of pioneers swarming over the Indian homeland. However, the more external qualities of the plant were utilized by a small number of American herbalists. Samuel Thomson used it, and it received some attention in the literature of physio-medical doctors. They noted that it was a gallbladder remedy. *Apocynum androsaemifolium* occupies a minuscule niche in the homeopathic materia medica. It received a brutal proving in the late nineteenth century. Massive doses (up to 600 drops) where used. These efforts did not bring out the subtle genius of the plant and it is hardly used in homeopathy today.

The Square and Pincers

Ojibwe medicine people considered the "elbow of the root" to be the most powerful part of the plant, according to anthropologist Frances Densmore. The T square-like root, and the pincer-like seedpods, are the distinctive shapes produced by the plant. It is noteworthy that these are the symbols of Freemasonry, which is an analogue to the Grand Medicine Lodge in white society.

"Nature abhors the square," it is said. It usually appears as a result of human activity. Nature is better represented by the circle, a symbol of wholeness and harmony, while mankind is represented by the square and pincers, symbols of conscious artifice. The right angle indicates the appearance of a kind of consciousness which is at right angles to Nature. It represents the conscious mind, the ego, and the characteristic building habits of the human race. The pincers represent the focusing, limiting, and ultimately egocentric fixation of the mind. The square and pincers stand for the characteristic nature of the human mind and will.

As a medicine, Medicine Lodge Root addresses problems which arise from the juxtaposition of the ego and the spirit. When the ego is too strong it fights against the natural order of things. When it is too weak it gives way to natural processes—death and unconsciousness.

Medicine Lodge Root is the remedy for people who are fighting against natural and divine order, or who are losing the battle to remain a separate, conscious individual. The personality, ego, or spiritual will is weak; they are battered down by outside influences and too easily dominated. They need to make a ninety degree turn or they will die—spiritually or physically. These are the times when nothing will do except total transformation. One can never return to the past.

Going further, Werewolf Root is a shape-shifting medicine. The human mind is usually fixated on an accepted, common reality. However, Werewolf Root can knock that focus flat, so that a different reality can be experienced. This progresses from small changes to profound transformation. One does not need to shift into the shape of an animal to feel the effect. It is more a matter of seeing the world in a radical, new way. The test imposed on the initiate of the fourth degree in Grand Medicine is that they be able to move objects at will, in front of their peers.

I was never able to call this plant Spreading Dogbane. The name Werewolf Root came to me instead, and I believe it was the plant itself which gave me that name. At the same time a phrase came to me which I believe is the motto of the plant: "I will never be the same again." What this meant to me was that Werewolf Root is for changes that are complete, so that one cannot go back to the old life one was living. To experience this is to begin to learn what it means to "shape-shift." The mold has been broken and one can more easily shift from one life to another.

Gallbladder Medicine

In folk medicine, it is not the brain but the gallbladder which is credited as the residence of the ego. When a person is willful in an appropriate or inappropriate fashion, they are said to have "a lot of gall" in English. There is a similar expression in China. A person with courage is said to have a "big gallbladder." A person lacking courage has a little one. We have a similar idea. A coward is called a "yellow belly." In Traditional Chinese Medicine, it is said that the conscious will is stored in the gallbladder, the will of the spirit in the kidneys.

In Western astrological medicine, the gallbladder is ruled by Capricorn. This sign is associated with the conscious ego, the desire for social prominence and social climbing, the need to rule and organize and the mountain goat. This animal climbs up the slopes making switch-backs at right angles, just as the gallbladder meridian climbs up the body and head, making switchbacks and angles. (Right angles and switchbacks in the pattern of plant growth are signatures for gallbladder remedies—see *Chelidonium* as well as *Apocynum*.)

In Traditional Chinese Medicine it is said that the will of the spirit resides in the kidneys. This power manifests on the physiological plane as the "kidney yang," or the powerful, fiery part of the kidney organ system (what we would call the adrenals). In the older texts, the kidney yang was called the "life fire gate." There is debate about what this means, but this seems to correspond to the idea that the basic spark of life, the pilot light so to speak, resides in the kidneys. Hence, the kidneys are called the gate of life and death, the source of fire and water, the foundation of yin and yang. When a person has "low adrenals," they lose the spark of life, the desire to life, the will to stand up for themselves, for the spirit.

Many of the ideas about the life fire gate are obscure, but if I may give my own free translation of the concept, I would say the following: when it comes into incarnation the spirit lends a part of itself to the temporal, material person. This is like the basic spark or fire of life and spirit. It has to be located somewhere, because spiritual realities are practical, so its location is the "life fire gate." All our experiences and decisions are run through the kidneys, the judging part of the body (see *Solidago*), and are resolved down into their quintessential spiritual lessons. These are then registered on the "life fire gate," which is like a little circle within which the fire sits. It is like the knights and maidens of the Grail Castle, whose names were engraved in the lip of the Grail. When the life is over, the spark of life goes back to the spirit, bringing with it the sum total of spiritual experiences. For better or worse, that is the sum accomplishment which the spirit derived from the life lived in time and space.

The kidneys also store the primal water or yin. This is the essence (*mercurius* in Western alchemy or *jing* in the East). The essence is the genetic-hormonal blueprint for the life. For this reason, profound experiences impact not only the life fire gate, but the kidney essence, causing a genetic change. This principle is described in the Genesis cycle of stories in the Hebrew Torah, where the cultural figures and ancestors are changed by their experiences—changes which are then carried down to their descendants.

Strengthens the Gallbladder and Expels Bile

The early root doctors used *Apocynum androsaemifolium* (which they generally called Dogbane) as a remedy for a weak gallbladder. "It is one of the greatest correctors of the bile," wrote Samuel Thomson in his materia medica (1842). "For regulating the bowels and removing a costive state, its operations are admirable." He also mentions its use in edema, but this is due to his inclusion of *Apocynum cannabinum* in the same batch. "We have gathered the two indiscriminately, compounded them together, and dealt them out as one and the same thing." This is quite a mistake. The *cannabinum* is a strong diuretic, while the *androsaemifolium* is not. Nor does the former possess the psycho-spiritual depth of the latter.

Werewolf Root was hardly used by the eclectics, allopaths, or homeopaths, but its properties were developed by Thomson's followers. A precious account is rendered by Dr. William Cook, in *The Physio-Medical Dispensary* (1869). "Most of its action is expended upon the gall-ducts, gall-cyst, and tubuli of the liver," he writes. It stimulates the strength of these structures, so that they can excrete better, rather than stimulating the manufacture of bile. It is not a cholagogue, but improves tone. "By its action on the biliary passages, it secures a free discharge of the bile, thus unloading the gall-cyst and relieving turgescence of the liver." It is useful "in all cases where a sallow skin, clammy and yellow tongue, and clay-colored or dark faeces, indicate deficient excretory action of these ducts." He says one would think of using cholagogues in such cases, but these are inappropriate. "Most of these cases, with their long train of gastric and nervous symptoms, usually pass under the general term of 'biliousness,' and are treated by hepatics." But this is not appropriate, he says. The need is for tonification, placing the emphasis on strengthening the gall ducts, rather than on bilious purges which would weaken them further. Cook also notes the strengthening effects it has on the muscles and mucus membranes coating the stomach and bowels. He gives excellent general symptoms upon which to prescribe the remedy. "It is best fitted for sluggish cases, where the pulse and the sensibilities are below normal; and this class of jaundiced patients some-times need no other article. When feverishness, a hard pulse, and pain, are present, it not an appropriate agent."

Homeopathic Literature

One of the few homeopaths who gives evidence of having used this rem-edy was Dr. Samuel Lilienthall of New York. In his *Special Therapeutics* (1880) he mentions "Apocynum andro." as a remedy for arthritis and rheumatism. This is certainly an area where it has important properties, especially in the sort of rheumatoid arthritis which borders on lupus, where there are great pains, changing from one part of the body to another, amid general deterioration of the system. Boericke gives a sum-mation of the homeopathic knowledge, but it is so slight that these symptoms need hardly be mentioned here. A better collection of symp-toms was obtained from accidental provings on myself and a patient.

When I first became interested in Medicine Lodge Root, I inad-vertently smeared some sap on my hands while picking the plant. The effect was almost unbelievable. In a short time I felt a splitting in my head, as if a wedge had been driven down through the vertex into the center of the brain. In a few hours this symptom had progressed to the level where I felt as if the "pincers of the mind" had been twisted com-pletely out of shape by the enormous force entering my head. Increasingly, I could not exercise the "pincers of my mind." I could not focus on anything without increasing the pain. At the same time, I could not focus my eyes. It felt as if the bones of my face were being bent at ninety degree angles. I had a sensation in the elbows and knees, as if I had fallen on a hard surface—the way one feels after falling on an elbow on the hard ice. The headache became stronger and stronger over the next twenty-four hours, until I was incapacitated. I lay motionless with my head between the bed and the wall, unable to think. Suddenly, a thought flashed across my mind. "I will never be the same again." Just then, the headache started to improve. All the symptoms disappeared after several days, except that my eyes never went back into focus. I had to get a new prescription for eye wear.

The first person I used *Apocynum* on was suffering from what was then diagnosed as lupus. Blood tests eventually showed that she had

Lyme Disease. I'm really not sure what the real problem was, but it was killing her. She had severe rheumatic pains, and was allergic to just about everything, including her own hormones. Unfortunately, she was addicted to cortisone, which she was periodically trying to get away from. She had a wrinkled, yellow complexion, so that she looked much beyond her years. She was suffering from total exhaustion. She experienced tremendous aggravation on trying to reduce the cortisone by half a milligram. We both felt, without saying as much, that her days were numbered, unless the adrenals kicked in. I had an intuition about *Apocynum*. I had tried to obtain it from a homeopathic pharmacy, but after a few unsuccessful tries I gave up. I had only a flower essence I had made when I proved the plant on myself. Even this was too powerful, and produced severe aggravation. The patient survived and was able to get off the cortisone completely in a few months, with the help of a single dose. Her adrenals kicked in and seven years later she is relatively healthy and functional. Several times since I have seen *Apocynum* prove helpful in cortisone dependence and collagen disease.

Here are the symptoms produced during the aggravation. She took one drop of the flower essence, into which some of the sap had exuded. Lack of control of the mind. Strange confusion, as if she didn't know whether she should breath in or out. She had to distract her mind so that she could breath. Feared she would die, thought "I will never be the same again." (This phrase came to her independently.) Thought the medicine would kill her. She had a headache, felt dull-minded, confused, and despairing. Dull but intense headache focused on the center of the brain, so that she could not think. Pressure and burning in the throat. Feeling of despair emanating from the throat. Neck felt as if grasped by a hand. Stiff, tense, rigid. Tightness, pressure in the chest, with difficult breathing, felt as if the wind was knocked out of her lungs by a sudden blow. Sensation of edema around heart, with occasional attacks of cardiac arrhythmia. Nausea in the stomach. Urination more than usual, followed by scantiness and retention. Stools moderately loose, then dry. Chills alternating with heat. Broke out in a sweat, like an adrenaline rush. Three days of prostration following the dose, during which she felt like she was not in her body. Burning, stiff, sore joints, muscles, and bones, especially of the forearms. Tingling of hands and forearms. "Buzzing" in all the joints.

"The High Impact Remedy"

These symptoms suggest that Werewolf Root should be of value in high impact injuries: blows to the head, falls on the ice, impacts on elbows and knees, and having the wind knocked out of the lungs. I have verified all of these uses since the "provings" mentioned above took place. Here are several case histories.

A twenty-two-year-old man complained of headache, as if there was a wedge in the middle of his head. The sensation reminded him of how he felt when he fell on the ice and hit his head, six months earlier. He was standing on the rink when his feet suddenly went out from under him. The side of his head caught the full impact of the fall. The next thing he remembered was standing, talking to his friends. Since that time he experienced this headache at different times. *Apocynum androsaemifolium* 6x, one dose, cured permanently.

A twenty-eight-year-old woman who had been chronically ill for nine years took a dose of homeopathic *Medhorrhinum* 10m (not administered by myself). She experienced a terrific reaction: headache, difficulty concentrating, had to concentrate on her breathing in order to make sure that it was taking place, felt tightness in the chest as if the wind had been knocked out of her. The condition had been going on for seventy-two hours. *Apocynum androsaemifolium* 12x, one dose, stopped the ill effects within an hour.

A fifty-seven-year-old woman was becoming progressively debilitated since a fall on the ice six months earlier. Now she suffered from total prostration, splitting headache, profuse perspiration. The skin was slightly yellow. When the fall occurred she dragged herself up, feeling it was "a miracle" that she was still conscious. "I had to control my mind," she said, "in order to remain conscious," so that she could walk the six blocks home with her granddaughter. *Apocynum androsaemifolium* 30x, several doses, aggravated the perspiration and exhaustion. It also brought on a slight fever. After three days she was much improved, and was able to return to work for the first time in two weeks. No return of the problem.

A fifty-four-year-old woman complained of swollen glands in the posterior chain of lymphatics under the right ear. She had conjunctivitis of the right eye with gummy, yellow exudate the day before. Some pain in front of the right ear. The lymphatics were becoming very painful. I was quite surprised when I took the pulse. In inflammatory conditions one would expect a fast pulse, but hers was weak and slow, so I suspected that there was some unusual etiology behind the condition. The only remedies I know of which have this type of pulse are the two *Apocynums,* but the *cannabinum* usually has edema with pitting around the vein as well. I asked the patient if she had fallen on the side of her head. Twenty years previously she had been in a car accident, in which the right side of her head came to rest against a telephone pole. When she woke she felt a dent in the temple. I asked if she feels like she is undergoing a profound change at the present time? Yes. *Apocynum androsaemifolium* 6c was given with prompt removal of physical symptoms. It also helped her make the profound change.

The highest impact of all occurs "when death enters the aura." (I don't want to give the impression that I see auras. This is merely the phrase I thought best to describe the feeling I get.) Medicine Lodge Root is indicated in persons who have been so deeply impacted that death sets its pincers into them. They may go on for years, or they may be headed for a quick termination, but the Grim Reaper has put his hand upon them. (The Grim Reaper is another symbol associated with the right angle.)

My friend Susan suffered for many years from Crohn's disease, which was slowly working its way towards a fatal conclusion. Among other things, her insurance company racked up one hundred and fifty thousand dollars in medical bills, she lost a third of her small intestine, and was in a coma for three months. She was hemorrhaging daily from the intestines and the doctors said there was nothing they could do when she dragged herself into Present Moment Herbs, in Minneapolis. Bob Gallagher, the owner of the store, suggested she consider a cold decoction of Calamus root. The bleeding was completely stopped in twenty-four hours. Susan needed many other remedies, but whenever the bleeding started up, she took Calamus. It did not fail for about seven years; then we had to switch to Gravel Root.

Susan still felt "like a shadow," like a piece was missing, for years afterwards. She had to make a complete and total change in her life. At one point I gave her *Apocynum androsaemifolium* 6x. I don't really know if this helped her. She was slowly returning to health. But it made me feel better. One day we were having lunch and a strange feeling came over me. I knew death was leaving my friend. I exclaimed, "Susan, death is coming out of your aura right now." She was in denial about how sick she really was, so she complained about this statement for a long time. "Some bedside manner you have," she remarked. "When I got back to work everybody said I was as pale as a ghost." Years later Susan finally understood what I meant. She was at a hospital visiting a seriously ill patient when she was struck by the fact that she herself had been far sicker than most of the people there. She knew it was a miracle she had survived and she knew that death had been her companion for a while.

Another strange story occurred when I was visiting some friends in Michigan. One of them had a horrific asthmatic attack. Ellen had been having them since childhood and I had never been able to get the right remedy because I had never been able to see an attack. My eyes almost popped out of my head when I saw how bad she was and I had that nasty old impression again, "death is in her aura." Once before, she had almost died when she was in this state. I gave her *Apocynum androsemifolium* 12x. Her husband commented, "I have never seen anything stop Ellen's asthmatic attacks as fast in fifteen years."

The longer we talked, the more bizarre the story became. Ellen said she had been having these symptoms ever since a bizarre occurrence in her childhood. One moment she was lying in bed, the next moment she was at the window, looking at a small fox-like figure standing on two hind legs, dressed in a little vest, with crossed arms. The being turned and looked at her with gleaming yellow eyes. Ellen was shocked. (A chill ran up my back as she was talking.) From that time on she experienced severe asthmatic attacks. She also determined that the fox-being was standing in a location that was not observable from the window, and she suspected an "out of the body" experience.

I saw Ellen two months later and something had changed in her. She was more relaxed and comfortable. The asthma was less bothersome, though not completely cured. Now she needed Agrimony because she was struggling to catch her breath. She took it in various homeopathic potencies. From the first day, it brought up mucous. This continued for months, until the lungs were cleaned out. "Nothing has ever helped me like those two remedies," Ellen commented to me years later. Except for occassional, fleeting discomforts, her asthma was virtually eliminated.

We did, however, have to use the Agrimony again. After a business partner married a domineering, hateful, greedy woman, Ellen and her husband found themselves attacked by a foe who bragged that she intended to destroy their life and livelyhood. We used both Agrimony and Cinquefoil. The motto for these plants is: "keep your hands off my stuff."

People who have been through life and death experiences have an easier time believing in magic. They can believe that plain, ordinary plants (i.e., those little green things) can transform the psychic environment around them, change their lives for the better, and drive harmful people away. For their part, plants like people who have a just cause.

Preparation, Toxicity, and Dosage

All parts of this plant are dangerous. I have had no problem digging the root, which is the part used by the Indian people. I only recommend that people "hold on to it." *Apocynum androsaemifolium* can be safely used in the homeopathic potencies: 6x to 30x and 6c to 30c. The material plant should not be taken internally.

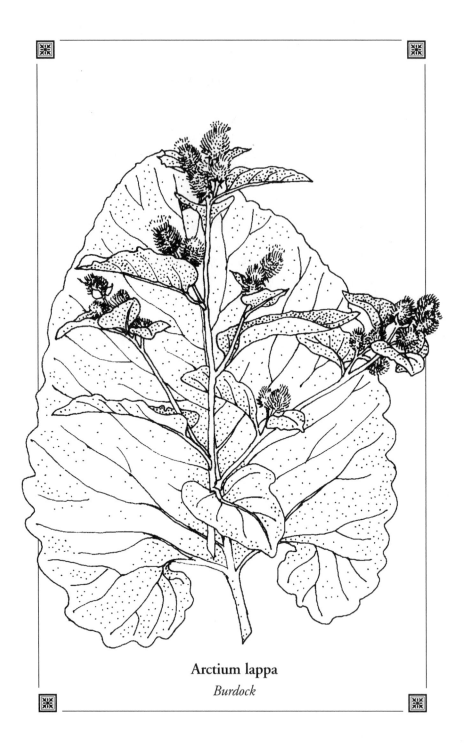

Arctium lappa

Burdock

Arctium lappa

Burdock

In tracing the history of medicinal plants I have seldom been surprised. One can often guess from how a plant is used, the cultural milieu within which it originated and was brought to prominence. With Burdock, however, I was taken aback. I expected it to be a timeless fixture of popular herbalism, an "old granny" remedy used as a comforting tea on vague indications as some kind of "blood tonic." It is described in contemporary literature as an "alterative" that "cleans the liver and kidneys," ridding the system of toxic waste materials. However, it turns out that the use of Burdock as an alterative to cleanse the liver and kidneys dates only to the late seventeen hundreds, and that it was introduced by allopathic doctors, of all people! It was almost completely ignored in North America until the late nineteenth century, when it was introduced by (again) professional physicians. From here it crept into popular herbalism, where it is now widely prescribed, though on rather vague indications, as a "blood purifier" and "liver cleaner." However, it appears that the old tradition particularly dwelt upon the resemblance of the seeds to urinary calculi and placed more the emphasis upon the influence Burdock has over the kidneys.

Burdock is a common weed native to Europe and Asia. The burs get caught in people's clothing—or dog fur—and, as a result have migrated in all directions. The plant is suited to a wide range of climates and is now naturalized on every continent. Burdock is a member of that adaptable family, the Asteraceae. There are two species which are used interchangeably: *Arctium lappa* and *A. minor.*

Dioscorides knew this plant under the name *Arcteion,* meaning "Bear Plant" in Greek. This hints at very ancient shamanic uses. When Burdock was brought to the Americas, the Indians latched upon it as a Bear Medicine. The dried brown burs look much like bear fur.

Plinius, another Roman author contemporary with Dioscorides, called this plant *Lappa,* which derives from a Greek word meaning "to hold fast." This name is also related to a word for mucus. Galen (150 C.E.) knew it under the name *Phasganion,* which Gerard considered to be a corruption of the name "Herb Victory." (The plant has spread everywhere and is certainly victorious in that regard.) The old English name is "Herrif" or "Aireve," from the Anglo-Saxon *hoeg* (hedge) + *reafe* (robber) or *reafian* (to seize). We can certainly appreciate the name "Hedge Ruffian."

I was surprised (again) to find that the name Burdock, which sounds like old English, is actually of recent, hybrid origin. It encorporates an old English word for a large leaf, *doc,* together with the French word for a bur, *burre.* The middle English and Renaissance authors generally knew the plant under the name "Clot Bur," which is related to the old German name, *Klettenwürzel.* The word "clot" reflects an English root word related to clinging, clotting, and cloying. Finally, about the time of Culpeper, the name was standardized as Burdock.

This widespread plant has found a niche in the herbal pharmacopoeia of nearly every culture where it grows. It is used in Europe, India, China, and Japan. Upon its arrival, the North American Indians adopted it into use.

Turning back to the original sources of our tradition, we find that Dioscorides recommended "the decoction of the root…together with the seed, against the tooth-ache, if it be holden awhile in the mouth." The seeds possess the same nerve-tingling, diffusive taste found in Echinacea, which is also used in this way. Dioscorides adds that Burdock is also useful for "strangury and paine in the hip." Several other Roman authors elaborated slightly on the uses of Burdock.

Medieval and Renaissance herbalists followed this impoverished tradition without making significant additions or changes. Gerard adds little to the classical sources, but speaks highly of Burdock as a food. "The stalke of Clot burre before the burres come forth, the rinde pilled off, being eaten raw with salt and pepper, or boyled in the broth of fat meate, is pleasant to be eaten." But, he cautions, "being taken in that manner it increaseth seed and stirreth vp lust."

It is Culpeper, writing fifty years after Gerard, who gives a more confident and detailed account. This shows evidence of personal experience with the plant. Many of the indications he gives are traditional, but some new ones appear and his decided preference for using the leaves is an idiosyncrasy showing no relationship to the received tradition.

Culpeper classifies the leaves as "cooling, moderately drying, and discussing," i.e., dispersing. They may be applied to places troubled with shrinking of the tendons, giving much ease. (This is not a use reported elsewhere.) The juice of the leaves drunk in old wine, "doth wonderfully help the bitings of serpents" (an old usage), or taken with honey, provoke urine and cure pain in the bladder. "The leaves bruised with the white of an egge, and applied to any place burnt with fire, take out the fire, give sudden ease, and heal it up afterwards." A decoction of the leaves placed on "any fretting sore or canker, stayeth the corroding quality." The root may be used to similar purpose. "The seed is much commended to break the stone, and causeth it to be expelled by urine, and is often used with other seeds, and things to that purpose." (The doctrine of signatures seems to be making a play for attention here, since the seeds look like little stones.)

One completely new addition that Culpeper makes to the discussion, and one which is most peculiar, relates to the uterus. "Venus challengeth this herb for her own," he writes. "By its seed or leaf, you may draw the womb which way you please, either upward by applying it to the crown of the head, in case it falls out, or downward in fits of the mother [uterine cramping], by applying it to the soles of the feet; or, if you would stay in its place, apply it to the navel, and that is likewise a good way to stay the child in it."

It seems almost certain that Culpeper picked up these curious ideas from folk practitioners. Excluding his astrology, this kind of openly magical element is almost never found in his writings. He does not rant against "vaine superstitions," as Gerard does (holding his venom for "papists.") Nevertheless, this kind of concept is rare in Culpeper. The validity of this usage has long been borne out in popular herbalism and even in professional medicine. We find *Arctium* used for uterine prolapse by such a pragmatic doctor as William Boericke.

After Culpeper, the professional doctors and apothecaries increasingly began to distance themselves from the common weeds and herb manuals which were easily obtained by the population. In an effort to raise the prestige of their profession, they concentrated on exotic and poisonous medicines. These also fit with emerging doctrines in chemistry which looked to valuable properties in small, refined concentrations of often poisonous material. Herbalism was relegated to poetry and the poor. It is therefore surprising that during the height of the Enlightenment, in the late eighteenth century, Burdock was brought back into popularity, on new and improved indications, by the professional doctors.

John Crellin and Jane Philpott trace this development in *Herbal Medicine, Past and Present* (1990). In 1719, John Quincy, a London writer on pharmacopoeia, noted that Burdock is "much in use among the country-people." The leaves are used "for burns and inflammatory tumors," the seeds are "esteem'd extremely diuretick and some reckon them effectual in carrying off by those discharges, what is very much the occasion of arthritick pains when 'tis once deposited upon the joints." At this point Burdock was still used much as it had been, though this is a rather more positive account than one often reads about the diuretic and antilithic properties of the plant. Later in the century, another London *Dispensary* written by George Motherby (1785), stated that Burdock was useful "in all cases in which China and sarsaparilla roots are used." These exotic plants were used as tonics which alter the whole organism by a generalized action through several systems of the body (hence "alterative".) Crellin and Philpott note that here, for the first time, the concept of Burdock as an "alterative" begins to appear. (Burdock hitched a ride on the back of other herbs to get to its new position.)

By the time Thomas Green wrote his *Universal Herbal* in 1820, the old and new pictures of Burdock were starting to be compressed together. "Some eminent physicians think a decoction of the root equal if not superior to that of sarsaparilla," he writes. It is a diaphoretic, "useful in fevers," but in "operating by urine is its greatest value." It clears gravel and stone from the kidney and bladder, and is useful for dropsy and venereal disorders. In addition it acts against jaundice, consumption, and "asthmatic habits."

During this period, Burdock was virtually unknown in America.

Thomson (1820-40) and Cook (1869) do not mention it at all. O. Phelps Brown (1867) dismisses it as overrated and unreliable. An Appalachian herb dealer noted in 1870 that he only purchased Burdock if a buyer asked for it. However, about this time Burdock began to enter back into American medicine. It was the eclectics who began to use "Lappa," as they called it: we find mention of it in the writings of Scudder, Locke, and King. The appearance of a patent medicine called "Burdock Blood Bitters" may have contributed to its reputation.

Scudder writes, "It acts directly and very kindly upon the urinary apparatus, increasing secretion, and removing irritation. Its action in this respect is especially beneficial in chronic disease, where old tissue is to be renewed, and the saline diuretics can not be used. It may also be employed to relieve bronchial irritation and check cough, there being the general indications for the class of remedies known as alterative." It may be that Scudder, rather insistently using this word alterative, was responsible for its widespread acceptance under this category of classification in the twentieth century.

Dr. John King (1898) offered a detailed compilation of the properties of "Lappa" in his massive *Dispensary*. Although he classified it as an alterative, he emphasized the action on the kidneys and downplayed or ignored the idea of its action on the liver or blood. In fact, he uses the phrase "alterative diuretic." He writes, "The action of the seeds upon the urinary tract is direct, relieving irritation and increasing renal activity, assisting at the same time in eliminating morbid products." The seeds are beneficial for dropsy, renal obstruction and painful urination. "It is of marked value in catarrhal and aphthous ulcerations of the digestive tract," including dyspepsia. It also relieves broncho-pulmonic irritation and cough. "Skin diseases, depending upon a depraved state of the cutaneous tissues and less upon the state of the blood itself, are conditions in which lappa has gained a reputation." It is particularly praised in psoriasis, sometimes requiring long continuance to effect cure. It can also be used in chronic erysipelas, dry, scaly eruptions, milk crust, eczema, scurvy, scrofula, obstinate ulcers, venereal, and leprous disorders. "The cutaneous circulation is feeble in cases requiring burdock seeds," he adds. "Rheumatism, both muscular and articular, when previous inflammations have left no structural alteration, are said to be benefited by the seeds."

By about this date Burdock was starting to become widely known. Generally, it was looked upon as a "blood cleanser" or "liver detoxifier." Although the definitions for these words were rather vague and folk-medical, Burdock had found its niche. The idea is that the liver, the seat of the metabolism, is not burning cleanly enough to remove all catabolic waste products, while the kidneys and the skin are overburdened or are themselves incapable of removing these waste products. The lymphatics, which assist all these organs, also enter into the picture. They may be pictured as getting slowly congested as, perhaps, a sort of haze of incomplete metabolites float around in the tissues. The scientific doctors were unsatisfied with such vague intuitions of how the body worked, so they called this class of remedies "alteratives," meaning a medicine that alters the system in some unknown way.

Arctium lappa was given a brief homeopathic proving. A short but useful account is rendered by William Boericke. It is "very important in skin therapeutics," he says. And he continued to recommend it in uterine prolapse. Cyril Boger also gives a useful account of *Arctium* in *A Synoptic Key of Materia Medica*.

Dr. Edward Shook summed up the history and properties of this valuable plant in his lectures in 1947. "Throughout the centuries, this majestic remedy for human ailments has stood the acid tests of human inconsistence, prejudice and ignorance and is still today one of the most extensively used herbs by country folk and herbalists throughout the civilized world. To our certain knowledge, it has cured syphilis after all other treatments had failed. For the successful treatment of chronic skin diseases, especially eczema, burdock has no equal, while for furunculosis [boils] its quick alterative and curative effect is truly remarkable."

The Medicinal Virtues of Hedge Ruffians

It has taken me a long time to come to an understanding of Burdock because I tend to like definite, specific indications for herb uses, rather than general ideas. Many other herbalists, more trusting than I, have attached themselves to the remedy with less to go on, and along my path of education I had to ask many of them about the plant.

"It is deep-rooted and strong-rooted," observes herbalist Kate Gilday of Coldbrook, New York. "Burdock grows up through the cracks in the sidewalks. It is a strong plant with a slow, steady, hardy influence, rejuvenating old chronic conditions. It helps frail people develop hardiness. It acts primarily on the liver, kidneys, and skin. The leaves are unusually good for itchy, sore rashes, eczema, and poison ivy; the seeds for adult acne."

Herbalist 7Song of Ithaca, New York, gave a similar report. "Burdock is especially suited to old, chronic cases where there is a lack of vigor and momentum. The person is caught in the slow, downward drag of chronic disease." And one of my students says, "Burdock helps the body remember what it was like to be healthy" and is suited to chronic cases "where the thread of health has been lost."

Mier Michel Abeshera, one of the early teachers of Macrobiotics with George Oshawa, gave his view in a lecture I attended. "Burdock is an interesting plant. You can kick it around, hit it and cut it up, but it always heads straight for the liver."

The action of Burdock is complicated and still not completely known. By looking at each structure of the plant, we can gain insight into different affinities and uses. The seed (or fruit, actually), bur, leaf, and root of the plant have all been used in herbal medicine.

The Root. Burdock is a biennial with a deeply anchored tap-root. However, the root rots out from the core after the first winter, so it needs to be harvested during the first summer. The root has a moderately bitter and sweet flavor, but a heavy, cloying property, due to a high oil content. This contrasts with the sharp, diffusive, tingly impression of the pungent seed. It is traditionally served in French cuisine with rich, oily food, to assist digestion of fats and oils. It is used the same way in Japanese cuisine—an application which comes down to us through macrobiotics. The bitter and sweet mixture point to stimulation of the digestive function.

The "mangy" appearance we find in the rotten roots of Burdock reminds us of the other great "blood and liver cleaners," Dandelion and Yellow Dock Root. They are rather mangy in their above ground parts. However, it also reminds us of how the structure of the body may be broken down, the blueprint for health lost, the essence which governs and gives form weakened and dissipated.

Burdock root acts more slowly than the seed, and has therefore been used for chronic conditions, where a slow, persistent stimulus is desired. "It slowly but steadily influences the skin, soothes the kidneys and relieves the lymphatics," wrote Dr. R. Swinburne Clymer. "It is of great value in the treatment of all skin diseases and in scrofulous affections. It is very soothing to the mucus membrane throughout the entire system and hence is valuable in irritated conditions." The fats, oils, and starches are lubricating and coating. "Its soothing character is also extended to the serous membrane and is valuable in rheumatism and also in venereal diseases."

The Seed (or Fruit). The tingly, diffusive impression given by the pungent flavored seed catches our attention. It speaks of something penetrating, provoking, diffusive, and sharp. Salivation is noticeably increased and secretions are promoted further down in the digestive tract and all the way out through the kidneys and skin.

Because of these combined influences, the seed has the capacity to penetrate to the core, stimulating metabolism and digestion, promoting waste removal, moving waste products towards the periphery and out through the sweat pores, urine, and stool. We have already seen how it was conceived to be a good kidney remedy, used to remove dropsy and gravel, as well as waste products which lodge elsewhere in the system due to poor kidney function.

Clymer preferred to use the seeds over the roots when there was active inflammation and fever. "In hot infusion [the seeds] influence the sebaceous glands, and are of superior importance in scarlatina, other exanthema, and also in typhoid fever." Here he combines the seed with Echinacea, one part each. "The roots will act in the same manner, though less actively."

Burdock seed is used in Chinese herbalism for "wind heat" fever, as seen in acute sore, red, swollen throat, and cough. It "releases the periphery," opening the sweat pores, relieving fever, and bringing out the rash.

I find that Burdock seed (or root) is beneficial for both profuse sweating and lack of perspiration. Dr. Cyril Boger (1931), one of the few homeopaths who seemed to have used *Arctium*, gives the symptom "axillary sweat" in large type. Both Burdock and Elderberry are suited to these two extremes. Both are suitable for acute or chronic skin conditions—here are a few case histories.

An old customer brought her new husband to see me. They were just about to leave on their honeymoon to the Riviera, but he was a bit sick and she wanted to make sure he was well. He was suffering from a great deal of perspiration on the face and elsewhere and had a worried look. He held a position of importance in city government, so I figured he had a lot to worry about—and then there was the wedding and the honeymoon. Burdock seed removed the worry, the sweating, and the hint of fever right away and they left in peace.

Another time, I was teaching a class in Indiana. During the lunch break I noticed a woman who had profuse sweating and a worried look on her face. I asked if she was O.K. "No, as a matter of fact," she exclaimed. "Thanks for noticing." She was suffering from a sore, hot throat. The worry had been going on for a long time, so seriously, that she would wring her hands from the anxiety. We went out in the barnyard, found a clean place up towards the house, and dug up a huge Burdock root. It was more than an inch in diameter. She nibbled on this and the sweat went down; eventually it cured her completely. She was not only grateful for the herb, but for the fact that someone noticed that she was sick. The true physician should have a therapeutic eye, which notices disease whenever it appears, not just when the time clock is running.

Another woman was going through stress at work. She was an anchor in her field, but felt unsupported in her work and was worried and anxious. She took homeopathic Calcium carbonate 30x (which has insecurity, feeling unsupported). The next month these symptoms were much better, but her skin was dried out and rashy, especially at the wrists. Burdock root tincture released the pores, the skin returned to normal, and she felt much better.

Recently a mother brought her fifteen-year-old son to see me. He was suffering from great anxiety and worry. He was on Prozac. After taking a long case the only thing that seemed distinctive was the dry skin. Otherwise, I would not have thought of Burdock. It proved to be a beneficial remedy for the skin, but the fears remain.

The hair is an important element related to the skin. As far back as Dioscorides, our stick-to-it-ive Hedge Ruffian was used for loss of hair. The bur looks like a little head with hair standing out. The homeopathic provings bear out a relationship to the scalp.

I saw one case where Burdock stopped hair loss associated with an unhealthy scalp. The client was a twenty-eight-year-old man who was in good health, except that he had been losing hair from the top of the head, "in handfuls," for about a month. It did not seem to be a true balding, but some kind of temporary condition. He had not had it diagnosed by a doctor. The scalp was mildly itchy. Skin generally moist and in good health. The pulse was superficial and wiry, the tongue somewhat dry, with tiny red points on a pale pink background. There was a little redness across the zygomatic arch: a slight malar flush. He had headaches, generally dull, but occasionally sharp in the forehead and temples, accompanied by sinus congestion and irritation. Also, a rash under the right axila, which was quite itchy. There was excessive sweating in both axila, but not elsewhere. (Rash, boils, profuse sweating, and lack of sweat are usually good indications of clogging in the lymphatic glands.) I asked if he experienced flushing, but he thought not. A little later he commented, "now I feel flushed," and his face looked more red in the malar area. He complained of feeling tense, but I thought he looked worried. Raw Burdock seed, a pinch as needed, brought glossiness to his hair, stopped the loss, removed the rash, and all the rest of the problems. After the first dose he felt relaxed, the pulse was decidedly reduced and the tongue was obviously wetter and felt less painful (he hadn't mentioned that it was painful before.) The hair grew back nicely.

I would like to comment that this person showed some symptoms of what the Chinese physicians would call "kidney yin deficiency," such as hair loss, the malar flush, and the sudden uprising of heat. This is due to the fluids in the kidneys being too low to sedate heat and nourish the hair. (See Water Lily and Goldenrod for a discussion of kidney yin deficiency.) I believe that Burdock is similar to Goldenrod. The fluids are too low and they do not sedate the heat of the liver. However, I do not believe that this is the total picture for Burdock, but only an element. Burdock also seems to act on an overfull liver, which is incapable of handling all the waste products sent its way for processing. The fire burns too hot and this may dissipate the fluids, the kidney yin. Or it may be that both things are happening simultaneously. Herbalist 7Song made a comment which is significant in this regard. He said that Burdock is for "liver acne," when the pimples are singular, large, and nasty, while Goldenrod is for "kidney acne," when they arise in little sheets of fine pimples accompanied by a general patch of reddish, dry, irritated skin.

The Leaf. Large leaves are a signature for the skin and the lungs. Plants with large leaves "perspire" a lot. That is to say, they transpire carbon dioxide and water vapor through the abundant pores in the leaves. The leaf is analogous to the skin and lungs in the human body, which exchange gases through the pores. These are the organ systems which especially depend upon a massive surface area to accomplish their activity. All the large-leafed plants, such as Burdock, Mullein, Comfrey, and Elecampane, have strong actions on the skin and lungs. Burdock leaves are generally not used for internal problems, but are widely applied as a salve or poultice on the skin.

Shook relates a case from his practice where the leaf poultices proved effectual for skin problems. "Some years ago, a man in his thirties came to us for help. He had suffered for nearly a year with boils on different parts of the body. He had nine of them on the nape of his neck. Some twenty-nine had been lanced by doctors previous to this flock of nine. His neck presented a most horrible sight. He had several more boils on different parts of his body. Two under one arm and one under the other. Several more were scattered about on his wrists, buttocks, and legs. It was the worst case of furunculosis we had ever seen. Fortunately, this happened in the early fall and we knew of a very thick growth of burdock not far away." Shook had the young man gather sacks of leaves that were not faded and dig up the first year roots. The leaves were to be made into a poultice, without heating, sprinkled with eucalyptus oil. The roots were boiled and a pint of the decoction taken every day. "In three weeks, the boils were all gone and in one month this young man was completely well." He had no relapse in seven years.

The action on the skin conditions in the armpits show an affinity to the lymphatic structures, which congregate under the arms. *Arctium* also has been used for skin problems in the creases and bends of joints, according to William Boericke.

Although Burdock is not greatly used at the present time as a respiratory remedy, it has a history of use in this area and should be considered. As we have seen, Burdock was used for bronchial irritation, cough, and asthma. (Through confusion in the reading of Dioscorides, where the herb *Arcion* is mistaken for *Arction,* it was also listed for consumption and blood spitting, but this does not fit the rest of the profile.)

There are a number of other organ systems that also need to maximize surface area in order to function. The kidneys crinkle up little capillaries in the nephron units in order to sort out and unload excessive salts and fluids. The liver bunches up venous tissue in order to maintain its structure and to process the combustible metabolic waste products coming up from the portal vein. The small intestine also requires surface area, as seen in the squiggling up of the guts in the abdomen. The brain seems to require extra surface area, hence the corrugated appearance. (Here, of course, we have a nice signature, since the bur looks like a head.) Unfortunately, we do not exactly know what Burdock does for the brain. However, some ideas on this subject have been offered.

The Bur. Besides being the inspiration for Velcro, the bur has a history of use in herbal medicine. The burs, more than any other part, remind us of the property of "seizing;" they also look like the head.

The Southern Indians used the bur as a remedy for improving the memory, according to "The Swimmer Manuscript," a manual of Cherokee medicine published by the famous anthropologist and friend of the Cherokee people, James Mooney (1932.) The idea is to make that memory like velcro, so that the things which pass by it will be seized or retained. A modern person might think that this is a superstitious and ridiculous way to use an herb, but on the other hand, such a usage may reflect the essence of the plant and allow it to express its true nature more fully. These magical uses often rely upon a rather literal interpretation of the doctrine of signatures. They also help us to view our faculties (in this case our memory) in a unique and unusual light. Collect the burs in the evening, when the mind is at rest. Make the tea in the morning, for several days in a row, when to stimulate the mind.

These insights point us in the direction of the kidneys, since they store the "essence," the genetic-hormonal material which provides the blueprint, "the original," for what the body should be doing. They are also the organs which "seize" most strongly, in their action on the blood. The kidneys grab the blood and take it within, where it is weighed out and judged. The useless part is shuffled off down the ureters, while the remainder is allowed to go back into the bloodstream. The kidneys, or sexual-urinary tract, are also the organs most likely to be damaged by syphilis (see Teasel). This disease directly breaks down the "essence," destroying the hard tissues, the frame, the blueprint. It was looked upon as a disease of the "essence," in Europe, India, and China.

We have already seen that Burdock is credited as a medicine for the uterus. I learned about the signature for this from a traveling herbalist. One day I was sitting on the roof of my barn putting on tar and shingles, when Adam Leibling, an herbalist from Cambridge, Massachusetts, pulled in the driveway. He joined me on top of the roof. "Yeah, I've spent time roofing with William LeSassier too," he commented. "That's one thing I like about herbalism. It's an occupation of diversity. One moment you're helping a person, another you're wildcrafting herbs in the woods, and then you're repairing the barn."

We talked about herbs as we laid down the dark adhesive. Adam said that large burs or thistles, such as we find on Burdock or Teasel, are an indication for the uterus. I tend to think of anything rather globe-like as a signature for the head, but he said it reminds us of the radiating, circulating influence the uterus has to maintain in order to nourish the fetus, and also to keep itself in order when there is no fetus.

The use of Burdock as a uterine medicine is also developed by Australian herbalist Dorothy Hall, in her fine book, *Creating Your Herbal Profile* (1989). I had one case which verified this use. A woman in her mid-thirties came to see me. She was suffering from a dragging, heavy feeling in the uterus which had been diagnosed as a prolapse. She didn't want a hysterectomy, if she could avoid it. Her whole personality seemed draggy, her feet tired. She was self-employed, ran a flower shop and was on her feet constantly. I wasn't the first person to recommend that she stay off her feet more, but I was the first person to give her Burdock seed. I ran into her six weeks later. Her whole personality was perkier. "How's the uterus?" I asked. "Hunh...Oh, I forgot about that," she said. It was fine now. She seemed to resent having nothing to complain about, or having to admit that she felt better.

Burdock also acts strongly on the prostate. Recently I saw a forty-three-year-old man who had been suffering with swollen prostate for about five years. I had helped him in the past, but the effect of the remedies wore off after a few years. I couldn't figure out the case based on the symptoms, but I recognized the pulse as a distinctive one calling for Burdock. (This is too difficult for me to put into words.) The remedy worked fine. Later I mentioned this case to my friend Margie Flint, an herbalist in Marblehead, Massachusetts. She said, "I use Burdock all the time for swollen prostate. Saw Palmetto [the fad herb for this complaint] sort of palliates, but Burdock goes to the core and permanently cures. It works for young men who have a swollen prostate from pumping iron incorrectly, as well as in older men." Now I understood why my client had prostate trouble at a young age—he mentioned that he lifted weights.

Let us bring our account to a summation. Burdock acts so widely on the system that it is somewhat difficult to pin down its exact affinities. Yet, we can say that it opens pores and promotes secretion from internal and external surfaces. It seems to act particularly through the liver, lymphatics, and kidneys. It stimulates metabolism through the liver, cleansing and feeding through the lymph, and waste removal through the veins. Thus, it strengthens, wrings out and lifts tissues and organs, including the uterus and prostate. It acts strongly on the skin, to promote or correct perspiration.

On the psychological level, Burdock helps us to deal with our worries about the unknown, the "Hedge Ruffians," the bears, which lurk in the dark woods beyond our control. It seizes upon deep, complex issues, penetrates to the core and brings up old memories and new answers. It gives us the faith to move ahead on our path, despite the unknown problems which may ensnare us along the way. It helps the person who is afraid become more hardy, while it brings the hardy wanderer back to his original path. It restores vigor and momentum.

Preparation, Toxicity, and Dosage

The root is picked at the end of the first season. It is difficult to store, because the high oil content tends to make the roots go rancid easily. A glycerinated preparation of the root is especially nice, as the sweet taste and heaviness of the root blends well with the glycerin. Brandy is the best alcohol for bringing out the sweet and bitter flavor. The fruit may be picked when they are ripe in the fall, but not long after, as they are consumed by insects. They should be run through a coffee mill or a food processor to remove the little splinters which cling to them from the bur. They should not be chopped. The black-brown "seeds" can be eaten without further preparation, a few at a time. They have a quick, sharp, salutary effect.

There is no known toxicity for Burdock, but a few cautions might be mentioned. Never chew on a bur or on a seed freshly removed from the bur, unless the little slivers that surround it have been removed. This might seem the most obvious observation in the world, but some people need to be specifically informed. I count myself among them. One time I tore a few seeds out of a bur and chewed on them. (I chew on virtually anything out there in the wild.) Little slivers drove themselves in my tongue and remained there for several days. I put Plantain leaves on to try to draw them out.

I thought nobody else was this stupid, but I mentioned it in my classes from time to time. I was surprised when one of my students posted me a note. "I have been receiving orthodontic," he wrote. "I have been trying all summer to get my molars to erupt with elastics attached to appliances on my teeth. They would not budge or move at all. A few weeks ago I was out in the field hunting pheasants and decided to eat some burdock burs, only to sliver my tongue severely in the process. For two nights, I was miserable and slept with plantain leaves covering my tongue to draw out the slivers. My tongue got better, but also my molars shifted and erupted quite dramatically."

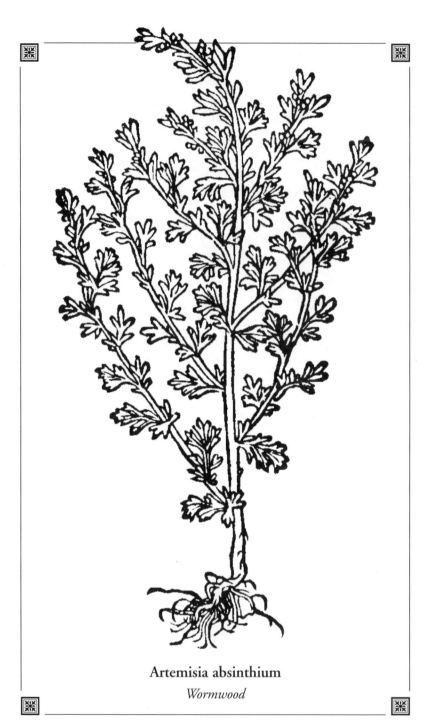

Artemisia absinthium

Wormwood

from *Herbarium Imagines Vivae*, published by Christianus Egenolphus, 1535

Artemisia absinthium
Wormwood

The *Artemisias* or Wormwoods are a distinctive clan belonging to the Aster or Composite family. They are generally very bitter, harsh tasting plants with a gray fur on the leaves, which usually look gray, silver, or dark green. They tend to grow in wastelands, deserts, and areas which have been devastated, such as road-cuts, quarries, and overpastured grassland. I discussed them as a family in my previous book, *Seven Herbs, Plants as Teachers*: they are nature's promise that out of devastation life will spring up anew. They are remedies for people who have been through rough, brutal, dehumanizing events or harsh environmental stress, resulting in emotional and physical coldness, lack of somatic activity, suppressed psychological affect, with stiff, cold extremities.

Artemisia absinthium, or Wormwood proper, is perhaps the archetypal representative of the family in Old World medicine. It is native to Europe and Asia, where it grows in desolate areas, but has been cultivated in gardens since antiquity, and is available worldwide as a garden herb. It is mentioned in the Bible as a metaphor for harsh, bitter experience and Shakespeare refers to it as the most bitter herb.

Wormwood was known to the ancient Greek and Roman practitioners. Dioscorides gives an extensive account which has not been much improved upon over the centuries. He used it principally for its stimulating influence on the stomach, gallbladder, and digestion. He classified it as warming and binding, with a "digestive facultie" capable of "taking away ye cholerick matter sticking to ye stomach, & ye belly." Taken with Cicely and French Nard, "It is good also for inflations and ye paines of the belly & of ye stomach." Taken by itself, "the dilutum or ye decoction of it doth heale want of appetite & ye ictericall," or jaundice. It can be externally "applied to ye Hypochondria, & ye liver, & a pained stomach." It protects against surfeits at the table, taken beforehand, and poisonings by hemlock and mushroom, not to mention "the biting of the shrew mouse, and of the Sea Dragon." It also proves "ureticall, hydropicall and splenicall," and "expells ye menstrua." A few little details are mentioned as well, such as matterings in the ears, ear pain, toothache, eye pain, and sugillations or outbreaks on the skin.

The reputation of Wormwood as a medicine specific to the stomach and liver continued down through the centuries. Gerard (1597) gives an account which builds a little upon the detail of Dioscorides. "It is very profitable to a weake stomacke that is troubled with choler, for it clenseth it through his bitternesse, purgeth by siege and vrine: by reason of the binding qualitie, it strengthneth and comforteth the stomacke, but helpeth nothing at all to remoue flegme contained in the stomacke, as Galen addeth."

"It is oftentimes a good remedie against long and lingring agues, especially tertians: for it doth not onely strengthen the stomacke and make an appetite to meat, but it yeeldeth strength to the liuer also, and riddeth it of obstructions or stopping, clensing by vrine naughtie humours."

"Againe, Wormewood voideth away wormes of the guts, not onely taken inwardly, but applied outwardly: it withstandeth all putrifactions; it is good against a stinking breath; it keepeth garments also from the Mothes; it driueth away gnats, the bodie being annointed with the oile thereof." It is used externally "to binde and to drie" and to remove "swartish markes that come vpon bruses."

Wormwood was also used in Europe to make vermouth or absinthe, but because it causes mental deterioration and insanity in addicts, it is no longer legal to use as an ingredient. Toxicological reports provided the basis of a homeopathic pathogenesis. These show that it acts strongly on the sensorium and nervous system, causing spasms, twitching, epilepsy, and night terrors. Unfortunately, the subtle and more useful characteristic symptoms relating to the digestion, stomach, and hepatic sphere were not brought out in such literature. "Absinthium," as it has been called in homeopathy, is little known or used in that school, though occasionally a case will come up where it will prove effective in night terrors. I have had cause to use it here, and it has proved palliative, but it is much more often indicated on the old guidelines inherited from herbal medicine.

Deadness and Coldness in the Stomach, Liver, and Gallbladder

"Wormwood ranks among the best known stomachics," wrote Father Sebastian Kneipp, the famous nineteenth-century German healer. "It leads the wind out of the stomach, improves the stomach juices, and so effects a good appetite and good digestion." He particularly recommended it when the breath was foul, especially "if it proceeds from the stomach." The other organ he mentions is the liver. "The decreasing yellowness of the skin will soon show the improvement of the gall, and the patient, whose breath has been, as it were, laced up by the foul air and often still more of foul juices—real dung-hills of the stomach—will breathe more freely again." He recommends the tea, powder, or tincture. "Travellers who are much troubled with indigestion and nausea should never forget to take with them as a faithful companion, their little bottle of wormwood tincture."

Our good father gives a dramatic case history. "On my return from a journey I visited a parish-priest of whom I had heard on the way that his end was expected. I entered and found the gentleman sitting in an arm-chair." He had twenty-five sores on his body, five on his face, which discharged a foul, brown fluid. "If I put on a plaster it will stick to the pustule for a day," the poor man commented. "When taken off, some putrid flesh will come off with it." He did not expect to recover, but sought palliation for the most disturbing symptom of all. "A foul taste in my mouth which is disgusting beyond description." Kneipp recommended a tea of sage and wormwood, four to six spoonfuls every two hours. "Then I left him, convinced that I should only see him in Heaven."

A messenger arrived after five days, reporting "the news—not of the priest's death—but that the tea had effected the desired change in the priest's taste, and that he even felt appetite for food." He felt confident enough to ask for a cure for the entire condition. Kneipp recommended whole body baths and washings. "After a fortnight the priest said Mass for the first time after a long interval." Hayflower baths were added. "The good priest's recovery was a perfect one, and he lived for twenty-four years after this cure cheerfully attending to his office as pastor."

If we look at the herbal literature, we find that Wormwood is primarily used as a bitter tonic to stimulate the stomach and hepatic tract. It is one of the most bitter herbs in the pharmacopoeia, along with Gentian and Barberry. Wormwood and Gentian are traditionally associated with the stomach and liver, the former with inactive conditions, the latter with heat and irritation.

The Wormwood conditions arise as a result of coldness and deadness in the stomach, solar plexus, and gallbladder. It is particularly suited to patients who have a lack of affect, a deadness in their personality, have suffered from brutal circumstances, and have the potential to be brutal themselves. "Brutal, insane, idiotic," say our homeopathic sources—here quoting from J. H. Clarke. On the other hand, some Wormwood people appear to be very animated. More often, however, the jaw is clenched, the expression guarded or artificial. From personal experience, I have learned that the most common pulse calling for Wormwood has a dead, masked feeling under the middle finger on the right hand of the patient, sometimes on the left. This corresponds to a condition where the solar plexus is guarded and the gallbladder reflexes are cold and dead. The liver, which should be the seat of warmth and animation, is cooled off.

Intermittent fever and jaundice may occur. These, we remember, are often associated with a deep chill to the system, and with the liver, which registers tension. Epileptic seizures and night terrors are possible in more advanced cases. Such conditions represent an advanced condition of liver stress. In Traditional Chinese Medicine they would be associated with cold suppressing the liver, resulting in "liver wind stirring," or spasmodic conditions in the muscles and tendons. Wormwood is used externally on sore, stiff muscles and cold extremities.

This is a very valuable remedy and I wish I could provide more in the way of case histories. However, over the years I have gotten in the habit of prescribing it when I run across the characteristic pulse (hard in the middle position on the right hand) and I seldom take much of a case or record much in my notes. It usually cures. The above portrait is the impression rendered by experience.

Preparation, Toxicity, and Dosage

Herbalist Michael Moore urges that Wormwood should not be used internally at all. It is banned for internal consumption in food in Europe and the United States. However, it can be used in small doses. I recommend it in doses of one drop, once or twice a week. Even a much larger dose would not make a person sick, but I find that giving Wornwood more often will often cause depression.

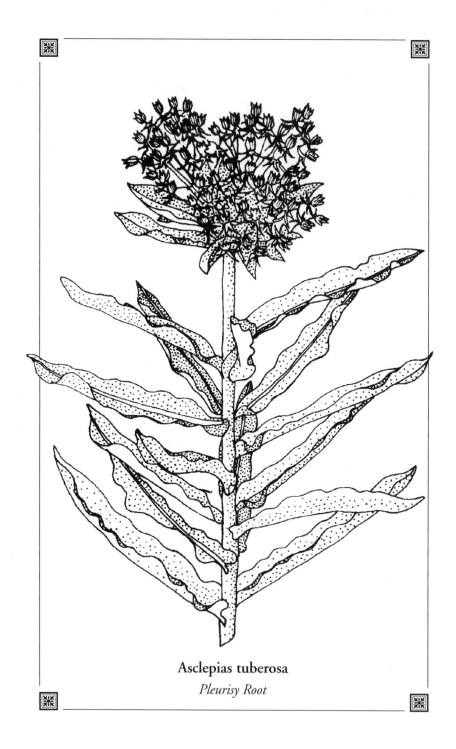

Asclepias tuberosa

Pleurisy Root

Asclepias tuberosa
Pleurisy Root

This is the most important member of the Milkweed family used in herbal medicine. The Indian people selected it from among the many members of that family as the most profitable, and it was adopted at a very early time by the English settlers as an herbal medicine. They called it "Pleurisy Root," after its main use. By 1800 it was quite popular with both the "root doctors" and the "regular physicians." It was considered to have a special relationship to pleurisy. It was later used by members of all schools, physio-medical, eclectic, and homeopathic. It is still popular today.

Pleurisy Root, or Butterfly Weed, is a handsome occupant of open meadows and roadsides in North America. It prefers light, sandy soil. It is distinguished by its bright orange flowers, but does not have the milky sap common to other members of the family.

Asclepias tuberosa is a good remedy for pleuritic complications, as the name suggests, but its sphere of influence should not be overemphasized. Acute inflammation of the pleura is better met by the homeopathic remedy Bryonia. *Asclepias* is suited to patients where the pleura have been damaged by inflammation, leading to adhesions and poor dissemination of fluids out of the pleural cavity. It is suited to acute conditions which have settled on the lungs and to chronic inflammation in other cavities, especially the bursa.

Diffusion of Fluids and Chi from the Lungs

Samuel Thomson classified this remedy as a diffusive. He noted that it dispersed fluids out of the lungs and brought perspiration to dry skin. He realized that these were related activities, and that *Asclepias* had the affinity to diffuse fluids through the tissues of the body generally. This insight captures the physiological essence of the plant.

In Traditional Chinese Medicine the lungs are said to disperse and disseminate fluids and chi. They maintain an open, misting activity, so that the tissues are permeable and substances are gently diffused outwards to the skin and downwards to the kidneys. If this process gets blocked up, we have a condition called "nondiffusion of the chi and fluids of the lungs." This usually results when the lung is invaded by exterior pathogenic factors (such as wind and cold), binding up and fettering the diffusive capacity. The principal symptoms are cough with varying amounts of mucus, scratchy throat, loss of voice, and lack of perspiration. Nondiffusion of lung chi usually occurs in acute respiratory infections, but it can linger and become a chronic condition.

This perfectly describes Pleurisy Root. It is a remedy which disperses the chi and fluids of the lungs to the skin and disseminates them downwards to the kidneys. It increases the perspiration in acute diseases and brings up phlegm in chronic cases.

For many years, I used to wonder what the strange appearance of the milkweed pod represented as a signature. One day I realized, simply, "Oh, it is a picture of a lung diffusing in all directions." This is one of those cases where the signature is almost cartoon-like in the literality of its picture-making.

Asclepias is suited to people who get an acute respiratory infection that settles on the lungs and becomes chronic. There is a feeling of oppression and tightness in the chest, impinging on the heart, so that they feel as if they might be having heart problems. Fortunately not. One herbalist teaching a class at my house commented that he was afraid to mention this herb. Whenever he did, someone in the class would need some. Sure enough, at the end of the day, one of the students said, "I think I need some of that Pleurisy Root. I feel just like that." Her pulse was a bit oppressed and irregular. Pleurisy Root quickly brought relief.

Asclepias is indicated in persons who have suffered from a severe bronchial infection, such as bronchitis or pneumonia, which has remained engrafted on the lungs. The pleura—the lining of the lungs—get dried out and the surfaces stick together, causing the "pleuritic stitch," a sharp pain which worsens from movement. At the same time, the dispersive capacity of the lungs are damaged, so that they cannot release and circulate fluids. The top of the lungs gets dry, the bottom collects water as the diffusive quality stagnates. This gives what I consider to be the characteristic *Asclepias* cough: "moist below and dry above." There is seldom any expectoration. One person spoke to me of bringing up profuse, gummy, white mucus after being on the remedy for a week. This seemed to be some kind of clearing. The skin is dry, the heart and circulation are oppressed, respiration is constricted. Occasional, sharp, stitching pains occur in the lower reaches of the lungs. The characteristic pulse in some cases is a thick, oppressed, full feeling. It feels as if the artery is not able to release or breathe.

Asclepias establishes the free flow of fluids to the surface, takes the burden off the heart and lungs, moistens the skin, removes effusion and adhesions, and settles the cough reflex. Here's a typical case. A woman in her mid-forties was suffering from bronchitis. The tongue was bright red and dry, indicating the fever was causing contraction of the muscles and bronchial tubes of the lungs. She had just entertained seventy relatives for a large wedding and was feeling harried. I gave *Lycopus virginicus* tincture, a drop on the wrist three times a day, and the inflammation and coughing subsided. However, shortness of breath settled in. "This always happens after the bronchitis," she reported. The tongue was much less red and not at all dry, the pulse felt "thick and hard," oppressed but not fast or slow. Like many asthmatics, she was perspiring, not profusely, but in a manner that suggested the perspiration was blocked. The entire system seemed to be compressed or oppressed. *Asclepias tuberosa* tincture, a drop on the wrist, as needed, removed the oppressive feeling, asthma, and perspiration.

Diffuses Fluids in the Joints

Asclepias tuberosa is not much used in homeopathy. Some important indications have, however, been noted. The patient is worse in cold and damp weather. This aggravates the chest symptoms, but also points to the use of the medicine in arthritic problems. Boericke gives the symptom, "Rheumatic joints give sensation as if adhesions being broken up on bending." Several times I have had people rub the tincture into a joint suffering from adhesions and clicking and clacking as it is turned. The sound disappears immediately and the condition is soon removed. *Asclepias* helps lubricate the bursa of the joints, just as it does the pleura of the lungs. Here again we think of *Asclepias* in relation to *Bryonia,* the foremost remedy for acute bursitis, as it is with pleurisy. However, *Bryonia* has active fever, while *Asclepias* has stagnation.

Sometimes *Asclepias* may be needed in more active, inflammatory cases. Here is an excellent case history from the practice of Dr. John Scudder (1870), the great eclectic. The patient was a forty-six-year-old man who was suffering from an inflammatory attack in the right knee. He averaged one attack a year, for the last five years, running a usual six week course. Scudder was called to attend him on the third day of the attack, and found the following symptoms. "Tongue clean, mucus membranes of normal color; bowels regular; pulse 110, full and oppressed; some difficulty in respiration, and oppression in praecordia, requires to be propped up in bed; the disease is localized in right knee, which is very much swollen, very painful, and exquisitely tender to touch; the most prominent symptom, as well as the most singular one, is constant profuse sweating." Scudder tried various remedies including *Aconitum, Cimicifuga,* Sodium bicarbonate, Potassium acetate, *Veratrum,* and *Colchicum,* but the symptoms grew much worse. "Eighth and ninth days a placebo; patient is suffering intensely, and talks of changing doctors." At this point Scudder had to take a new look at the case. "Reading up the treatment of phthisis a few weeks since I noticed the recommendation of a diaphoretic for night-sweats—have tried it in one case with advantage—why not give a diaphoretic for this prodigious sweating." Scudder decided on *Asclepias,* a strong infusion in tablespoonful doses. "There was a decided amendment the first day, and by the fifteenth day of the disease the patient was convalescent."

Notice Scudder's description of the pulse: "full and oppressed." The profuse perspiration resulted from a blockage or oppression interfering with the diffusion of fluids, and did not result directly from fever—hence, the appropriateness of a diaphoretic to clear the channels of perspiration.

Preparation and Dosage

This plant prefers to grow on sandy and gravely soil. Dr. O. Phelps Brown (1867) stated that the *Asclepias tuberosa* grown on sandy soil is twice as effective as that grown on fertile soils. This has been attested by others. It should be picked where it likes to grow, not from a garden. Make an infusion by pouring a cup of water over one-half to one teaspoon of the rhizome and steep for ten minutes. The tincture can be made by chopping the rhizome and macerating it in brandy. The dose need not be much—three to five drops is sufficient.

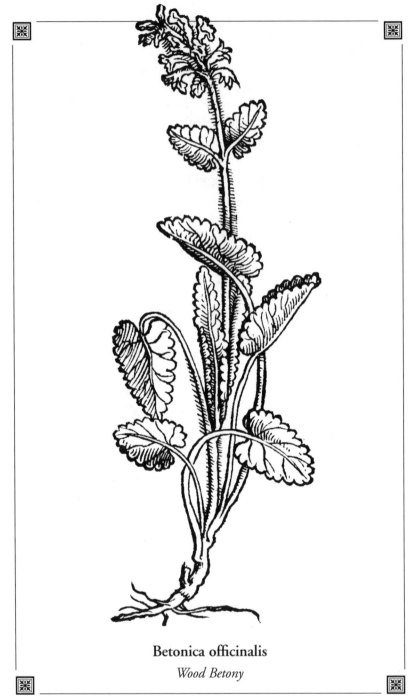

Betonica officinalis

Wood Betony

from *Herbarium Imagines Vivae,* published by Christianus Egenolphus, 1535

Betonica officinalis
Wood Betony

This was one of the most popular herbs in the Greek and Roman period. Antonius Musa, physician to the Emperor Augustus, wrote a book about Wood Betony, describing forty-seven uses. Most of these revolved around the stomach and digestive tract. Two hundred years later, another Graeco-Roman physician, Menemachus, summed up the basic idea. He said every formula for the stomach should include this plant. That is still worthy advice today.

Betonica was also considered to be one of the best medicines for the bite of the European viper. "Of betony above all the rest there is made a most sovereign salve to be laid upon the place that is stung," wrote Plinius in 70 A.C.E. "And such a contrariety in nature or antipathy there is (by folks' report) between them and this herb, that if the leaves thereof be stewed in a circle round about them, the serpents within will never give over flapping with their tails, and beating their own sides, until they have killed themselves."

Wood Betony continued to be held in high esteem down through the centuries. In the Middle Ages it picked up an additional use which may be related to the fabulous account by Plinius. Wood Betony and St. John's Wort were the two most essential herbs to used drive away "wycked spirits." Not surprisingly, Wood Betony was one of the most important remedies of the Middle Ages. It is mentioned in the works of Aemilius Macer (eleventh century) and Hildegard von Bingen (twelfth century). One medieval herbal happily reports, "It is good whether for the man's soul or for his body." Rychard Banckes (1525) adds, "It shields him against monstrous nocturnal visitors and against frightful visions and dreams." And in a more mundane vein, "If a man become tired in mickle [much] riding or in mickle goings let him take betony." Fabulous ideas continued to circulate at an even later date. The *London Pharmacopoeia,* translated by Nicholas Culpeper in 1653, states that, "The scull of a man that was never buried, being beaten to pouder and given inwardly, and quantity of a drachm at a time, in Bettony water, helps palsies, and falling sickness."

Wood Betony was still considered a general panacea in the Renaissance. "You should have as many virtues as Betony," was a popular saying of the time. Nicholas Culpeper (1652), writing in his own herbal, says, "It is a very precious herb…most fitting to be kept in a man's house, both in syrup, conserve, oil, ointment, and plaister." William Salmon (1710), writing at the end of the period, still speaks highly of *Betonica.* The decoction in wine is "Stomatick and Cephalick, comforts the Nerves and Brain, refreshes the Spirits, opens Obstructions of the Liver and Spleen, and is said to kill Worms, ease the Gripings of the Bowels, and the Colick." The syrup is "Pectoral, and causes an Expectoration of Flegm, and other tough Viscous Humors out of the Lappets of the Lungs, and other places adjacent. It may be taken with a Liquorice stick." The saline tincture is used for obstructions of the veins and the oil is applied externally on "Blows, Bruises or other weakness of the Limbs and Joints," on the head for headache.

Unfortunately, herbs are subject to fads, and like many other famous plants, Wood Betony passed into oblivion and was virtually forgotten. During the eighteenth century, when doctors began to turn away from common folk medicines, they distanced themselves from this popular little herb. (Perhaps they wre trying to live down the skull formula.) It continued to be used by herbalists, but even within the profession it has fallen into some degree of obscurity.

Wood Betony is a medium-sized mint native to sandy, sunny slopes and dry forests in central and southern Europe. It can be grown in most temperate regions as a garden plant and sometimes naturalizes in North America. The name *Betonica* is of ancient and uncertain origin. Originally the plant was classified as *Betonica officinalis,* but modern botanists changed the name to *Stachys officinalis* to show the affinity to the rest of the *Stachys* (or Woundwort) section of the Mint family. The old name is still sometimes used in herbal literature, and I give it preference here. European Wood Betony is not related to the American Wood Betony or *Pedicularis,* which is a member of the Foxglove family. The plants look similar from several feet away, but are exceedingly different in character and properties.

Our Betony grows in a neat clump, close to the earth, the leaves radiating forth from the ground. After it has established itself securely, it sends up long, slender flower stalks. This is the signature: Wood Betony is a remedy which helps establish rootedness, connectedness, earthiness, and groundedness. It is a plant for people who are cut off from the earth or their bodies. It strengthens the solar plexus—the place which helps us feel connected—and through the solar plexus it strengthens the stomach and the rest of the nervous system, including the brain. Through this general strengthening property, Wood Betony enhances the actions of diverse organs—lungs, liver, gallbladder, intestines, kidneys, and uterus. By strengthening the solar plexus and helping people to feel grounded, it has an impact on psychological health which helps to explain its magical uses.

If we can understand the nature of the solar plexus, we will be able to take in why this is such an important and powerful remedy, innocuous though it may seem. The solar plexus is one of the most significant nerve centers in the body. It is the switchboard for digestive functioning and gut-level instincts and reactions. As such, it is a terribly important center, and any medicine which acts upon it is liable to be constantly needed. So closely is Wood Betony associated with the solar plexus, that it is impossible to separate the two. It serves as an archetypal medicine plant illustrating this nerve center.

The Solar Plexus

The solar plexus is located at the lower end of the stomach, near the pyloric sphincter, just below the end of the sternum. We often feel it when we have a strong emotion or instinct which causes a "thump" in the belly. The solar plexus is "the brain of the stomach," coordinating the visceral functions associated with digestion and nutrition, but at the same time it is the instinctive brain or "gut-level instinct" center, giving hunches and "body knowledge" about different situations.

As the coordinating nerve center, the solar plexus is the master switchboard of the digestive tract. When food is eaten, the nerves of the solar plexus are stimulated. Signals are sent to and fro, causing the mouth to secrete saliva, the esophagus to begin peristaltic action, the stomach to squeeze and churn, the cardiac and pyloric sphincters to open and close, the gall bladder to release bile and the intestines to move with peristalsis. The mucus membranes from the mouth on down the alimentary tract secrete juices to promote digestion. All of this is coordinated by the solar plexus, so that the timing and activities are completely integrated and sensible, from beginning to end.

A wide array of problems are due to debility of the solar plexus. Here we turn to folk tradition and experience, because Western scientific medicine does not notice, describe, or attempt to treat anything like "debility of the solar plexus." Herbal medicine, on the other hand, rising as it does directly up out of the soil, is attuned to patterns in the natural world.

When the solar plexus becomes run down, the digestive processes are not as strong. Nervous stimulation, peristalsis, tissue and organ movements, nerve signals, coordination between functions and in fact all digestive functions, are affected by this weakness. The gallbladder does not excrete as well, the sphincters do not open and close, substances are not sent along at a nice clip, the cells are less active and secrete less, and so forth. The appetite and digestion become sub-par in a subtle sort of way that is hard to pin down—from a conventional medical standpoint.

In addition to these physical problems, there are some serious psychological problems as well, since the solar plexus is the center for "gut-level instincts." The sense of groundedness, instinctive wisdom, and self-confidence in subjective impressions is adversely affected. In such a state, one may indeed be susceptible to visits by "wycked spirits." Instincts and mental processes are weaker. Sometimes this comes on late in life, due to aging as the cerebral circulation and nervous system as a whole decline in strength. Occasionally a head injury will dissociate an individual. Wood Betony not only increases nervous strength and circulation in the solar plexus, "the brain of the stomach," but in the brain itself.

Because the solar plexus is such a large nerve center, debility and decline often affect the nervous system as a whole when it is affected. Through lack of stimulation and coordination of function, the nervous system becomes susceptible to atrophy and decline. There is also undernourishment of the tissues from lack of digestion. Weakness gives rise to an inability to deal with stress, and this creates nervous and muscular tensions. These interact to create high blood pressure and arterial tension—symptoms associated with Wood Betony today.

Distress in the solar plexus seems to particularly affect the brain. There is a reflex relation between the "brain of the stomach" and the "brain of the head." Diminished cerebral blood flow and nerve activity are the likely result of debility in the solar plexus. There is also a problem on the psychological level. When the solar plexus is functioning strongly, a person's inner life is enriched by intuition, instinct, and zest for life. This brings into play a more complete array of emotions and thoughts, which is healthy for the brain and thought-life.

Ancient and traditional medical systems placed a strong emphasis on the solar plexus and its attendant physical structures, especially the stomach, pyloric sphincter, and duodenum. Ayurvedic medicine visualizes the duodenum as "the seat of the *agni*," the primal fire of the body. The same idea is found in Western alchemy. Paracelsus said the "archeus," or innate intelligence of the body dwells in the stomach. A hundred years later, J. B. Von Helmont believed that the "sensitive animated soul" had its residence in the pyloric sphincter. Samuel Thomson, the folk doctor from New Hampshire, thought the stomach was the residence of the vital force. He visualized it like a stove in which a fire of heat and vital force burned, radiating in all directions, warming and vitalizing the body. In Traditional Chinese Medicine many of the physical problems described above would be classified as "stomach chi deficiency" or "deficient chi of the gallbladder." The stomach is not given as much credit as a psychological center in the official chinese medical tradition of today, but there are different strains of thought, some of which value the stomach more highly. In Taoist folklore, the image of the round-bellied, jovial little wise man reflects the idea that the belly is the seat of basic, down-to-earth wisdom.

A Specific and a Tonic

When we appreciate the wide array of functions associated with the solar plexus and the central position it occupies in the organism—like a brain—we begin to appreciate the importance of a medical agent which acts powerfully upon the solar plexus. We can also see why this herbal agent is not only a medicine with specific properties but a general tonic. This explains the prominent position Wood Betony held in ancient and traditional materia medica.

Wood Betony leapt to my awareness when I was musing over a difficult case. A thirty-year-old-man came to the chiropractic clinic where I sometimes see people, on a workman's compensation claim. He injured his back while lifting and was now unemployed. Nobody seemed to be able to get a fix on his problems. "I feel guilty treating him," said the assistant chiropractor. "I can't figure out what is wrong." The neuromuscular therapist countered, "Well, he does have lesions in the muscles." She was a fine therapist, with long, bony fingers like a schoolteacher from Iowa. It was hard for any problem to elude her grasp. He was thin, a bit pale, and sort of hard to connect with. I'd just sort of sit there and wait for him to respond to my questions with some sort of intensity, but even when he became interested in something, there was a frailty in his expression. I tried a few remedies without success. I felt there was some weakness of the solar plexus, some inability to really be in the body, present. I even resorted to telling him to rub Goldenseal on his stomach! A week later I was reading about Wood Betony in *Herbal Medication* by Priest and Priest. They only gave a few succinct indications, but it was clear that this was a remedy for the stomach and the brain. Somehow, that said *solar plexus.* Something seemed to resonate and I felt I had the right remedy. I recommended Wood Betony and our patient did wonderfully. He put on weight, his complexion improved, he seemed to engage in life more deeply, the chiropractic adjustments started to work and he got a new job. After three months he no longer needed to see us.

The influence of Wood Betony is subtle but significant. The person feels more alert, more "in the body," better grounded and physically stronger. Plinius wrote that Betonica gives the countenance a good color, removing the wan or leaden aspect. Appetite and eating habits are improved. The thin person tends to take on healthy weight and build up flesh, while the tendency to eat poorly and irregularly is combated. "I always prepare a lunch now," said one of my friends who started taking it. "Before I didn't think about it, so I ate junk food." After improving the appetite, Wood Betony helps the digestion. Macer writes, "a bean's weight of the powder of betony eaten with honey after supper greatly helps the stomach to digest meat." It settles the stomach, eliminating gas, burning, and discomfort. It is used for eating disorders, emaciation, stomach pain, and weak nerve reflexes of the stomach, gallbladder, and intestines.

A thirty-two-year-old woman came to see me for pain, burning, and gas in the stomach. The doctors said she had mild ulceration and she had, from time to time, taken the regular medicines for ulcers. Although she appeared to be quite present—no pale, leaden aspect here—the friend that came with her said she was a bit of a space cadet. They both laughed in agreement. Wood Betony not only removed the digestive problems rapidly, but improved her ability to function. I heard about this repeatedly from the friend, who was quite impressed.

The influence of Wood Betony extends from the solar plexus into the nervous system as a whole and thence to many other organs. Like so many good nervines, Wood Betony both relaxes and strengthens—building nerve force while reducing nervous and muscular tension—so that the person is better able to deal with stress and tension. The organs are likewise tonified.

Wood Betony has a potent effect upon the brain and mental functions. It promotes cerebral circulation and enervation in the head, opens the arterial blood supply, and is thought to reduce high blood pressure. It has been used in the past to correct vertigo, headache, loss of memory, difficult comprehension, and facial neuralgia. *Betonica* is an important medicine for migraine and headache which produce severe pain or frenzy. It is one of the best "general remedies" for headache; it dilates the cerebral arteries. One of my students started using it for sinus congestion—which it admirably cured in several cases. It acts on the eyes and vision, removing irritation and wateriness. (In ancient medicine, *Betonica* was combined with *Ruta* in ocular complaints.)

It is easy to see why Wood Betony has been used for old people or frail persons with poor circulation in the head and body generally. While I was down in Rochester, Minnesota, visiting my friends, students, and clients, I shared Wood Betony with a ninety-two-year-old man who was suffering from weakness, debility, pallor, lack of interest in his surroundings, frailty, and the sorts of conditions incident to great age. "Wow," he exclaimed. "What is this stuff?" It gave him a lot of energy, but it did not improve his basic problem. His wife and all his friends were dead. He wanted to die. Wood Betony put him in his body, but unfortunately, he didn't really want to be there. Another time I was called to assist an eighty-nine-year-old woman in St. Paul. She had a perky mental attitude and a considerable love of life. She was very stiff, but still exercised. When I put a drop on her wrist, she exclaimed, "I feel life flowing into my arm." She loved Wood Betony. A friend massaged it into her poor, stiff, cold feet, and it brought back warmth, feeling, and activity.

Wood Betony is just an excellent remedy for the elderly, and they will feel its action more readily than many. It has a similar action to Ginkgo, the modern "fad herb" for improving cerebral circulation. I find it ironic that this Chinese herb was introduced by German pharmaceutical companies, when they could have used Wood Betony, if they were aware of their own herbal tradition. I use Wood Betony, Rosemary, and Ginkgo in equal parts as a general tonic for older people. It is a "precious remedy," to quote Culpeper again. Rosemary is warming and activating to the circulation, and was considered a "heart tonic" for the elderly by Sebastian Kneipp and a remedy for the memory by Shakespeare and the herbal tradition. (It is surprisingly effective in removing serious deposites of fluid from the chest in advanced cases of cardio-pulmonary failure.)

According to traditional authorities, Wood Betony will prevent strokes or will stimulate improvement when given shortly after a stroke. Macer wrote in the eleventh century, "a plaster made of betony leaves ground well will heal an eye which has been damaged by a stroke. Make certain the plaster lies still against the eye all night." *Betonica* is still used for these purposes today.

By strengthening the entire nervous system and improving digestion and nutrition, Wood Betony builds up the tone of the flesh and muscles. It strengthens the lungs in wasting diseases and weakness. It has been used to stop the expectoration of blood, nosebleed, shortness of breath, chest pain, copious white or yellow mucus, and coughing or wheezing when associated with debility and lung weakness. It also acts on the liver and intestines. They are made more efficient in action. The bile is expelled more effectively, jaundice eliminated, and constipation reduced. By tonifying the system in general, it strengthens the kidneys, increasing urination and eliminating edema. By improving nervous and muscular tone, it can reduce high blood pressure. Wood Betony also exerts an influence over the female system. By improving the circulation, enervation, and muscular tone of the uterus, it has been used to remove uterine prolapse, menstrual pain, weak labor, and excessive bleeding. Because it is a mild uterine stimulant, it is contraindicated in pregnancy, unless carefully administered by a well trained herbalist.

Through its influence on the nervous system, Wood Betony is useful for various kinds of fever which either imbalance or burn out the nervous system. It has been used for chills, fever, and the ill-effects of high fever. It is one of the remedies which rebuild the nervous system after the damaging effects of fever (also think of *Verbena, Cypripedium,* and *Scutellaria.*) I used it myself once, in a bad case of food poisoning.

I was out in the country on a house call, at a little farm in the middle of a bog in the middle of nowhere. The four kids had food poisoning. I was thoughtless enough to stay for lunch. (Not following my instincts.) The next morning I had severe stomach cramps and explosive diarrhea. I took the standard homeopathic remedy for food-poisoning, Arsenicum album. This seemed to help the cramping pain for the diarrhea, but some discomfort continued for two days. On the afternoon of the second day I was visiting in the garden of an accomplished herbalist, Kate Gilday, in Coldbrook, New York, when I spied her little planting of Wood Betony. I was attracted to it, took it that evening, and felt much better. It relieved the exhaustion, slowed the diarrhea, settled the stomach, and returned the color to my face. The next morning I was pretty much back to normal.

Wood Betony is a specific when there is nerve pain associated with a tendency to disconnectedness, hysteria, or frenzy. It is one of the remedies for severe pain (also refer to *Agrimonia, Hypericum,* and *Zanthoxylum.*) It is also a traditional and important medicine for head injuries. Aemilius Macer (eleventh century) says it is good for a "fractured skull." Rychard Banckes (1525) goes so far as to describe how it is good when the cranial bone is pushed into the brain. This may seem like the unsophisticated musings of absurd old herbalists, but it is well to remember that people can survive terrible head wounds—like gunshots and so on—if the wound is kept clean. I have already mentioned a case where it was used in conjunction with Yarrow for a brain aneurism.

A friend called me in a state of great concern. Her three-year-old nephew had been operated on for a congenital heart condition. The operation went fine, except that he did not regain consciousness. After five days, the surgeons thought he probably would not revive. The next morning my friend applied Bach Rescue Remedy and Wood Betony. He immediately reacted; within three days he was back to full cerebral function.

Those Old "Wycked Spirits"

If it is still not clear what a "lack of groundedness" means, perhaps the following case will help. A forty-four-year-old man came in complaining of low energy, a serious ulcer in the stomach, severe depression, and anxiety. He was on a prescription tranquilizer and antidepressant. The pulse was full, rapid, somewhat flooding and tympanitic (indicating heat driving towards the exterior and gas). The tongue was very red and dry (a common occurrence in psychiatric cases since heat agitates the mind), slightly swollen around the edges, and coated yellow at the back. He stated his symptoms. The low energy occurred in conjunction with the depression. He tired easily after a few days of work, felt "rough," low motivation. "I don't have the normal range of affect," he commented. "People think my emotions are controlled, but actually I don't have enough energy...and I'm a little scared." I noticed what he was describing. He was sitting a little hunched up, like he was protecting himself, particularly the solar plexus. He had had the ulcer for the last two years, pain in the stomach area extending up the esophagus, sharp, "gas can't get out," the ulcer sometimes bleeds. I asked him about the depression. "I've had several setbacks during the past ten years," he said hesitantly. "I...I don't usually talk about this, but I suppose it would be O.K. I'm a UFO abductee victim."

My head was swimming. I didn't know what to say, but I wasn't going to invalidate his view of reality—especially as I believe in aliens myself—so I let him talk. "I've been abducted several times over the past ten years. It's been a terrifying experience. They also abducted my girlfriend. We were members of a UFO abductee support group." Eventually, she committed suicide. "I don't understand much about who they are, or what they're doing, but I do know that they...don't care about us at all. They are terrifying and violational. I try not to think about them or they draw close. I'm getting anxious...like they are...operating in the area right now." I didn't know what to say, so I asked what he thought would help? "I need to be better grounded on the earth."

The light went off in my head, and also in the head of an apprentice sitting in on the consultation. We were both thinking of Goldenseal and Wood Betony by this time. The former is the remedy for the physical lesion: heat in the stomach, ulceration, and loss of energy from the solar plexus. The latter is the true remedy for the disease, as it promotes groundedness. Dose, one drop of *Hydrastis* tincture, once a day, five to ten drops of *Betonica,* three times a day, or as needed.

Our friend felt and looked much better after the first dose. As we anticipated, Goldenseal helped with the ulceration and pain in the stomach. In a month he was cured. But it was the Wood Betony that really helped the basic problem. He became much more confident, capable of emotional interaction and more easy with people, felt more energy, and ceased to fear alien abduction. The tongue became less red and dry. He reduced the psychiatric drugs, but—last I heard—still continued to use them.

The real proof of cure was shown in the fact that he was able to move from a job as an orderly at a hospital to a position at a University. I later sent him Wormwood which is the remedy for "lack of affect," but I have not heard back as he lives out of state.

A few years after seeing this person I was interested to read that Wood Betony was the principal remedy used in the Middle Ages to exorcise demons. I could well understand this. It works, not by artificially removing "demons," like an exorcist in a movie or on a revivalist stage, but by strengthening and grounding the patient so that they are not threatened by distortions in thinking that may result from weak instincts and mental lapses. Their energy field is stronger and they repel these evil powers.

And this was not the last case where I used Wood Betony for an "unwilling UFO abductee." A thirty-two-year-old woman who had been a Satanic cult abuse victim as a child and who was now on heavy psychiatric drugs was induced to try an herbal remedy by her lover. "She just can't get over this UFO stuff," said her girlfriend. "I wonder if she's been abducted or something, or maybe it is some damage from the cult." She regressed to a little, childish voice and felt very intimidated and afraid when talking about "the aliens"—it reminded me of the man who worried that they might come around while he was talking about them. "They hurt me," she said.

"Well why don't you tell them to go away?" her lover asked.

"Well, they're trying to help people," she replied. How so? "When the planet is destroyed they are going to pick people up and take them away." That is not a good excuse for abusing a person.

We gave Wood Betony and our friend immediately began to change to a different state of mind. She was grief-stricken. "I don't want to feel this," her little child voice complained.

"What do you feel?" her lover asked.

"I feel sad about how people are treating the Earth," she said in a much more adult voice.

Wood Betony helped this woman to cope with the very real sadness that so many people feel about the terrible way our planet is brutalized by human exploitation. This made her more grounded and the alien abduction phenomena went away. I cannot say that the remedy solved all her psychological problems. She continued on the psychiatric drugs, but over the next few years she really began to improve in many ways. She continued to feel strengthened and helped by the Wood Betony all during this time. Both of them felt that nothing helped as this plant did.

In closing, I would like to bring before the mind the image of these "beings from outer space," totally alienated from earth, claiming they are going to "take people away" when the earth is destroyed. What better metaphor could we have for a lack of groundedness and earthiness. And they say modern people lack imagination. When these beings appeared after World War II, they were just replacing older, necessary images of alienation from grounded reality.

Preparation and Dosage

Wood Betony is usually picked before flowering. The fine vanilla-like flavor is best in the spring and early summer, before the flower stalks shoot up. The leaves are the part used. A simple infusion is made by pouring a cup of boiling water over one to two teaspoonfuls of the dried herb. A tincture can be made by chopping the fresh herb and macerating it in good quality brandy. This helps bring out the vanilla-like taste of the coumarins. A sufficient dose is one to two drops, one to two times a day. I have also used the flower essence with success.

Conservative modern literature considers Wood Betony to be contraindicated in pregnancy, due to the tendency to mildly stimulate uterine contraction. In the hands of a skilled practitioner it would probably be quite beneficial. It is used during labor to improve the contractions. It is a mild agent and it is not likely that it would produce startling changes in the pregnant condition when well indicated and used in moderate doses.

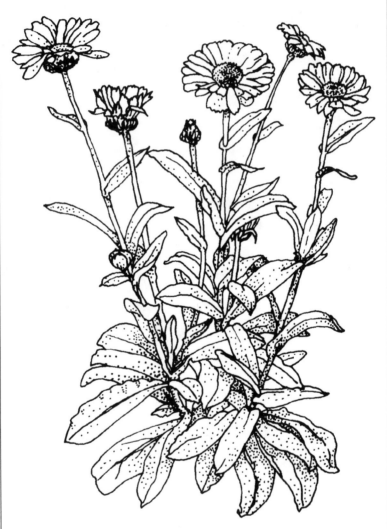

Calendula officinalis

Calendula

Calendula officinalis
Calendula

This cheerful flower is a member of the Aster family native to Europe, but widely cultivated for its beauty and sometimes naturalized. The golden-orange flowers look like a piece of the sun fallen to earth. By a happy plan of Mother Nature, these flowers remain in bloom for almost the whole length of the summer. Indeed, this is the origin of the name Calendula. As Gerard explains, "It is to be seene in floure in the Calends almost of everie moneth."

Calendula was used in German folk medicine as a remedy for wounds and glandular problems. The medicinal properties are resident in the resin which are concentrated on the underside of the flower heads, less so on the petals, leaves, and stems. They make the plant a bit sticky. In England, Calendula flowers were picked and dried. During the winter time they were thrown in soup with the belief that they helped a person fight off colds and fevers. These three uses: as (1) a wound medicine, (2) a remedy for affections of the lymphatic glands, and (3) a general "immune tonic," as we would call it today—are interlocking and bring out the true genius of the plant.

The reputation of Calendula as a wound medicine in German folk practice came to the attention of Hahnemann, the founder of homeopathy. In 1828 he assigned the study and "proving" of this plant to one of his students, Dr. Franz. As a boy, Franz had been caught in some mill wheels, suffering lacerations and scar tissue on the legs. I think we can see that Hahnemann anticipated the direction in which Calendula would express itself. He knew it had been used as a wound

medicine and he was hoping it would produce symptoms in a susceptible "prover." After a few doses of Calendula the scars became sensitive and sore and Franz began to suffer from fever and chills. When the
scars threatened to suppurate and discharge pus, he discontinued the
experiment. In this way, Calendula was added to the homeopathic
pharmacopoeia.

It was, however, a few years before homeopaths began to appreciate what they had. Shortly afterwards, another German homeopath,
Dr. Thorer, learned about Calendula from laypersons. His work was
translated by Charles J. Hemple's *Jahr's Symptomen Codex* (1848), one
of the first large homeopathic materia medicas published in the United
States. Up to Thorer's time, homeopaths had been using Arnica as the
remedy for all recent wounds. It was Dr. Thorer who first suggested
that Arnica was a specific only for bruises, strains, and contusions
without laceration, with Calendula as a specific for external wounds
and lacerations. This is the modern viewpoint in homeopathy. Thorer
used Calendula in terrible wounds, even in amputation of arms and
legs caused by machinery or surgery. He found that it routinely prevented the suppuration of pus and helped the wound heal cleanly. He
also considered it a remedy for swollen glands.

"From that time to this Calendula has always been used in
homoeopathic practice to promote the healing process in wounds,
ulcers, burns, and other breaches of surface," wrote Dr. Richard
Hughes (1880). "It was used on a large scale by our American colleagues in the treatment of the injuries arising in the course of their
civil war; and it obtained ... their warmest commendations. No suppuration seems able to live in its presence."

Calendula is one of the few remedies used in material doses in
homeopathy. The tincture, succus (fresh juice extract), salve, ointment,
or cream made from the flowers are all used. It is now widely used by
herbal practitioners as well.

Modern research shows that Calendula in material doses is not an
antiseptic, but bacteriostatic. That is to say, it does not kill bacteria, but
contains them, keeps the wound clean and thus helps the body to cure
itself. Dr. Hughes was on the mark when he said, "no suppuration
seems able to live in its presence." So often, we see these flashes of intuitive understanding in the old doctors. Some day, perhaps our modern
doctors will again trust their intuition and imagination.

Herbal Sunshine

One of my colleagues, herbalist Chris Hafner of Minneapolis, coined the name "herbal sunshine" for this plant. He adds that Calendula is the remedy "for places where the sun doesn't shine." This points the finger at the lymphatic structures, for they lie like a vast netting under major structures of the body—under the chin, under the arms and breasts, in the armpits, and in the inguinal crease.

Calendula is not only suitable to lacerations which threaten suppuration, but also to lymphatic glands which become swollen and stagnant, where the immunity is compromised and there are lingering remnants of infection. Calendula has been used as an herbal deodorant. The presence of unpleasant perspiration under the arms may indicate incomplete cleansing in the adjacent lymphatic structures. It is also used for vaginal discharge where the inguinal glands are swollen.

An unintentional proving by a nineteenth century homeopathic pharmacist showed just how far the doctrine of signatures can be pushed. After spilling some of the tincture on his hands, he experienced melancholy and depression, significantly worse when the sun went behind a cloud. This gives additional insight into problems associated with Calendula. The sun clears away clouds and dries up moisture. The presence of dampness is a pathological sign calling for Calendula. This remedy is used for conditions where there may be some excess dampness in the wound or in the tissues: thrush, swollen lymphatics, and vaginal discharge. Calendula is not a strong or forceful remedy, but when it is specifically indicated, it will clear lymphatic stagnation.

Dampness in Wounds

Calendula has been used by external application as a dressing for wounds which are tender, red, swollen, and tending towards the production of pus. They may be open or closed, with or without loss of flesh. It is used as a general remedy for inflamed conditions of the skin from lacerations, burns, sunburns, irritations, and chaffing.

The timely use of Calendula may prevent the formation of unsightly scar tissue. Here is one of the cases cited by Dr. Thorer. "Miss A. had a fall down stairs. She had several contusions on the chest, a deep hole on the forehead, and another hole much larger on the tip of the nose and on the back. She complained of great pain and was very much worried about her mutilated nose. Calendula was applied, and the healing of the wounds was so perfect that no one would suspect that there has ever been a wound of any kind." Dr. Thorer also used Calendula for cases where fingers or parts of flesh were torn off by mechanical injury or removed in surgery. In all cases, it prevented formation and suppuration of pus, kept the wound clean, promoted granulation and healthy scar tissue and removed the exhaustion which attacked patients laboring under a wound infection. The affinity to wound fever is seen in the original proving by Dr. Franz.

There are several ways to visualize the kind of wound to which Calendula is remedial. I like to say it "looks like a cat scratch"—red, swollen, tender, puffed up, infected. A holistic veterinarian from Atlanta, Georgia, heard me say that in class and made a big bottle for her clinic. It worked excellently for the staff. Here's another way to describe the Calendula wound. If you have ever canoed or boated a lot, you know that cuts that are repeatedly exposed to water get red, tender, and swollen. Calendula is particularly good here. It seems to take out the fluids (or "humidities" as the old authors would have put it) and keeps the wound clean.

Careful observation of the type of wounds most readily healed by Calendula leads us to the conclusion that it must clean the wound "from the inside," in other words, through the lymphatics beneath the skin. This explains why it works so well on wounds that are closed up and ones that are exposed to water. "Herbal sunshine" helps dry up and disinfect stagnant puddles of water or "humidities" under the skin. This points us in the direction of the traditional uses of Calendula as a remedy for the lymphatic and immune system.

Lymphatic Stagnation

Calendula is suited to people who have had swollen glands for some time, without signs of active inflammation, but with some dulling of immunity. Although it produced fever and chills during the homeopathic provings, I have never used it for active cases, but always for people laboring with unresolved lymphatic stagnation. Even then, one might expect it to produce fever as part of a detoxification, but its action is often gentle and it manages to remove swollen glands without much disturbance.

I have fond memories of cases where Calendula worked to remove swollen glands. A thirty-four-year-old auto mechanic came in with his wife and son, aged one and a half, to get a remedy for the little boy. He had a relapsing cough with rattling of mucus. The slightly blue complexion around the eyes and the disorganized cough reflex led to the selection of Antimonium tartaricum 30x. That remedy is perfectly suited to little children and old people who have weak cough reflexes. The cough hits in a different place each time and just rattles the mucus around without bringing any up. They seem a bit disorganized mentally or emotionally. As they were going, the father mentioned that he had a rib head that kept popping out of place—it was attached to the sternum. A naturopath (four-year-school graduate) kept adjusting it, but it continued to pop out of place. Our mechanic seemed to be very tired—bone weary. There was a bit of yellow around the eyes. I speculated that there might be some swollen glands congesting the chest. I could feel them through his shirt as a matter of fact. He and his wife got quite scared. Three years previously he had lymph glands in the neck removed due to Hodgkin's disease. He had not been back for his last yearly checkup. "Well go," I insisted. I'm afraid it ruined their Christmas. "In the mean time, take Calendula. Maybe it's just swollen glands because of the burden placed on the remaining glands or a tendency to lymphatic troubles. Even if it's something worse, Calendula will help." Fortunately, it turned out that there was no return of the malignancy and the Calendula cleared up the swellings, the exhaustion, and the yellow around the eyes.

Another case was that of a fifty-five-year-old nun who was holding the weight of the world on her shoulders, doing a lot of important work for the poor. Her entry complaint was "heart palpitations," but I noted the yellow color around the eyes and the weariness and sent her off with Calendula. This, in concert with some chiropractic adjustments, removed all the problems.

Finally I had a case that brings us back to an earlier comment. A somewhat modest woman in her late twenties took me aside at the herb store to say that she had a problem "where the sun doesn't shine." What she meant was a vaginal discharge with swollen glands but little irritation. I saw Chris up on a ladder putting some remedies away on the shelves. "Hey Chris, this woman has a problem 'where the sun doesn't shine,'" I called out in a tone somewhat louder than our customer had been using. We gave her Calendula and she forgave us when the problem disappeared.

Low Immunity

We can now begin to appreciate the old English practice of putting Calendula flowers in soup in the winter time. The idea was that this would increase resistance to colds and fevers. England has a damp winter with little sunlight. This plant may be particularly suited to that locale or it may be a good idea which is universal. I know I would be cheered up to have some Calendula flowers in my soup (but I use them all for making tinctures at this point). It is tempting to think that Calendula is a remedy for Seasonal Affective Disorder Syndrome, when people get depressed during the winter. I used it this way myself last winter and felt I had positive results—but who knows, it is easy to go through mood swings. At any rate, by mildly cleansing the lymphatics, Calendula probably does provide increased immunity, because the lymphatics are the vehicle for so much immune activity.

Preparation and Dosage

The flowers are picked and dried for use as a tea. They are prepared as an infusion by pouring one cup of boiling water over a tablespoon and steeping for ten minutes. The tincture can be made from the fresh or dried flower, and is used in doses of one to ten drops. Externally, it is often used as a cream or salve. Some people have wondered whether it would be possible to pick and use the entire plant, which is covered with the medicinally active resin.

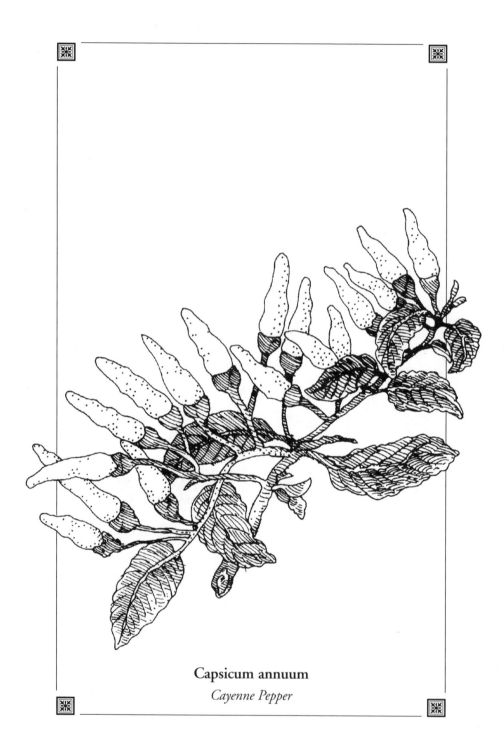

Capsicum annuum

Cayenne Pepper

Capsicum annuum
Cayenne Pepper

Hot Pepper originated in the Americas but spread throughout the world shortly after the voyage of Columbus. It quickly became a staple of diet and medicine in Africa, Asia, and the Indian subcontinent. It acclimatized so well to life in Africa that the hottest pepper comes from there, rather than Central America! It was so deeply incorporated into East Indian culture that the early botanists wondered if it was not indigenous to Asia, as well as the Americas. More lately, Cayenne has come to be appreciated in cooler climes—Europe and North America.

Cayenne Pepper was probably used by Afro-American slave doctors in the New World, but credit for the introduction of Cayenne Pepper into the literature of Western herbal medicine belongs to Samuel Thomson. For several years he had been looking for a medicine which acted on the blood the way that Lobelia acted on the nerves and muscles. He wanted something to disperse and equalize congestions of blood, as well as the thermic imbalances which follow when the blood is confined by local congestion. What he particularly wanted was a remedy which would "hold the heat in the stomach" after it had been evacuated by an emetic like Lobelia. On a trip to see patients in Massachusetts, he came down out of the mountains of New Hampshire. At a farm house where he was staying, he happened to see a string of red peppers hanging on the wall. He inquired after their nature and tried a piece. He quickly realized that he had the remedy for which he had been looking.

187

Thomson preferred the imported article, but also emphasized that the garden variety grown in the north could also be used.

"First, Equalize the Circulation"

Wooster Beach, the founder of eclectic medicine, deserves credit for another idea which gives insight into the conditions where *Capsicum* is the required remedy. In the treatment of cardiovascular problems, Beach said that one should "first equalize the circulation." What he meant by this is that the distribution of blood in the vasculature can become unequal. Due to weaknesses in the system, there could also be disparities between different circuits of the vasculature. For example, overeating might cause an excess blood supply to the digestive organs, smoking to the lungs, drinking or drug-abuse to the liver, constipation to the large intestine, or there might be stagnation around the heart itself, or in the surface, the capillaries. When this inequality occurs a burden is placed upon the heart. In treating cardiovascular conditions, one had first to equalize the circulation to remove this burden. An orderly approach to cardiovascular disease, according to Beach, was to first relieve the inequality in the circulation, so that the burden is removed from the heart. After this has been accomplished, it is possible to see the real condition of the heart, and to treat it with heart-specific remedies, if necessary.

Beach's idea is highly compatible with Thomson's concept of diffusion of the blood. In fact, Thomson's followers readily picked up Beach's motto and incorporated it into their practice. No other concept leads more directly to a core understanding of this remedy.

The highly stimulating and heating properties of Cayenne Pepper rouse the circulation, move the blood to the surface, and engorge the capillaries. As a general stimulant and corrector of circulatory problems it has no equal. I find it to be the single most useful cardiovascular remedy in my practice. It is suited to patients who are flabby, lazy, self-indulgent, or simply getting middle-aged, where the heart muscles are starting to become lazy and the circulation is getting stagnant in places. *Capsicum,* in either the herbal or the homeopathic preparation, will rouse the dilapidated organism, tonify the heart muscles, and clean out circulatory inequalities. It is a member of the Nightshade family, which gives us so many remedies with cardiovascular effects (*Belladonna, Hyoscyamus, Datura,* and *Tabacum*).

Capsicum was proven and introduced into homeopathic materia medica. However, homeopaths did not have the insight into its properties that the followers of Thomson and Beach had. They developed a comprehensive schedule of symptoms upon which to prescribe *Capsicum,* but no understanding of what it really does in the interior of the body. Not surprisingly, this symptom-picture corresponds to the type of patient and conditions which occur as the result of unequal distribution of the blood. By placing the Beachian/Thomsonian explanation of *Capsicum* along side the homeopathic symptom-picture we have a picture of this remedy which does not deceive.

According to homeopathic literature, *Capsicum* is called for in patients of lax fiber and flabby muscles, who don't exercise and eat the wrong foods. Has a red face, yet the face feels cold to the touch and is generally chilly. At times he or she gasps for breath, or can't catch the breath. Worse from slight drafts, cold air, cold water, uncovering, dampness, bathing, drinking, and eating, better from continued motion and exercise. These symptoms describe a patient with poor circulation.

One of the most characteristic symptoms, in my experience, is what I call the "unequal pulse." This can appear in several different ways. The artery is flaccid in some positions, but sharp as a knife blade in others. Sometimes the beat is not synchronized from one arm to the other. Another characteristic symptom is the facial and skin color, which is not just "red," as the homeopathic literature explains, but a reddish-purple—like the hot pepper itself. One quickly gets the picture of stagnation in the capillaries. This is especially evident on the cheeks.

Here are a few case histories which illustrate the use of *Capsicum* from the Thomsonian point of view. I prefer to use the 3x and 6x potencies, rather than the material dose used by Thomson. (1) A twenty-eight-year-old woman was in the third month of her second pregnancy. She was flabby, lax-fibered, lazy, and red-faced. The pulse was unequal and the doctors had told her she had a heart murmur. *Capsicum* 6x removed the murmur in less than a week and she went full term to a successful conclusion. (2) The patient was a twenty-eight-year-old woman with flabby muscles, lax-fiber, and red cheeks. She had suffered with a heart murmur since adolescence, for which, of course, no cure was offered. Pulse unequal. *Capsicum* 6x, repeated when she felt shortness of breath, control led the symptoms. Three years later, she is on her third bottle of the remedy, so the cure is not complete, but it improved her life greatly.

Capsicum also has an application in more precipitous cardiovascular problems. Thomson reasoned that during a heart attack the blood pooled in the interior and congested around the heart, while it was absent in the extremities—which were cold and blue. As a consequence, Cayenne was his remedy of choice in the treatment of acute heart attack. The late Dr. Christopher said that Cayenne never failed him in over thirty years of use as a remedy for heart attack. Here the crude substance should be used, rather than the potencies.

Capsicum was used by Thomson and his followers to stop bleeding and remove blood stasis following injuries. Here is a case history which illustrates the use of *Capsicum* to remove stagnant blood. The patient was a thirty-seven-year-old woman who had just delivered her first baby. The pregnancy had been difficult, there was extensive postpartum bleeding and hematoma in the vagina. 500 cc of blood was removed surgically. She was given antibiotics. Two weeks later a vaginal culture showed a "beta-strep" infection. She felt slight itching, was a little hot, cheeks red, especially the left, fatigued. This was a case where it was necessary to consider the nature of the condition, in order to arrive at the correct remedy. Obviously, there was still "stagnant blood" in the birth canal. The superficial vessels, the capillaries, were likely to be glutted with coagulated and slow-moving blood. This would result in inflammation, and this (with the antibiotics) would produce a condition where bacteria could flourish. The unevenly reddened cheeks indicated some disharmony in circulation. There is no way one could have arrived at *Capsicum* through the use of homeopathic symptoms and repertory, but the remedy fit the pathological state. *Capsicum* 3x, a few doses a day cured promptly. Four days later, no red cheeks, no itching, little fatigue.

I cannot close out this account without reference to the doctrine of signatures. The reddish color of the red pepper, with a slight purple undertone is a good indication of the properties of this plant. The fruit is shaped somewhat like a heart. Even more interesting, however, is the interior, which is divided into four "ventricles," just like a heart. *Capsicum* integrates the four quadrants of the body and strengthens the corresponding chambers of the heart.

Preparation and Dosage

Some of the active ingredients of this plant are destroyed by heat, so the full medicinal value cannot be had by eating it as a food. The material substance can be a bit overwhelming when it is taken by itself, so it can be used in a capsule form in order to be palatable. Some people seek stronger and hotter Cayenne, but this is not usually necessary. I have gotten all the best results from the use of the homeopathic potencies (3x to 30x).

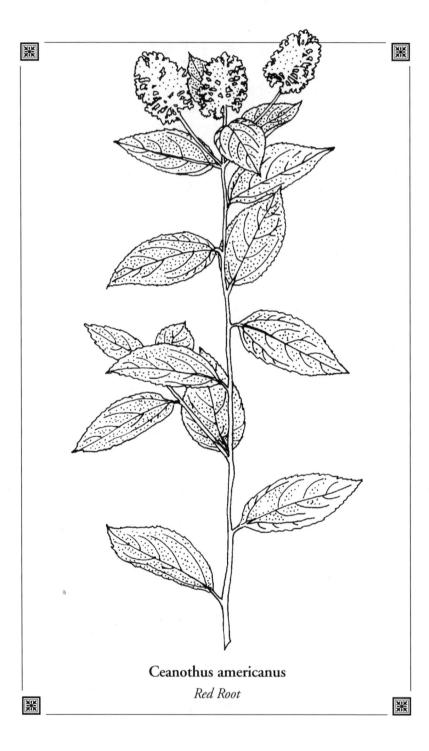

Ceanothus americanus

Red Root

Ceanothus americanus

Red Root

This little shrub is native to glades, openings, and prairies in east-ern North America. The leaves impart a taste similar to black tea and were used for this purpose during the Revolution. The roots are the part used in herbalism. They are covered by little nodules which vividly suggest a picture of lymphatic nodes. Red Root is a member of the Rhamnaceae or Buckthorn family, many of whom act on the intestinal tract.

Ceanothus received scant notice in professional medicine until 1835, when it was discovered to be an antihemorrhagic astringent by allopathic physicians. It was used by surgeons in Boston and the big cities to stop bleeding during operations. During the Civil War it became a popular medicine for "ague cake"—the swollen spleen associated with malaria and intermittent fever. The affinities to glands, the spleen, and lymphatics remained unappreciated by professional doctors for some time yet. William Cook commented in 1867 that it is "not very powerful or reliable." Shortly afterwards, Dr. Edwin Hale described *Ceanothus* in his *New Remedies,* a book intended to introduce indigenous American herbal remedies to the homeopathic audience. Even this account was overlooked for many years, until an English homeopath, Dr. J. Compton Burnett, went searching for a spleen-specific medicine. He found what he was looking for in Hale's account of *Ceanothus.*

Burnett was a colorful writer who tended to obscure the lines between the schools. Consequently, his works were appreciated by all schools—allopaths, homeopaths, physio-medicalists, and eclectics. After his little booklet on *Diseases of the Spleen* (1898) appeared, *Ceanothus* was adopted into the pharmacopoeia in every school. It is widely used in American herbalism at the present time as an "alterative" or general cleanser. It is slightly known and used in homeopathy as a specific for swollen spleen. Neither of these ideas bring out its full essence.

In 1900, a homeopath, Dr. J. C. Fahnestock gave *Ceanothus* a homeopathic proving. This verified Burnett's conception of the remedy. Fahnestock wrote, "To my surprise the first symptom noticed was a sticking pain in the spleen, and after the continued use of the remedy, there was quite an enlargement of that organ, worse by motion, but at the same time unable to lie on the left side; following this there was pain in the liver, a congestion and enlargement, with sticking pains worse by motion and touch."

Despite the clear affinities pictured here, it is a mistake to place too much emphasis on the relationship of *Ceanothus* to the spleen. It actually acts on the entire lymphatic system, of which that organ is only a part. Let us begin our account, however, with the spleen.

The Archetypal Spleen Medicine

According to Traditional Chinese Medicine the primary function of the spleen is to separate the pure fluids from the turbid fluids, sending the pure upwards and the turbid downwards. The "spleen yang" is the fire which does this job of separation. It causes a gentle circulation of the fluids, so that nutriment is transported to the sites where it is used and transformed into flesh, while waste products are removed from the system. By uplifting and flesh-building, the spleen "holds up the organs." It also holds up the blood vessels and "binds the blood in the vessels." When the spleen is not capable of doing its job, lymph stagnates, edema results, dampness precipitates into mucus, swollen glands appear, the blood is not adequately nourished and extravasates from the vessels, the tissues are not well nourished, and emaciation may set in.

What Chinese folk medicine is describing under the name "spleen" is the lymphatic system. Through the lymphatics nutriment is taken up from the digestive tract and distributed throughout the body, while waste is absorbed and removed. From a holistic perspective, pathologies of the lymphatic system would include stagnation of fluids, precipitation of turbid lymph into mucus, poor nutrition of the blood and tissues, swollen glands, etc. The spleen is a part of the lymphatic system, originating from the same embryological tissue and having important relations with lymphatic functions. When it is swollen there are often problems in the lymphatics.

Burnett's idea that *Ceanothus* is an organ-specific remedy for the spleen was handicapped by the limited view of that organ held in his time. Not only is this an excellent remedy for a swollen spleen, pure and simple, but it has an application in all the problems which touch upon the lymphatic system.

From the best of the old authors (herbal and homeopathic) we learn that *Ceanothus* is a remedy for swollen glands, lymphatic stagnation, edema, pelvic congestion, enlargement and inflammation of the spleen, violent shortness of breath caused by a swollen spleen, chronic bronchitis with profuse mucus secretion, and pain in the liver or back, from congestion or fluid retention. It is useful for loss of appetite, loss of flesh, general weakness, pain and weakness in the umbilical region, anemia, pallor, diarrhea, bearing down pains in the abdomen and rectum, constant urging to urinate, profuse menstruation, extravasation of blood, and leucorrhea. Symptoms are worse in damp, cold weather.

According to the Fahnestock provings the tongue is swollen and covered with a dirty white coating. I have verified this many times; it is one of the best indications for the remedy.

Herbalist Tommie Bass of Alabama says Red Root is almost a specific for a swollen sore throat. He also introduced it into use as a medicine for swollen prostate. They make sense since *Ceanothus* is useful for congested glands. It is also sometimes used for problems in the breasts.

All of these symptoms correspond with what the Chinese would call a spleen disease. The fountain head of splenic disease is "spleen yang deficiency." This is a condition where the "yang of the spleen," the heat and power which allow the spleen to transport and transform fluids and food, is low so that these substances stagnate. Dampness builds up, heat disappears, and there is a cold tendency. The typical symptoms are cold extremities, a moist, swollen, pale tongue, a slow, frail pulse, watery stools containing digested food, abdominal distention or pain (ameliorated by heat and pressure). From this condition there is a progression as dampness builds up, causing the pulse to get soggy or slippery and adding more of a coat to the tongue. In addition, there may be lack of appetite and loss of taste, watery stool, nausea, fullness in the chest or head, and skin eruptions containing fluids. This is called "dampness distressing the spleen." *Ceanothus* seems to be suited to this progressive development. Although there are sometimes local symptoms of heat, the emphasis in *Ceanothus* is upon stagnation. Calendula is better suited to splenic conditions where heat joins the dampness, or "damp heat collecting in the spleen."

There is also a connection between the spleen and the blood. Traditional Chinese Medicine says the spleen "binds the blood in the vessels." We would expect this of a great spleen remedy too. Red Root originally got its start as an antihemorrhagic. This usage may have had something to do with the doctrine of signatures. A cross section of the root shows a pink-reddishness suffusing through a pale, serouslike tan-yellow coloring. It looks like blood suffusing through a piece of liver. A tincture made from the predominantly tan-yellow roots slowly gives off a deep, blood red. The allopathic surgeons who introduced *Ceanothus* into medicine did not believe in the doctrine of signatures, of course, but this pictures the kind of bleeding one would come up against in an operation.

Michael Moore, the "grand-daddy of Southwestern herbalism," has gone a step further with this aspect of *Ceanothus*. He mixed some of his blood with some juice from the plant and put it under the microscope. From the observations he made, he was able to demonstrate that *Ceanothus* acts on the electrical charge which separates the red blood cells and blood proteins from the wall of the artery. This charge enhances the ability of the vessels to keep the blood cells inside them, while at the same time allowing for easy transportation of the lymph through the sieve-like walls of the artery. The result is that the blood is better able to receive and give nutriment, and the lymph is better able to receive and remove waste material. See his *Medicinal Plants of the Desert and Canyon West* for a more detailed discussion of this phenomena.

One of my friends had surgery for ballooning in her intestine. It was successful, but after two weeks her pelvis was full of blood. She was bleeding internally and starting her period. Lucky her. She was lying on her back, virtually incapable of movement. A few doses of Red Root tincture and she up and about in a few hours. The next day there was no sign of the extra blood.

Melancholia

According to traditional Greek medicine, the emotion connected with the spleen is melancholia. The word "melancholia" means "black bile" and refers to a substance which is supposed to be stored in the spleen. An excess of "black bile" or "melancholia" causes the corresponding emotion.

The Chinese attribute the same psychological disorder to the spleen, although they have no concept of the "black bile." In ancient Chinese medicine it was stated that the spleen "stores the ideas" or images. Excessive thought, brooding, and introspection is an imbalance associated with the spleen. This turns to pensiveness, brooding, and melancholia.

Herbal literature does not contain much information about the emotional state associated with Ceanothus. However, Dr. R. Swinburne Clymer considered *Ceanothus* to be specific for swollen spleen accompanied by melancholia.

There is no mention of emotions specifically associated with *Ceanothus* in homeopathic literature. The late Edward Cotter, an English homeopath, did give a case history which might suggest melancholy. A woman suffering from swollen spleen and "depression" was cured by him with *Ceanothus* 3c.

The word melancholy is not well understood at the present time. Generally, we use the word "depression." Actually, these two words do not mean exactly the same thing. Melancholy is associated with a lack of direction, purpose, creativity, with an artistic funk or an inability to think oneself out of a predicament. Depression, while it may include this, is more often associated with grief and loss. *Ceanothus* is very much the remedy for melancholia.

I was comparing notes about how we used Red Root with my friends Mimi Kamp and Halsey Brandt, of Bisbee, Arizona. "I consider it a remedy for artistic funk," I said. Mimi responded, "That's interesting; we use it for people who seem to be unable to think their way out of a problem."

The psychological faculty most closely associated with the spleen is the imagination. Images flit too and fro through our imagination, sort of like the particles circulating in the lymphatic fluids. An image comes to rest from time to time, alighting on some filament of consciousness and arising into our everyday awareness, just as a particle of nutriment comes to the cell that needs it and is absorbed within.

In both Greek and Chinese medicine the spleen is associated with the earth element or phase. In one sense, the earth is associated with feeding and nutrition. In another, it is the doorway through which the images come, from the unconscious to consciousness. The spleen connects us to the Underworld, the spirit residing inside the earth.

According to myth, there is a cauldron or grail in the Underworld, the source of light, life, and renewal. Images arise from this cauldron up to our conscious mind. We are enriched by this communication. Our body is made strong and grounded. Our life is given purpose.

When the spleen is strong, the imagination flourishes. Life is happy, well-adjusted, vibrant, and meaningful. This is an important organ indeed.

Preparation and Dosage

The root is the part traditionally used in herbalism. The taste and properties differ slightly from the leaves, which some people prefer. The root needs to be chopped when it is still fresh because it dries to rock-hard consistency. It is then boiled to release the active ingredients. A tincture can be made by chopping it finely and macerating it fresh in alcohol, sometimes heated. It takes several weeks to mature.

Ceanothus is commonly used in material doses by herbalists. However, Burnett found that such doses can cause aggravations. I have seen this myself. For instance, I gave a friend *Ceanothus* tincture, three drops, three times a day. The next day he complained that his tongue was massively swollen and the taste buds were swollen and elevated. Generally this remedy is used in homeopathy in the lowest potencies— 3x and 3c.

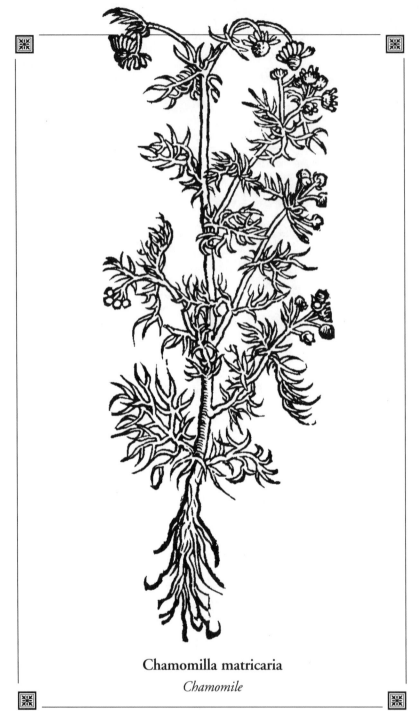

Chamomilla matricaria

Chamomile

from *Herbarium Imagines Vivae,* published by Christianus Egenolphus, 1535

Chamomilla matricaria
Chamomile

There are a half dozen plants going by the name Chamomile, all belonging to the Aster family. Two of them are used in herbal medicine, *Chamomilla matricaria* and *Anthemis nobilis,* sometimes called "German" and "Roman" Chamomile. Both contain a blue volatile oil which is the active ingredient responsible for the medicinal properties. They have been used interchangeably since antiquity and their uses are not well differentiated in traditional or modern literature. Even homeopathy has not been able to substantially differentiate their properties.

Both Chamomiles are extremely popular in European medicine. They are given for nearly every minor complaint: fever, indigestion, dyspepsia, tension, nervousness, sleeplessness, and pain. They are well suited to a wide variety of simple problems. More especially, Chamomile is suited to the problems of babies: teething, colic, whining, etc. In Germany, Chamomile is an indispensable item in the medicine cabinet of many mothers. In England it is used to a lesser extent. Readers of Peter Rabbit with remember that, after his terrifying adventure, Peter's mother put him to bed with a cup of Chamomile tea.

Samuel Hahnemann, the founder of homeopathy, resolved to prove *Chamomilla matricaria,* in order to determine, first, if the continuous effect of drinking Chamomile tea had a negative influence, and second, if it was a valuable medicinal remedy. He found that repetitive overdoses of Chamomilla produced symptoms, which meant that both propositions were true. He therefore opposed the overenthusiastic use of Chamomile tea and attempted to establish specific indications for its use. In this way *Chamomilla* became a specific remedy of great utility in homeopathic medicine. It is associated with a distinctive personality which every homeopath (or mother of young children) is quick to recognize.

Anthemis nobilis was also given a homeopathic proving. This showed that it had properties virtually identical to *Chamomilla matricaria*. As a result, it has not been used much in homeopathy.

"The baby remedy"

Chamomile has a long history of use in folk medicine as a sedative for cross, whining, irritated babies, and the problems incident to babyhood, such as teething, earaches, and intolerance to pain. The child is peevish, whining, complaining, angry, demands attention and petting. He demands a toy, receives it, then throws it on the floor. *Chamomilla* is suited to this kind of behavior at any age. Therefore, I like to say it is "the remedy for babies of any age." Whatever the age, the behavior is unmistakable. Petulant, self-centered, intolerant of pain or not having their way, inclined to pick quarrels, or averse to being touched, soothed, or spoken to. (*Sambucus* is the "infant remedy," *Chamomilla* the "baby medicine," and *Chicorium* is for "childishness.")

Here's a case history which is rather typical of the experience of many homeopathic practitioners. It was related to me several years ago by an eighty-seven-year-old, life-long adherent of homeopathic medicine. His father, a New England clergyman, had been a lay-practitioner. One time, while traveling on a crowded train before the turn of the century, there was a baby crying uncontrollably. The whole car was disturbed, as happens in such cases, the mother was embarrassed, and so forth. The Reverend could hold himself back no more, so he finally asked the woman if he could give the baby something that would help. She agreed, "as long as it isn't an opiate." He gave *Chamomilla* and the baby instantly stopped crying. She shot back, "you gave him an opiate!"

A nineteenth century homeopath, Dr. Temple Hoyne (1879), collected numerous *Chamomilla* case histories. His description of the personality is worth examination:

He seeks a cause for quarreling; he inclines to be angry and out of humor; he leaves out whole words in writing; very impatient, can hardly answer one with civility; contrary to her condition in health, she is always out of humor, particularly at her menstrual period, when she is headstrong, even unto quarreling. Children are quarrelsome, want to be carried; child is exceedingly fretful, must be carried about all the time; child wants different things and repels them when getting them.

Tension Combined with Heat

Chamomilla is suited to conditions where there is both heat and tension, or where inflammatory conditions combine with constriction and irritability. This leads to the characteristic pain and tenderness of *Chamomilla*. The characteristic fever is "incomplete," as the tension interferes and limits the expression of the heat in a uniform manner. Dr. Carrol Dunham, a homeopath of the mid-nineteenth century, describes this tendency in the fever of *Chamomilla*. "Though marked by excitement and increased sensibility, it is, nevertheless, not a well-developed inflammatory fever. The prostration is likewise represented. The heat is partial, confined, for example, to one cheek, and is conjoined with profuse sweat of the head. The fever does not last long, but often recurs."

Here's a case where tension quite literally caused an inflammatory condition. "A gentleman was attacked with a violent sore-throat, from substituting a thin cravat [collar] for a heavy one. The velum, uvula and tonsils were much inflamed; fauces covered with little ulcers; deglutition was excessively painful. Cham. 30. Better in five minutes, and well on the second day" (Hoyne). Here's a case where the inflammation caused the pain. "Girl aged thirteen, of weak constitution, obstinate, had been suffering for several days with toothache, a rending pain in the head and face, stitches in the ear, and profuse salivation." Dr. Gustave Gross administered *Chamomilla* 200c by olfaction—a method worked out by Hahnemann—and the next day she was well (Hoyne.)

Certain structures of the body are more susceptible to maddening irritation and pain than others. The ears, eyes, teeth, and sexual organs seem to be the principal organs. Many cases of earache and toothache have been cured by homeopaths. "Girl aged five, tension, tearing and jerking pain in the ear, increasing in intensity with every recurring attack, so as to cause the child to cry out suddenly. Cham. cured perfectly in five minutes. Dr. Henry B. Harris" (Hoyne.)

Tension and Heat Affecting the Liver

In terms of Chinese medicine it may be said that *Chamomilla* corresponds to a condition of "constricted liver chi," giving rise to "liver fire." In other words, tension in the circulation causes irritation (or maybe it is the other way around.) There is "irritated fiber," to use the old-fashioned expression. This irritation rises (because heat rises), creating mental tension, irritability, headache, facial redness, and inflammation of the eyes. In addition, constriction causes irritation of the stomach and digestion, resulting in indigestion, acidity, bloating and a bitter taste (from bile.) This condition corresponds to what the Chinese physicians call "liver attacking the stomach." Observations by nineteenth century homeopaths give us the tongue and pulse indications for *Chamomilla*. The tongue tends to be irritated along the sides and coated white-yellow in the middle, according to Dr. William Bayes, showing a combination of heat, tension, and accumulation of debris in the lymphatics. The pulse is small, tense, and rapid, according to Dr. Adolph Lippe. This corresponds to a condition where there is constriction of the artery and heat.

Hahnemann described a disease to which *Chamomilla* is suited which would have been recognized, either by the physicians of his era, or the Chinese doctors, as a "bilious" or hepatic condition. "The sometimes dangerous illness resembling acute bilious fever, that often comes on immediately after a violent vexation causing anger, with heat of face, unquenchable thirst, taste of bile, nausea, anxiety, restlessness, etc., has such great homoeopathic analogy with the symptoms of chamomile, that chamomile cannot fail to remove the whole malady rapidly and specifically, which is done as if by a miracle by one drop of the above-mentioned juice."

Here is a case history given by Temple Hoyne, demonstrating typical symptoms of "constricted liver chi" and "liver attacking the stomach." "Mrs. A. has headaches from time to time, caused by changes in the weather. She, although usually of sweet disposition, is then a perfect tyrant, stamps and scolds; has a bitter taste in the mouth, and vomits bile. Cham. 12 cured her."

When the liver chi becomes constricted, intermittent fever may result, or again, intermittent fever may cause constriction in the arterial circulation and "liver chi." This condition has also been cured by *Chamomilla.* A thirty-year-old woman came to see a Dr. A. L. Fisher with an intermittent fever. She had a light chill, lasting three hours, with red cheeks, no thirst, followed by a high fever, with one red cheek and vomiting of bile. There was much perspiration. She was "very cross." *Chamomilla* 200 every three to four hours, during the intermission, cured her (Hoyne.)

Chamomilla causes—and cures—profuse perspiration. Hence, it is a remedy for fever with perspiration. Chinese medicine recognizes a condition where heat (fever) depletes the "liver yin" (fluids, especially those lubricating the tendons and sinews). This gives rise to "liver wind stirring" (convulsion or spasm). Here's a case history collected by Temple Hoyne which demonstrates this condition. A twenty-five-year-old woman had convulsions following measles. They occurred several times a day, steadily increasing in severity, assuming a tetanic form, throwing her from side to side, forwards and backwards. "Eyes protrude and rotate constantly in their orbits." Petroleum 200c and *Secale* 200c helped somewhat; *Chamomilla* 200c in the hand of Dr. A. Puccinelli cured (Hoyne.)

When the yin of the liver is depleted, but the yang (or fire) is surging upwards, we have a condition of great uncertainty in the organism, where the balancing mechanism of the liver has been completely disturbed. This results in the appearance of extreme manifestations of tension and heat, such as rage and abscesses. (This is called "arrogant liver yang ascending" in Chinese medicine). The homeopathic remedy Hepar sulphuris calcarea corresponds the most closely to this condition, but *Chamomilla* can sometimes develop this far. Dr. Bayes said, "*Chamomilla* has appeared to me to promote the formation of pus in chronic abscesses where Hepar has failed to act promptly. It also appeared to relieve the pains to some extent, and to make them more bearable. In some cases, threatened abscess of the face or jaws has dispersed under Chamomilla 3[x]" (Hoyne.)

When heat penetrates to a deep layer of the blood it tends to infect the blood (cf. *Echinacea, Achillea,* and *Baptisia*), producing a condition called "heat in the blood" in Traditional Chinese Medicine. This corresponds with what the old Western physicians would have recognized as "septic fever." Skin rashes may appear, boils, abscesses, and putrid, purulent processes. These conditions lie on a continuum with the preceding syndrome. Homeopathic literature records a number of such serious conditions cured with *Chamomilla*. In one case, there was an erysipelas of the face and scalp, with enormous swelling of the tissue, swelling of the submaxillary glands with abscesses forming there and on the skull. There was intolerable headache, abundant suppuration of pus, and denuding of the bone of the skull. A decoction of *Chamomilla* cured in three weeks (from *Raue's Record;* quoted by Hoyne.)

Constriction of the arterial circulation associated with liver tension can cause tightness and tension in the tendons, ligaments, muscles, and extremities. The enervation is interfered with, hence, *Chamomilla* causes—and cures—paralytic pains, with numbness and tearing, in the extremities. It is, therefore, suited to various kinds of convulsion, spasm, tightness, rheumatic pain, and neuralgias.

The liver tends to have a regulating influence on flow, as we have seen, and when disturbed, is associated with tension, spasm, and pain. The release of the menstrual flow is associated with constricted liver chi in Chinese medicine. When pain and cramping are associated with great tenderness or cannot be borne with any patience, *Chamomilla* may be indicated.

Dr. Thomas Skinner gave a dramatic case in which *Chamomilla* cured an extremely painful period in a twenty-four-year-old woman, who had had them since puberty. "One week before menses, when her irritability begins, she has pains like those of labor, always in the morning before breakfast, with sickness and vomiting of her meals. Headache, with throbbing in both temples, with a bursting feeling in vertex, relieved by pressure and cold; aggravated by reading, by bright light, and by looking at an object fixedly. Her sufferings eased off generally on the second day after the flow was established." She had been examined and treated by several doctors. Skinner observed that "she was very irritable when spoken to, both before and during the flow of the menses." He gave *Chamomilla* 3x and 10m and there was complete cure (Hoyne.) Although the principal complaint is menstrual pain, the symptoms (irritability, headache, stomach pain, menstrual cramping) point to the liver as the ultimate source of the illness.

Although *Chamomilla* is often recommended as a female remedy and for menstrual problems, a doctor reported in the *Homeopathic*

Recorder in 1934, "When the husband complains of the wife's being cross and irritable, and he can't get along with her, give him a dose of Chamomilla." This approach had "worked many times."

Chamomile as an Antidote and a Poison.

Hahnemann writes, "A very small dose of *Chamomilla* seems to moderate excessive sensitiveness to pain, or the disturbing influence which pain exercises in some persons upon the mind; for this reason it relieves many of the morbid symptoms produced by the excessive use of coffee and narcotic substances, and is on the other hand, less beneficial to those who remain patient and composed during their sufferings."

Here is a case illustrating the use of Chamomilla as an antidote, related by Dr. Grimmer. The patient was a young woman suffering from strychnine poisoning due to overmedication with an allopathic drug. She was in the throes of convulsions; her teeth clenched, head drawn back, face pale. No stomach pump was available, nor would it have worked, for the poison had been taken cumulatively, over a period of time. "I started to ask a few questions and she said through her teeth, 'Why don't you do something? I can't bear this any longer. Do something!'" That was all he needed to hear, to give *Chamomilla*. He gave the 1m potency, "and I want to tell you no chemical antidote would bring the results that that did." She soon relaxed, in five minutes vomited and a few minutes later had a bowel movement. By morning she was better, except for muscular soreness and a rash around the mouth. Grimmer gave *Rhus tox.* and these symptoms quickly abated.

Chamomilla can produce symptoms. This is recognized both in homeopathy and in conventional medicine. Temple Hoyne relates a case from a Dr. Van Cutsem. He was called to see a woman of "nervous temperament, very irritable and subject to headache." He "found her extended on a bed in disorder, her face red, hot and covered to her very hair with a profuse perspiration." She was very anxious and excited, "scratched at the walls with her hands," while "her cries could be heard through the whole neighborhood." After twenty minutes, the face grew pale, the pulse small and rapid. "I was thinking of sending for a priest, when I learned at last that…her husband had prepared her a strong infusion of the flowers of chamomile," for her headache. *Coffea* 3 "relieved her in a few moments."

Preparation and Dosage

The same conditions are met by the material herb, the tincture, and the homeopathic potencies. The fresh herb has considerably more virtue than the dried. The taste is quite different. The homeopathic preparations are made from the fresh juice of the plant. In herbal medicine, Chamomile is often associated with the other nervines such as Skullcap, Valerian and Passionflower.

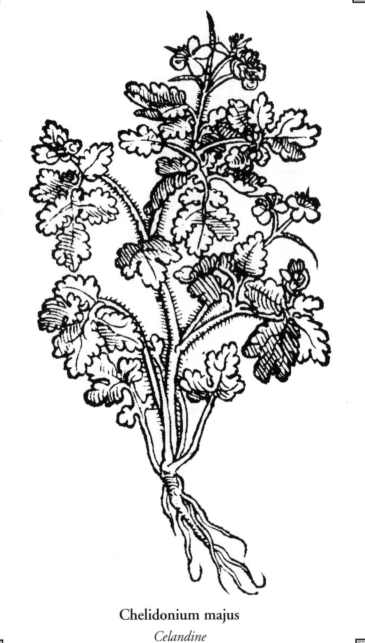

Chelidonium majus

Celandine

from *Herbarium Imagines Vivae,* published by Christianus Egenolphus, 1535

Chelidonium majus
Celandine

This unusual plant is a member of the Poppy family. It has a bright yellow-orange sap, about the color of an acrylic paint—quite unique in the vegetable kingdom. This suggested its use in jaundice and bilious problems. "The use of the greater Celandine in jaundice has trickled down to us through the ages from the primary source of the doctrine of signatures," comments Burnett. Another idea about its use came from the observation of animals. Classical writers claimed that the mother swallow would rub *Chelidonium* on the eyes of their babies to improve or restore their sight. This statement is also made about Eyebright. The name *Chelidonium* means "of the swallows." It was sometimes called "Swallow Wort" or "Kenning Wort" (seeing plant).

Chelidonium has long been popular in European herbalism. Johann Gottfried Rademacher, the great "organopath" who did so much to determine the specific "organ-affinities" of some of our most important herbal medicines, said that *Chelidonium* had an affinity to the "inner liver," or that part of the organ responsible for the consistency of the bile. (As we shall see, it is actually the gallbladder which rules this aspect.) The contemporary Gascon herbalist, Maurice Messegue, uses *Chelidonium* extensively as a deeply cleansing agent with a strong affinity to the liver and gall.

Chelidonium was brought to America, where it flourished both in the field and in use. John Josselyn recorded it in the gardens of New England in 1676, but it quickly jumped the fence. A hundred years later Manasseh Cutler noted that it was "common by fences and amongst

211

rubbish." Celandine was widely used by American lay and professional doctors. The Pennsylvania Dutch taught the Delaware Indians to use it as a liver medicine.

Samuel Hahnemann, the founder of homeopathy, gave *Chelidonium* a proving and it was reproven by a Dr. O. Buchman sometime later. The provings verified the traditional indications, and *Chelidonium* is therefore used almost in the same way in both herbalism and homeopathy. It is generally classified as a liver remedy with an affinity to the bile and jaundice. The most complete account of *Chelidonium* that I have been able to find is by Temple Hoyne. He records many observations and case histories. The modern homeopathic writings on *Chelidonium* are not as rich.

The Gallbladder

When the liver is skipping along happily, it detoxifies the portal blood supply. Out of this toxic material the bile is created. Because bile is an irritant substance it is excreted from the hepatic cells as soon as it is created. The bile flows through little channels, is collected into the gall ducts, and finally arrives in the gallbladder. Here it is stored until the demands of digestion require it. When food is being worked in the alimentary tract, the solar plexus is stimulated and sends messages to the nerves of the gall sac and gall ducts, causing them to release their contents into the duodenum. The bile breaks up the oils into little pieces, so that they can be digested, then drifts with the digestate back into the bloodstream.

The sphere of the gallbladder begins at the wall of the hepatic cell, when the bile is excreted, and ends at the gall duct, where the bile is secreted into the duodenum. The principal structures of the gallbladder organ system are the ducts, which collect bile from the liver, send it to the gallbladder itself, and on into the small intestine, plus the gall sac or bladder, and the nerves which run between the solar plexus and the organ itself. The principal function of the gallbladder is the storage and concentration of bile. According to the length of time the bile is stored in the system, the bile will be thicker or thinner. The longer it stays, the thicker it gets, as the gallbladder, huddled under the liver, tends to warm the bile and drive off the fluid. Factors which influence the consistency of the bile are stagnation in the gall ducts and sac, weakness in the gallbladder nerve reflexes, heat caused by inflammation in the liver or gall-bladder, or sogginess caused by lymphatic stagnation.

The old authors thought that the consistency of the bile depended on the liver itself. The origin of bile is in the liver, but the condition of the bile when it is delivered to the small intestine is determined by what happens to it during its residency in the gallbladder organ system.

Chelidonium is one of the primal remedies illustrating the function of the gallbladder and acting as a gallbladder organ-remedy. It is suited to conditions where the bile is too thick and there is stagnation in the gallbladder tract. This leads to congestion in the gall sac, which causes irritation and inflammation of the walls of the gallbladder and thicken-ing of the bile into a mucus-like consistency. This thicker bile sometimes blocks up the gall ducts, causing a lack of secretion into the bowels, resulting in constipation. At other times there is an excess of bile in the digestive tract, resulting in "bilious indigestion," as the old timers called it (tension and bloating in the stomach and abdomen with jaundice usu-ally of a mild character.) The bile backs up into the liver and blood-stream, creating a swollen liver and jaundice. The tension controlling mechanisms of the liver are disturbed, so that intermittent fever symp-toms may appear (or conversely, intermittent fever and arterial tension can damage the gallbladder, resulting in the *Chelidonium* condition). Finally, the inflammation caused by blockage and stagnation in the gall ducts creates a heat which acts on the thickened bile to dry it out. This results in the formation of gallstones. All of these conditions are described by the Chinese as "damp heat encumbering the liver and gall-bladder." In addition to these conditions, the swelling and tension in the liver creates tension which reflexes from under the scapula up into the neck and head resulting in migraine headaches. The Chinese call these "gallbladder headaches," since they follow the course of the gallbladder meridian, up the neck, over the sides of the head, the temples, and into the eyes.

All of these conditions are met by *Chelidonium*. It follows through from the constricted chi symptoms of bilious fever all the way to damp heat, the formation of gallstones, and the appearance of gallbladder or migraine headaches. It has been used in herbal and homeopathic medi-cine as a remedy for fever, constipation due to lack of bile in the stool, bilious indigestion, migraine, jaundice, swelling and inflammation of the liver, and gallstones. Dr. Edwin Hale, a low-potency homeopath, suggested that *Chelidonium* had a "peculiar action on the hepatic cells, causing them to secrete a thinner and more profuse bile." As we have seen, he is somewhat mistaken about the liver making the bile thin.

The influence of *Chelidonium* extends from the gallbladder back up into the liver. A common symptom calling for *Chelidonium* is swelling and pain in the liver. The characteristic pain of this remedy is felt from the right hypochrondrium or back through on the underside of the right scapula. It manifests a sharp pain under the shoulder blade. By reflex, this pain can appear on either side, under the scapula, but it is far more common on the right side. With this swelling there will be the jaundice, seen as a yellow discoloration in the conjunctiva, face, skin, diarrhea, or urine. In severe case the jaundice approaches green.

Through this dull, occluding, thickened, bilious condition there tends to run a slight arterial tension, so that the bilious symptoms are ameliorated by the appearance of the fever and released with sweating, but return periodically. Due to the intermittent discharge of bile, constipation alternates with diarrhea—hard, knotty, whitish stools with yellow, watery ones. All of this is described by Hoyne.

Chelidonium was an important remedy in the treatment of gall stones in herbalism and homeopathy. Hale writes, "I have treated many intractable cases when the stones had remained in the duct several months—in one case a year—and where icterus was intense. The whole body, eyes, tongue, lips and vagina had assumed a greenish-yellow hue. Several of these cases did not improve until *Chelidonium* was given and under its use the calculi were discharged."

Swelling of the hepatic structure and glutting of the system with mucus tends to affect the lungs. This is especially true with the right lung, which is next to the liver. Thus, *Chelidonium* has an old reputation as a remedy for congestion and oppressed respiration, sometimes going so far as hepatization of the lung. Hoyne describes the characteristic cough: "Frequent paroxysms of dry, violent, hollow or short, exhausting cough (worse in the morning), excited by tickling in larynx, by sensation of dust in the trachea, throat and behind the sternum, not relieved by coughing; loose rattling coughs; bright-yellow stools; pain under the lower angle of right shoulder-blade." *Chelidonium* is therefore useful in rhinitis, laryngitis, trachitis, influenza, capillary bronchitis, and pneumonia. Swelling, inflammation, and glutting of mucus can also affect the heart, producing inflammation, heart pain, palpitation, and irregular pulses.

"Gallbladder Headache"

Chelidonium is a very important remedy for migraine. It should be put on the list next to *Sanguinaria,* but it is usually overlooked. Dr. Richard Hughes gives a good case history quoted by Temple Hoyne. A thirty-year-old woman was suffering from recurrent "sick headaches" (the old-fashioned word for migraines) over the preceding eight years. "Every fortnight regularly much pain in right hypochondrium, gradually increasing in severity; as it grows worse head begins to ache, especially in the right forehead and temples; when rising to its acme, nausea and bilious vomiting; gradual decline of symptoms after a few hours, attack lasting nearly three days; in the free intervals occasional feeling of headache and slight pain in the right side; secretions and menses normal." *Chelidonium* 3x cured.

In addition to the headaches, neuralgic pains in the head and face are found in the provings. Great pain in the eyes, worse from light, facial pain, ear pain, and pain in the area of the eyebrows. Until turning to Hoyne and Buchman, I had not realized just how prominent these symptoms can be. Here is a case history quoted by Hoyne from a Dr. C. C. Smith. "Mrs. S., third day after confinement, sever neuralgic pains across the eyes from left to right, accompanied with the most profuse lachrymation and dread of light; has to keep the room dark. All noises disturbed her; no sleep day or night. Attack lasted six days with no relief from apparently indicated remedies. Chel. tinct. one dose at first slightly aggravated, afterward no change. The second dose made her feel as if she would go crazy, and as though the 'whole top of the brain was caving in;' but she soon feel asleep and awoke well." These migraine symptoms remind us very much of *Sanguinaria,* as it is protrayed in homeopathic literature.

As a result of the appearance of the extra "mucus" in the bile (and then in the bloodstream), there is dullness and occlusion of the sensorium, resulting in lethargy, laziness, drowsiness, confusion and vertigo. On the other hand, there may be a terrible sharpness of thinking, with a sense of having committed some misdeed. This also results from the sense of an occlusion, of something hidden one cannot grasp.

In several cases I have used *Chelidonium* for people who were suffering from the side effects of legal or illegal psychoactive drugs. These substances, as well as the tensions which led to drug use, tend to irritate the liver. One case involved a thirty-five-year-old man. He had been on amphetamines for the last year, and had quit two months before. "They messed me up." They had been prescribed for depression following an intense, deep, but unsuccessful love affair. Two weeks ago he was suffering from anxiety and a poisoned sensation, which Arsenicum 30x cleared up. Now he felt dull and lethargic. Complexion a little sallow. Tongue is swollen and interferes with the speech. Large, swollen, flabby, especially about the edges. Coating scraped off this morning, but usually present. Pulse full, slippery, wiry, and languid. Dull-minded, pain under the right scapula, overcast weather brings on depression, stool loose. *Chelidonium* 6x cleared up these symptoms, but not the heartbreak.

As we saw in our discussion of Werewolf Root, the gallbladder is traditionally associated with the personal will or ego. It is probable that *Chelidonium* also acts in this sphere. We might expect it to treat some symptoms opposite to dull sensorium, especially associated with an inappropriate, overassertive personality, anxious of having committed some wrong. Buchman gives a case history that illustrates this side of the remedy. A twenty-two-year-old woman, who had always been well and looked robust, "came with an anxious, disturbed look: said she was not right in her head; feels as if she would get crazy; horrible anguish; day or night no rest, as if she had killed somebody." This anxiety takes away all pleasure from work. The symptoms had been getting worse for five weeks. "Is there any help for me? Shall I lose my reason?" The physical symptoms included soreness on pressure in the pit of the stomach and left hypogastrium. Her appetite was entirely gone, no thirst, bitter taste, stools hard, whitish-yellow, often has vertigo, as if she would fall forward; flushes of heat in the face; oppression of the chest, with violent palpitation. *Chelidonium* 6, every three hours, cured.

So often we find opposing tendencies running together in a single remedy or person. Boericke gives a symptom under *Chelidonium* which seems to unify the two diverse states of mind: "Averse to work or movement, but driven about by anxiety." *Chelidonium* seems to be rather similar to Arsenicum, the great homeopathic remedy for anxiety. Celandine is a member of the Poppy family, along with *Sanguinaria* and Opium. All of these plants display a general tendency to moral and spiritual apathy.

Herbal tradition has included *Chelidonium* as a remedy in traumatic conditions. This has been verified in the homeopathic provings.

Heavy, stiff, sore, paralyzed, dislocative, or broken feelings in the joints were produced. Buchmann recommended it as a supplementary remedy after Arnica. Unfortunately, few herbalists or homeopaths think of it in this relation, so the conditions under which it would be used have not been identified. It is also used externally for warts. Sometimes it figures in formulas for cancer. (The old authors would have placed these two conditions together happily, under the heading of "growths.")

Preparation, Toxicity, and Dosage

Since *Chelidonium* is moderately toxic in material doses, only small doses of the tincture or crude article should be used. The low homeopathic potencies would be well indicated. This remedy is seldom used in high potencies, since it has such a strong organ-affinity. The tincture should be made from the fresh herb, within a few minutes of being picked. A sufficient dose is one drop.

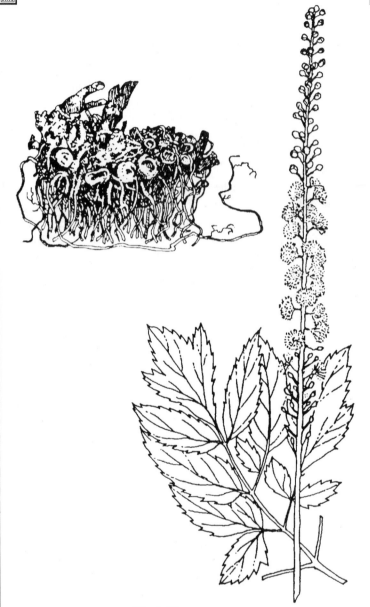

Cimicifuga racemosa

Black Cohosh

Cimicifuga racemosa
Black Cohosh

T his is one of my favorite plants. I associate it with the "Big Woods" of eastern North America, and the herbal tradition of the Eastern Woodland Indians. It was one of the many important and distinctive remedies which the pioneers learned from the Native Americans. It is an interesting medicine plant, for its qualities run in a deep psychological vein. Black Cohosh has an organ-affinity with the cerebrospinal system. The account of the plant given in my earlier book, *Seven Herbs,* is quite adequate, but a few additional points may be made.

The American Indians have given us ten times as many female remedies as any other culture. Black Cohosh was used for menstrual problems and as a parturient in the late stages of labor. The name "cohosh" seems to come from an Algonquin word associated with pregnancy. It was also called Black Snake Root. Another name is Rattle Root. J. I. Lightall (1880), the "great Indian medicine man," explains, "When the stalk is shaken the seeds will rattle, producing a sound like that of a rattlesnake." It was one of the "snake roots" used for snake bite and as a Snake Medicine.

The botanical name for this plant varied during the nineteenth century, between *Actea, Macrotys,* and *Cimicifuga,* but the last finally won out as the official designation. Black Cohosh was widely used in domestic practice for female complaints. Rafinesque introduced it to medical literature and it was adopted by the early physio-medical and eclectic physicians. Dr. C. J. Hemple gave it a proving in 1856, and it was adopted into homeopathy.

Cimicifuga is a member of the Buttercup or Ranunculaceae family, which makes it a cousin of Pulsatilla. These two remedies have many similarities and should be remembered together.

The Indian Woman's Medicine

Black Cohosh is to American Indian medicine what Pulsatilla is to homeopathy: the single most important herb for menstrual and female problems. Both are used for premenstrual moodiness, scanty menses, cramps, problems dating to the onset of menstruation, irregular menses in young girls, fluid retention, and menstrual spasm. There are also differences: Black Cohosh has a dark, brooding mentality, whereas Pulsatilla has a happy/sad, changeable, yielding disposition. Very often there is a history of intense emotional and sexual attachments or abuse in the Black Cohosh personality.

Here is a good case history describing the mental state from one of the old authors. A twenty-two-year-old woman who was depressed and suicidal after a matrimonial engagement had been broken off. She suffered from "extreme dejection of spirits; great desire for solitude; very timid; will not answer questions; at other times, extremely loquacious; shows a strong propensity to suicide." Dr. H.W. Budd cured with *Cimicifuga* in two weeks (Hoyne.)

Sometimes these mental states are due to dealing with abusive business problems. Here is another good case from Dr. Budd. A fifty-four-year-old tradesman, after the failure of his business was suffering from sleeplessness for five nights, with occassional moaning or crying aloud, constantly talking to himself. (The withdrawn, introspective qualities show up here.) *Cimicifuga* cured in eight days (Hoyne.)

Black Cohosh is an important old Indian remedy in parturition. It is used to ripen and descend the uterus, in the latter days of pregnancy, also promoting even contractions. It tends to encourage the uterus by unloosening the fluids and through this, the muscles. Herbalist Ed Smith of Williams, Oregon, points out how the unfolding, uncurling stalks in the spring, which look much like the unfolding fronds of ferns, remind one of a fetus.

"The Whiplash Remedy"

The long, slender stems which bear the racemes, or tufts of flowers, rise up above the bushier growth of leaves. They whip in the breeze. This is a signature pointing to the use of Black Cohosh in whiplash—a condition which I have seen it cure or palliate in dozens of cases. But our thinking should not stop here. Black Cohosh is a remedy for conditions in which the cerebrospinal fluid is "bunching up," as I like to put it. This is the core condition of the *Cimicifuga* problem, and all the characteristic conditions emanate from this situation. The dark, brooding state of mind, the neck and lower back pain, rheumatism, relief from fluid discharges, amelioration from menstruation, aggravation from their ceasation at menopause, the ripening and readying of the uterus late in pregnancy. The dark, congested, interwoven roots beneath the ground present a signature of the congestion, whether it be psychic or physical, which typifies this medicine plant.

I gave a considerable number of case histories for whiplash in my original book, *Seven Herbs;* more could be added. Nowadays the term "fibro-myalgia" has been introduced and is thrown around in a rather liberal fashion by medical practitioners. Many cases coming under this designation also repond to Black Cohosh, but one has to look at each case. The keynote symptom calling for *Cimicifuga* is tightness and hardness in the trapezius muscles, where they attach to the shoulder-blades.

Wind, Damp, and Cold

The word "rheumatism" comes from the Greek word for "dampness." Rheumatic sufferers are generally worse from exposure to cold and damp. In the old days, this condition was looked upon as a concretion of dampness in the joints and muscles. In Traditional Chinese Medicine certain types of rheumatism are classified under the heading "wind-damp." This also describes the Black Cohosh condition, for there is a combination of wind (tension, binding, changeable pains) and dampness.

A Dr. Drumm saw a patient who was lame and stiff, from the atlas to the soles of the feet, except for the arms. He gave the first dilution of *Cimicifuga* (one part in ten), two drops, two times a day. After one month the man could flex his legs and turn his head. Eventually he was completely cured (Hoyne.)

Rheumatic tendencies are found in all the conditions which we have just gone over, especially in the case of whiplash. The homeopathic authors noted that *Cimicifuga* was specific for rheumatism in the "belly of the muscle." That means the underside of the upper arm, the thigh, or places where the muscles "hang" from the bones. Whiplash creates a shock wave which runs along the muscles and which is pronounced when it hits the hanging muscles. Black Cohosh is also beneficial in sharp, shifting, neuralgic pains, and even convulsions and spasms.

Moving to a different sphere, Black Cohosh has an affinity for respiratory conditions associated with cold and damp, according to herbalist Amanada McQuade Crawford. This includes bronchitis. A peculiar thing about *Cimicifuga* is that the smell of the flowers (or a good tincture of the root) is stuffy, making one feel bound up or contained. This is a respiratory signature.

Through its action on the lungs and muscles, *Cimicifuga* exerts some influence on the heart and circulation. It unbinds the peripheral circulation and is beneficial in some cases of high blood pressure. Here is a case history from one of the old authors. An elderly lady would be aroused from sleep by violent throbbing of the heart, with flushes over the body, resulting in profuse perspiration and increased urine. Dr. J. C. Morgan cured this with *Cimicifuga* 200c (Hoyne.)

Fever

Because of its affinity for the spine, *Cimicifuga* has some reputation as a remedy in cerebrospinal fevers. I have not had extensive experience with such conditions. I saw one case where it cured side effects remaining after such a disease. A woman in her early thirties had suffered from meningitis two years previously. Although recovered, she was still beset by a tensive, terribly painful headache in the right hemisphere. This seemed to result from swelling of the meninges. She had had a hysterectomy, so symptoms could not be relieved by menstruation. Complexion, eyes, hair dark. *Cimicifuga* in homeopathic potency relieved the condition entirely.

Here is a case history from an old author, where we see the damage to the nervous system from febrile disease. "In a case of typhoid fever, after Bapt[isia] had acted well," the patient was "in a state of high nervous excitement difficult to describe, with headache, flying nervous pains here and there, and, above all, a tremor, accompanied by partial convulsions most painful to witness." Dr. J. J. Navarro cured the condition with *Cimicifuga* 2nd potency (one part in a hundred). This low potency seemed to work very well. Dr. A. L. Fisher noted that it worked in cases where the 200c potency failed (Hoyne.)

Cimicifuga was used to help bring out the rash in measles and eruptive disease (the same use is associated with its Chinese cousin, *Cimicifuga foetida*.) Homeopathy gets a similar usage from Pulsatilla. *Cimicifuga* is good for anyone who has ever had measles, as it clears the debris of this sickness out of the system. I have seen half a dozen cases where ill health was corrected on the premise that the patient had had measles and Black Cohosh cleared the system. Here is a case from an old author.

A forty-five-year-old, menopausal woman in generally good health, was "depressed and despondent, suspicious; lived in the most cruel doubts and fears, in constant terror and the lowest state of dejection." Here we see the rather characteristic depression of this remedy. Dr. Verdi gave *Cimicifuga* tincture, three drops, three times a day, and cured this condition in a few days. However, "her body became covered with an eruption of red patches, very slightly elevated," as the condition disappeared (Hoyne.)

Preparation, Toxicity, and Dosage

This plant is usually prepared from the dried root. Let me tell you, this does not compare to the fresh. When Black Cohosh root is fresh it tastes like the rich, damp forest floor where it grows. The dried root looses all of this and has a flat, wooden taste by comparison. So dig up your Black Cohosh, chop it up and macerate in good quality brandy or vodka. You can also prepare a fairly active flower essence by soaking the flowers in water during the month of July, when it is in bloom, and preserving it with brandy.

Black Cohosh, especially in herb teas and capsules, is a little bit too strong for many cases. Several times I have observed aggravations arising from this mode of preparation. For this reason I only use the tincture in small doses and the homeopathic potencies. In spinal problems and rheumatism, where calcification has set in, we would not want to stimulate the vital force before removing the material hindrances affecting the sick person. Therefore, in whiplash cases where the condition has been in existence for a long time, use the tincture and not the homeopathic potencies. One to three drops per dose, once a day, for about six weeks. Follow this with low to moderate homeopathic potencies, if necessary. In menstrual conditions either method can be used.

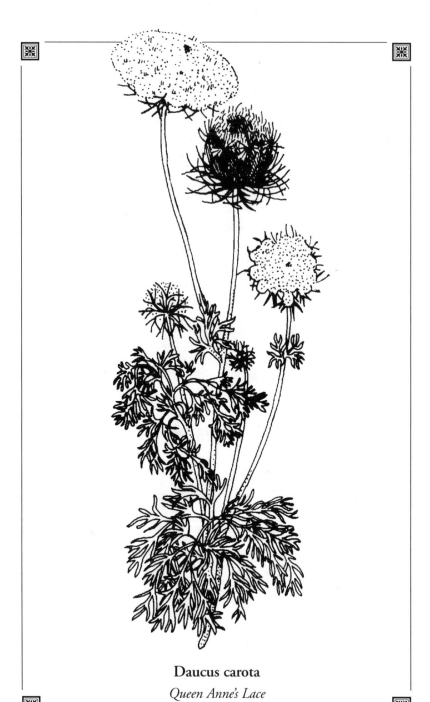

Daucus carota

Queen Anne's Lace

Daucus carota

Queen Anne's Lace

This plant is commonly called Wild Carrot because it is the wild relative from which the garden carrot was bred. The name Queen Anne's Lace refers to the lacey white flower. The first name is more commonly used in England, the latter in America. It is also called Bird's Nest, the flower very much resembling one at a certain point in its development (see illustration).

Queen Anne's Lace is a polymorphous species, capable of assuming many forms. Through selective breeding the garden variety (*Daucus carota sativa*) was developed over many centuries. The root became larger, sweeter, and less pungent, while the top became smaller. This is sometimes used in herbal medicine as a moistening poultice and a source of vitamin A, but it lacks the strong medicinal properties of its wild cousin. Queen Anne's Lace has a more pungent, bitter, and sweet flavor. It is native to Europe, but widely naturalized in North America.

All the way down to the Renaissance, herbal writers recommended the wild and domestic varieties for the same complaints, but until modern times there was little difference between them. Culpeper comments, "The root is small, long and hard, and unfit for meat, being somewhat sharp and strong."

Dauca carota is in the Parsley or Apiaceae family. Most members of this clan possess volatile oils that impart pungence and flavor, so that many are used for culinary and medicinal purposes. Even the domestic carrot is slightly pungent and bitter at times. "Wild carrots belong to Mercury," comments Culpeper. The aerial planet is indeed a fitting ruler for a plant with such aery stalks and flowers. It does seem to break up stagnant blood, remove gas and flatus, such as we would expect from a Mercurial rulership. However, it also has a strong connection to the procreative function, and hence Venus. Perhaps Culpeper, a doughty Puritan, missed this association.

Gerard summarizes traditional herbal literature going back to classical authors:

The root boiled and eaten, or boiled with wine, and the decoction drunke provoketh urine, expelleth the stone, bringeth forth the birth, and procureth bodily lust. The seed drunke bringeth downe the desired sicknes [menstruation], it is good for them that can hardly make water, it breakieth and dissolveth winde, it remedieth the dropsies, it cureth the collick and stone, being drunke in wine. It is also good for the passion of the mother [uterus].

Like many easily available, nontoxic herbs, Queen Anne's Lace was ignored by professional doctors from the eighteenth century onwards. The seed and roots are still, however, widely used by herbal practitioners at the present time.

The Lacemaker and the Drop of Blood

The lacy round umbel flower top looks like a net of white lace into which has fallen a single drop of blood, for there is a black-red point in the middle of the umbel. It seems to picture a piece of lace onto which a lacemaker has dropped a single drop of blood, after pricking her finger. An English writer, Geoffrey Grigson, suggested that the name Queen Anne's Lace should be traced back to St. Anne, the patron saint of lacemakers. There is also some additional justice in this, since St. Anne was supposed to be the midwife of St. Mary, and this plant is used in herbal medicine as a female remedy.

However, the name Queen Anne's Lace appears to be of American origin. It is not found in Culpeper and the popular seventeenth century herbalists, so some have associated it with Queen Anne, at the beginning of the eighteenth century, the only monarch by this name who ever ruled the American colonies. She would have had the wide white collar worn by the Puritans at that date.

There has been debate about the origin of the name and I even saw a letter to the editor of the *New Your Times,* printed on the editorial page, where a writer contested the association with Queen Anne as some kind of Protestant nonsense. A third theory is that the queen was Anne Bolyn. According to this scenario, the red droplet in the center of the flower would be where they cut off her head, while the white part corresponds to the big collar they wore in England in that era. There is also the point that Anne Bolyn was executed for witchcraft (this plant is sometimes associated with that subject), though in actuality it was infertility (a major usage). It may be that both Queen Anne and St. Anne contributed to the origin of the name. Ironically, Queen Anne's Lace survives only as an American name.

Strange to say, all of these ideas relate to the medicinal powers of the plant one way or another. Pricking one's finger is an ancient and powerful motif in fairytales and European folk imagination. It represents individualization of life experience. The character who pricks his or her finger is suddenly pushed unprepared into a new epoch in life. To some extent, it represents becoming open to or abused by powerful influences outside oneself. When the image appears in fairy tales it often relates to the awareness of one's sexual identity or vulnerability.

This motif matches the natural history of the plant. Wild Carrot grows in heavy grasses, where it is difficult for the little barbed seeds to penetrate the turf. And yet they do, so that the plant proliferates widely in heavy turf as well as bare ground. It is like a needle piercing through. The story also matches the medicinal use of the plant

I was first taught about this herb by one of my students, Lise Wolff. She says that Queen Anne's Lace seed helps slough the uterine membrane and regulate the menstrual cycle. It reduces heavy flow, excessive growth of the uterine membrane, and probably endometriosis. It seems to aerate the blood and prevent clotting and heavy flow in this manner as well. When used before, during, or after the period it prevents conception by sloughing the membrane. However, after its use has been stopped, it will encourage conception because the menstrual cycle and uterine membrane are newly toned. Herbalist Susun Weed testifies that she and her students have used Queen Anne's Lace seed successfully in hundreds of cases as a form of birth control.

Queen Anne's Lace is also a powerful diuretic. Here the seed or the root may be used. A good source of information about this use is herbalist Tommie Bass of northern Alabama, the subject of a study by John

Crellin and Jane Philpot (1989). He considered Wild Carrot among his top remedies for water removal, weight loss, gout, and rheumatism. "We have experimented with it and we've had more results with it for reducing than anything," he says. "Some lose fifteen to twenty pounds." He recounts the case of a man who "couldn't pull up his pantlegs," his legs and stomach were so swollen. He was a beer-drinker with an enormous stomach. The man drank more than two gallons of Queen Anne's Lace and was returned to normal in a few months.

Like so many kidney remedies, Wild Carrot is used, not only to eliminate water from the system, but to remove concretions through the urine. Hence it has a reputation in the treatment of kidney stone, gout, and rheumatism. I like to say that it "helps thread the urine through the kidneys."

We have been talking about the intimate details of bodily existence and procreation. The resemblance of the flower top of Queen Anne's Lace to an Elizabethan or Puritan collar is relevant here. It originated during a period of history in which English culture was moving away from the body, towards a more "puritanical" view of sexuality. It makes it difficult to look down at one's own body! The disconnection between the head and the body reached an apex in the story of Anne Bolyn. Queen Anne's Lace does not just "stir up bodily lust," as Gerard remarks, but operates on a subtle level to help one appreciate the body.

And, speaking of bodily processes, Wild Carrot contains volatile oils which promote the appetite and digestion, expelling flatulence.

Preparation and Dosage

Tommie Bass recommends using the tops, before they go to seed. Lise Wolff tries to get the seed before they are fully mature. An infusion is made by pouring a cup of water over a teaspoon of the tops or seeds. This is more active than the mature seeds or roots. Lise makes a tincture. Steep the immature seeds in high proof vodka. Brandy does not yield a good product. The high alcohol content seems to extract the volatile oils better. Of this, only a small dose, a few drops, is necessary.

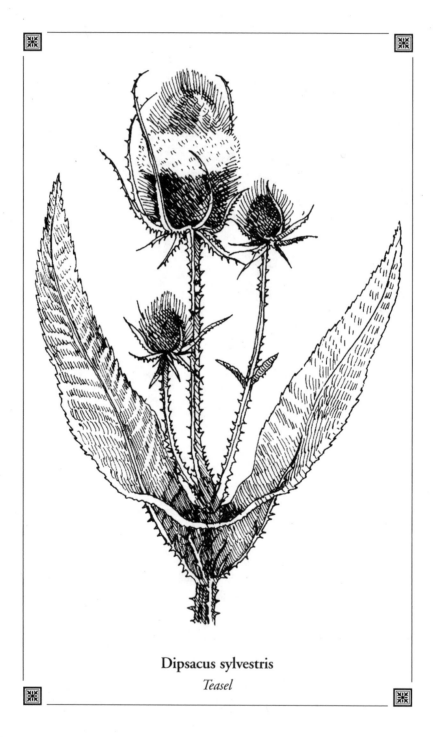

Dipsacus sylvestris

Teasel

Dipsacus sylvestris
Teasel Root

This tall, imposing thistle is a member of the Teasel family, closely allied to and resembling the Asteraceae or Sunflower family. It is native to Europe, but was introduced to America and is now common in many waste places, especially in the lower Great Lakes region. It is a biennial, producing a rosette of leaves next to the ground the first year, followed by a tall, rigid stalk surmounted by impressive, compact thistles the second.

Teasel is best known for its economic use (which persisted until World War II) as a sort of brush to card, sort or tease the fibers of wool in the fulling process. A special variety, *Dipsacus sativa,* was bred for this purpose. The wild kind is known as *Dipsacus sylvestris.*

There is little history of use of Teasel in Western herbal medicine. Dioscorides recommended the root for "chaps and fistulaes of the fundament." Pliny reported that the worms found in the seed heads were put into a bag and carried around the neck, as a cure for recurrent or intermittent fever. Gerard tried this and was sorely disappointed. "They are nothing else but most vaine and trifling toies, as my selfe haue proued," he says. "Hauing a most grieuous ague, and of long continuance: notwithstanding Physicke charmes, these worms hanged about my neck, spiders put into a walnutshell, and diuers such foolish toies that I was constrained to take by fantasticke peoples procurement; notwithstanding I say, my helpe came from God himselfe, for these medicines and all other such things did me no good at all." Yet, Teasel is a remedy for intermittent fever.

Since poor Gerard's exasperating experience with Teasel, few have attempted to use it medicinally. Teasel has virtually no reputation in European herbalism, nor among the American Indians. However, a similar species is widely used in China.

Despite this impoverished history, when I first looked at Teasel I was impressed with the potential of the plant as a medicine. The large, hard, tall stalks, which remain dead but still strong through the winter, seemed to indicate an affinity for bones. At intervals along the stem the opposite leaves merge together to form a cup which holds water after a rain. Surely, I thought, this must be a remedy for the joints and the kidney essence. Several months later I met William LeSassier, a remarkable and talented herbalist living in New York City. He had been using *Dipsacus sylvestris* based on the indications from the Chinese tradition.

Teasel is one of William's favorite herbs, and he had extensive experience with it. All he told me at first was that it was the remedy for joints that have been torn, stretched, or wrenched. I looked Teasel up in Dan Bensky's *Chinese Herbal Medicine, Materia Medica,* to fill out my knowledge. I was not surprised to find that it was considered a medicine for the kidney *jing* or essence.

In Traditional Chinese Medicine, the root of *Dipsacus japonica* is used. The Chinese name translates, "Restore What is Broken." It is used for trauma to the joints and muscles. It is understood that this action operates through tonification of the kidney essence and the liver blood, which are responsible for the strength of the joints and tendons respectively. When the kidney essence is deficient the lower back and knees are compromised. They become weak, stiff and achy. When the liver blood is deficient, the muscles and tendons are not nourished; they tighten and are more easily injured. Teasel also promotes the circulation of the blood and removes pain and stiffness in areas that have been bruised. It can be applied either internally or externally. It is also used to stop uterine bleeding, halt miscarriage, and calm a restless fetus.

Acting on these simple tips, I soon found that Teasel was an excellent medicine for joint injury. From my experiences and those of my students, plus the continued teaching of William, I began to learn more about this invaluable plant. Teasel is particularly beneficial for large, bulky people who throw joints out with special force, because they have a lot of momentum behind their movements. This does not disqualify it as a remedy for other people. Teasel is excellent for chronic inflammation of the muscles, with limitation of movement and great pain. Whole areas, like the girdle of the shoulders or the lower back become inflamed and difficult to use. Sometimes the entire body is affected. Teasel is well indicated in chronic cases where the person becomes arthritic, the muscles all over are stiff and sore and they are eventually incapacitated. "It is for people who had a use, but lost it," William explained graphically. "They stepped off the path." One of my students commented, "It is for people who jump in to things bull-headed, head first, and suffer the consequences." Slowly, I moved to a deeper understanding of the affinities of Teasel and began to use it in more serious problems.

If you have ever suffered from the experience of having something "broken" in your life, so that a major piece, a part of your path, does not come into play, cannot become manifest, then you know how important it is that there is a medicine to "Restore What is Broken."

The Three Precious Substances

In order to understand the nature of Teasel, we have to have an understanding of what the Chinese call the kidney essence. This is an old alchemical concept, found in the East and West. The ancients lumped together all phenomena which related to genetically determined pattern, hormonal regulation of the unfoldment of pattern and all kinds of pattern which were innate or fixed in a given species. They called this the essence. They conceived of it as a sort of primordial fluid out of which all life arose, and through which every species propagated itself. It was very much seen as a water or fluid, the source of sexual and bodily secretions. In old age, as the essence diminishes, the body dries out, the fertility decreases, the pattern starts to break down, and even, finally, the personal identity may deteriorate into a senile dementia.

In alchemy, the primal fluid is associated with mercury, because this is the metal which remains in a liquid form. The other metals have to be reduced to a liquid, malleable, fusible form in order to be refined, but mercury is already in this state at room temperature. Thus, mercury is looked upon as the "mother of metals," and as the substance most closely representing the essence. The essence was associated with mercury in both the East and the West. The common term in China, however, is *jing,* from a root which means to winnow wheat or sort through something to get to the essence.

The essence is one of the three precious substances which make up the primordial foundation of the body in Taoist alchemy. In China they are called *jing, chi,* and *shen.* In the West these three *principia* are called *mercurius, sulphur,* and *salt.*

In Traditional Chinese Medicine, the essence is said to be stored in the kidneys, the topmost organ of the sexual-urinary tract. A certain amount, containing the genetic blueprint, is supplied at conception. This is supplemented by nourishment throughout life, but the basic configuration cannot be significantly altered. Birth defects are classified as a serious deficiency of the kidney jing. Slow closure of the fontanels, development of teeth, delayed puberty, or problems with maturation and aging are associated with less serious deficiencies of the essence. These conditions are treatable.

The kidney essence is conceived of as the blueprint from which the form of the body develops. It creates and maintains all sexual and hormonal functions throughout life. In addition, it generates the marrow and bones. The bones are considered to be an extrusion of the kidneys. The skeleton is an analogue of the genetic blueprint. Developmental problems with the bones are associated with the essence.

The disease which particularly attacks the kidney essence is syphilis, since it destroys the hard, structural tissues of the body—bones, joints, cartilage, tendons—and the organs through which the hormones operate, the glands. At the same time, it breaks down the inherent integrity and structure of the psyche, producing syphilitic dementia. When syphilis first appeared in the Old World, after the voyage of Columbus, it spread with rapidity around the globe. In Europe, India, and China, mercury popped up spontaneously as the medicine for syphilis. It was, in fact, Paracelsus, the great alchemist, who introduced it into European pharmacy. He noted that the disease was not found in parts of Slovenia where it was mined. It was quickly noted that the symptoms produced by mercury as a poison were similar to those of syphilis. The homeopaths maintained that it worked by virtue of similarity.

The untreated syphilitic degenerates into a muscular-skeletal wreck; the cartilage of the nose deteriorates and breaks down along with the joints. The personality loses its integrity, its essence, so that it seems as if there was a piece missing. The logic of the person seems faulty. The characteristic syphilitic personality, in its extroverted phase, is famous in the history books. Henry VIII is believed to have been one, Idi Amin as well. After their actions and statements, one wants to ask these people: "Huh, what's the logic here? Why are you chopping off the queen's head?" It is not just the brutality, but the irrationality that marks the deteriorating syphilitic.

The three substances are held to be "precious" by the Oriental sages, because they are the basic building blocks of life. If we squander, ignore, or waste our internal resources, what kind of a life will we have? We will not learn from our experiences, we will not value the deep, internal feelings and strivings of the soul, we will not value or attempt to fulfill the path which the Creator has laid before our feet. This is called indulgence, and perhaps it is the chief cause of diseases which emanate from a spiritual level. That is not to say that all diseases begin on such an exalted level, or that we, as mere handmaidens of Mother Nature, can perceive the deep, interior mysteries of our patients, where they cannot.

Hahnemann, the founder of homeopathy, saw that the syphilitic taint was a wide reaching phenomena, sometimes associated directly with the disease, sometimes passed on as an inherited taint, and sometimes manifested as a pattern independent of the disease. His theory of the three chronic miasms directly reflects the alchemical doctrine of the three primordial substances. The three miasms, psora, syphilis, and sycosis (gonorrhea), are treated by three archetypal remedies, *Mercurius vivus, Sulphur* and *Thuja occidentalis* (Northern White Cedar). Since his time, *Natrum sulphuricum* (Glauber's Salt) has been introduced as a principal medicine for sycosis. The theory of the three chronic miasms is an attempt to describe and wrestle with the primal sources of disease.

Teasel and the Kidney Essence

As far as I know, Teasel is a superlative medicine for the kidney essence. The muscle and joint pain, the deterioration of structure, the helplessness and loss of purpose, etc., all relate to this pattern. The tall, hulking stalks, remaining through the winter, suggest the skeletal system and the cup-like leaves filled with water suggest the kidney essence and the lubrication of the joints. The large, thorny stalk is a signature for injuries and pains in large nerves such as the sciatic.

A common form of the syphilitic miasm at the present time is Lyme disease. This is essentially a form of "deer syphilis" carried by ticks. The spirochete stimulates the growth of antlers in the male deer, but it acts as a syphilitic infection in human beings. It is communicated from the deer to human beings by deer ticks. After entering the body through a tick bite, the spirochetes burrow into the muscles where they settle down to live. Here they produce chronic inflammation and pain, with destruction of muscles and joints. People become like the broken-down "tertiary syphilitics" described in old medical textbooks.

It turns out that Teasel is a powerful remedy for Lyme disease. For the last two years I have seen it cure five out of five cases of Lyme disease, either based on the blood tests or the persons own experience of the disease. Four of these were cases where medical tests showed clear or partial evidence of Lyme disease. One did not show up on any of the tests and may have been something else.

The first case was dramatic. For several years I had known a middle-aged woman who had been carrying the Lyme diagnosis for five years. She was at length reduced to collecting social security and living the life of a shut-in invalid. I tried to help her without success a few times. She pleaded with me for a remedy and gave me some hints. This set me to thinking about Teasel and she came out and picked some up at the farm. After two weeks on the tincture (three drops, three times a day) she developed a genital rash. "So you have deer syphilis," I teased. After three and a half weeks all four of her blood tests came up negative for the first time in five years. She felt much better. "This plant reaches to the very mechanism of the autoimmune system," she commented. "The Deer Nation thank you," added this Mdewakantan Dakota woman. "They don't like to be the carriers of this dreaded disease."

A month later I had another opportunity to use Teasel in a similar case where there was not a Lyme pathology. A thirty-five-year-old woman was suffering from extensive, chronic health problems that had also reduced her to living on social security. She had a large, farm-girl type frame and was increasingly obese in the last few years. Even walking around her apartment tore muscles. She was a multiple personality, had suffered from diarrhea for over a year at one point, been treated for syphilis at least once (one personality had liked to be a prostitute, she confided), had chronic vaginitis, massive adhesions in the abdomen from hernia and intestinal surgery, and a variety of problems which culminated in a congested and infected gallbladder. At one point she was devastated to learn that she did not test HIV positive. ("At least there would be a name for what I have," she explained.) After removal of the gallbladder, the diarrhea stopped for a while, but the wound discharged pus for eight months. There were at least four massive abscesses in the area and the wound left a huge twitched scar that you could put your fingers into up to the first knuckle. Adhesions covered about a quarter of her large, distended abdomen.

I thought of Teasel because of the torn muscles and brought her a bottle. Within a short time she felt the muscles "rearranging" inside her abdomen. Then she developed a burning genital rash. A layer of skin was excoriated off the genitals in twenty-four hours. "It feels like someone poured acid on me." The pain was unbearable and I had to give something (a dose of homeopathic Nitric acid 30x) to rein it in. The Teasel was continued and the results were prompt and amazing. Within a week the scar reduced one half in depth and the twist was removed, along with large parts of the adhesions: the muscles were repaired and actually changed in shape and location; she lost an inch off her waist and was almost reborn to mental clarity. The way she moved her body as she walked changed from an uncomfortable jerkiness to a flowing movement. The cure continued, she lost a large amount of weight, the adhesions virtually disappeared, and she looked and felt like a new person.

Several months later a woman called me up to ask about using Teasel for Lyme disease. She had been positively diagnosed, from the time she was bit on the thigh six years previously by a deer tick. She had the classic bull's eye rash around the bite and the usual treatment with massive antibiotics. At the place where the tick bit her there was a sore which had never gone away. She had the usual train of symptoms: muscle and joint pain, fatigue, and loss of mental clarity. In addition, she also had heart palpitations. She took the tincture, three drops, twice a day. After ten days the sore went away. She experienced some real aggravations until the symptoms reminded her of the worst episodes she had ever experienced. Then everything started to clear up, after a month she had a little rash of "blood blisters" on her thigh and she felt cured. She raved about the improvement and thanked God for the cure.

A year later I was asked to send a bottle of Teasel to a woman in Wisconsin, who had been suffering from Lyme disease to the point where she had to quit working at the head of her small company. She suffered the usual muscular-skeletal pains with terrible debility of the mind. After three months I heard back through her friends. The symptoms got better from the top down. First the head, then the torso down to the waist. She was able to return to work. That was the last I heard of this case through friends.

The ability for the muscles to move is dependent on little cross fibers which move the muscle cells or fibers. As the muscle tissue moves in a purposeful way, the muscle fibers straighten out and move in concert with each other. This reminds us of the way Teasel heads are used to "tease" fibers of wool.

Teasel Endorsed by the Deer Nation

A few weeks after my first experience using Teasel for Lyme disease I went out behind my barn to admire the plant. There, in the new fallen snow under the moonlight, I saw deer tracks coming to the little patch from all directions. I was astonished and recalled what my friend had said about the Deer Nation. A year later, I mentioned this observation during a conference in Boulder. Herbalist Terry Willard of Calgary, Alberta, noted with surprise that he had seen the same phenomenon. Teasel is rare in Calgary; the deer came to his garden from all directions to the patch of Teasel. Terry added that deer antler is used in China as a treatment for Lyme Disease. "It's great to share notes with other herbalists," he commented. "When they point out common experiences you were not even aware of until they spoke up ... you know you are looking at something that is true."

Preparation and Dosage

Teasel is a biennial, but the young plants spring up irrepressibly all summer long, so it is best to pick the large ones at whatever time of the summer the basal rosette of leaves reaches a large circumference. They may be dried by the usual methods. In Chinese herbalism the roots are roasted with salt to facilitate the action on the kidneys and toasted in vinegar to enhance the ability to reduce pain and circulate the blood. I make a tincture by macerating the fresh roots in vodka. I use only a small dosage, one to three drops, one to three times a day. In a serious, chronic case, even this may produce an aggravation. In this case, the dosage should be stopped or lessened for a while.

Dipsacus is closely related to the Asteraceae family and has many properties in common with members of that family. *Arctium lappa* (Burdock) has been used for syphilis. Boneset and Dandelion have also been suggested as cures for Lyme disease.

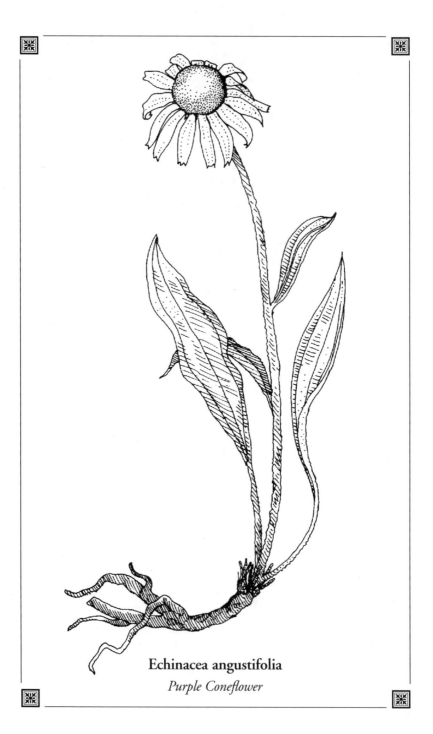

Echinacea angustifolia

Purple Coneflower

Echinacea angustifolia
Purple Coneflower

No contemporary herbal would be complete without an account of this popular herb, which now approaches the level of a household word. At the present time Echinacea is widely used as an "immune booster." This use depends upon the physical properties of the plant administered in large doses; it does not reflect the essential nature and specific properties, which require only a small dosage. In this book we will only be considering the use of Echinacea as a specific.

The name Echinacea is italicized when we are reflecting a botanical viewpoint, but not when we are referring to it as a common name. *Echinacea* is a genus in the Asteraceae family native to the United States. East of the Mississippi the principal representative is *Echinacea purpurea;* on the Western prairies it is *E. angustifolia.* The former is cultivated as an ornamental under the common name Purple Coneflower. It was not widely used by the Eastern Woodland Indians or the pioneers, though there was a slave doctor in North Carolina who used it as a snakebite remedy; it was called "Black Sampson" in his honor. *E. angustifolia,* on the other hand, is one of the most important medicinal plants of the Plains Indians. For this reason, Echinacea did not enter into popular herbalism and botanical medicine until after the settlement of the prairie states.

Modern pharmacological research has shown that these two Echinaceas possess similar constituents and properties. At the present time they are often used interchangeably. Several other varieties are now also used interchangeably, including *E. pallida* and *E. paradoxa.*

However, the fact that the Plains Indians favored *E. angustifolia* may be significant. The eclectics, who introduced Echinacea into professional usage, stated that *E. purpurea* would not provide the same results as *E. angustifolia*. The homeopaths proved and generally used this species as well.

Western Purple Coneflower, or Narrow Leaf Echinacea, is one of the most important plants in the medical tradition of the Plains Indians. It was used as a specific for the bite of the rattlesnake and the rabid dog, and as a general remedy in diverse acute and chronic diseases. It is still an important medicine today for traditional Plains Indians and may be considered a heritage gift from these people. As in most instances, the Indians prefer to use the root. The most common Indian name is "Toothache Root," but it is also one of the Indian "Snake Roots."

The Original Snake Oil

Echinacea angustifolia was first popularized in the 1880s by a patent medicine vendor in Pawnee City, Nebraska, Dr. H. C. F. Meyer. He learned about it from the Indians, bought it from them, and sold it on the market as a cure-all. Among other things, he claimed to have cured over six hundred snakebites. In fact, he repeatedly allowed himself to be bitten by rattlesnakes in order to demonstrate its efficacy. His preparation was literally the original "snake oil."

Meyer tried to interest serious physicians in Echinacea. He contacted Dr. John King and Dr. John Uri Lloyd, of the Eclectic Medical Institute in Cincinnati. Lloyd was highly prejudiced against the claims of a "quack" who offered to inject himself with rattlesnake poison, but Dr. King confirmed its value on a case of personal importance. Echinacea gave comfort and rest to his cancer-ridden wife. In 1887 King introduced *Echinacea angustifolia* into eclectic practice. Lloyd subsequently chastised himself for his prejudice. "My own delay in its general introduction is to me now a subject of self-criticism."

The eclectics developed an extensive portrait of the problems for which Echinacea is remedial. Dr. Harvey Felter (1927) described the characteristic symptoms as follows:

Echinacea is a remedy for auto infection, and where the blood stream becomes slowly infected either from within or without the blood, elimi-

nation is imperfect, the body tissues become altered, and there is developed within the fluids and tissues septic action with adynamia resulting in boils, carbuncles, cellular tissue inflammations, abscesses, and other septicemic processes.

We see how different this is from the modern use of Echinacea as an "immune boaster." Felter goes on to warn that Echinacea is "by no means a cure-all," a warning which should be remembered today.

Echinacea proved to be one of the most important remedies in the eclectic pharmacopeia and came to be identified with the school. As a consequence, the A.M.A. fought against its entry into conventional practice in the early part of our century. Nevertheless, by the 1920s it was the most widely used botanical agent in American medicine.

Echinacea angustifolia received a homeopathic proving in 1900 at the hands of Dr. J. C. Fahnestock, and was reproved in the 1950s. It is interesting to note that in the Fahnestock proving the tincture produced many pathogenetic symptoms, the 6x produced a few and the 30x potency produced none. This tends to indicate that *Echinacea* is a remedy which works well in the material doses, not in the potencies. We should also note that it accumulated its medicinal praise in the material doses and among low potency homeopathic prescribers like William Boericke and George Royal.

It was Dr. Royal who wrote the best account of *Echinacea* I have been able to find in homeopathic literature. Strangly, he used *Echinacea purpurea*, rather than the *angustifolia*, which was officinal. Dr. Royal gives specific symptoms for *Echinacea purpurea* from experience. He writes, "the most characteristic symptom is tiredness, whatever the disease may be named." Other symptoms included a fluctuating temperature, "from 97 to 105," flushed face, marked chilliness, offensive discharges, and mental confusion. "Echinacea presents changes in the blood simulating typhoid, pyemia, diphtheria, scarlatina, septicemia, also the effects of vaccination" with a contaminated serum. He compares *Echinacea* with *Arnica* and *Baptisia*. All of these are remedies which are suited to low-grade, septic infection, or "heat in the blood," to use the Chinese expression.

Boericke considered *Echinacea* to be almost a specific for boils and a constitutional remedy for people who chronically produce boils. Royal gives a detailed description of the kinds of boils he used it with. "The boils were small ('cat-boils'), very sensitive and seemed to come in crops, more about the neck and shoulders. For carbuncles [masses of boils] with profuse sanguino-purulent discharge [bloody-pus], marked prostration (the tired feeling), some rise in temperature and large sloughing [of skin]. They also come in crops and mostly about the neck, sometimes on perineum."

Royal used Echinacea for septic infections where the glands became swollen further up the limb from the sight of the injury, or where the veins were swollen and purple in the area leading from the injured part. He cites one case of a young bricklayer whose hand and fingers were so injured that he had been advised to have the fingers amputated because of sepsis. The glands under the arms were enlarged and there was fever. *Echinacea purpurea* 1x internally and externally, saved the fingers.

Echinacea was not widely adopted by lay herbalists and with the demise of eclecticism it almost lapsed into obscurity. Just as it was about to be forgotten, however, it was noted by a German pharmaceutical researcher who brought the seeds of *Echinacea purpurea* back to Germany with him. Research began, and Echinacea has since been shown to deserve the reputation it held among the Indians and professional doctors at the turn of the century. Pharmacological studies showed that Echinacea possesses a wealth of "immune-stimulating" compounds. It can raise the white blood count. In the last twenty years Echinacea was reintroduced back into the American marketplace from Germany.

Now that Echinacea is back in vogue, it is unfortunately overused. I have talked to people who take this remedy all the time, in the belief that it will "boost the immunity." Unfortunately, the excessive use of Echinacea can cause the very symptoms it is supposed to cure. After about two weeks it sometimes causes exhaustion. (This is the characteristic symptom it cures, so the reaction is essentially a homeopathic proving!) When Echinacea is properly indicated by some kind of exhaustion or depression of the immune system, it is indeed an "immune booster," but otherwise it may become wearing on the system or depression of the immune system, if it is indeed an "immune booster," but otherwise it may be wearing on the system. Research has also indicated several conditions where it may have a deleterious effect. It may interfere with drugs taken for HIV and TB. It is thought that it might not be advantageous in auto immune diseases.

There are two excellent books on Echinacea. Steven Foster,

Echinacea, Nature's Immune Enhancer (1991), gives an excellent account with relevant technical information from new and old sources. Christopher Hobbs, *Echinacea, The Immune Herb!* (1990), gives a shorter, more popular treatment.

Hobbs quotes herbalist Brian Weissbach of San Anselmo, California, who says, "Echinacea's primary indication is lymphatic stasis with inflammation and immune-depression." This is the traditional viewpoint. Weissbach also plays down the "cure-all" reputation of Echinacea. "Bear in mind that universal panaceas are mythical creatures."

Prairie Doctor, Farmer Remedy

If we remain true to the careful indications developed by the eclectic physicians, we will not have much trouble using Echinacea on specific indications. The affinities and properties are well described by King, Ellingwood, Felter, and others. We can also learn by direct examination of the physical properties of the plant—the flavor, temperature, impression, and signatures.

Echinacea possesses a unique taste. It is sweet, cool, and strongly diffusive (or tingling and numbing.) If Samuel Thomson had been alive when Echinacea came into prominence he would have ranked it among the top diffusives. These are the class of remedies which impart a strong, tingling impression to the tongue, indicating an immediate and powerful action on the nervous system. The diffusives tend to pick certain areas where they act most strongly: Lobelia on the muscles, Prickly Ash on the nerves, Bayberry bark on the mucosa, Cayenne Pepper on the cardiovascular system, and Echinacea on the lymph and blood. Foster quotes Felter on his view of the primal seat of action of Echinacea. It is, he writes, "A corrector of the depravation of the body's fluids."

As a diffusive with an emphasis on the lymphatic system and blood, Echinacea acts predominantly on low states of fever with exhaustion, lymphatic sluggishness, and septic materials in the bloodstream. The most characteristic symptoms are pimples and boils, dirty, dull skin tone, swelling and purple color of the veins or tongue, exhaustion, dullness of the mind and sensorium, swollen glands, and tired, dull eyes. The fever is continuous, not punctuated by intermittent chills, and may be high or low—but usually the latter. The remedy was well suited to the prostration of typhoid and septic fevers common in the late nineteenth century (for which Baptisia was also used.)

The doctrine of signatures also points to the properties of Echinacea. The flower petals are colored indigo-purple at the outer edges, changing to an intense red-purple towards the center. The color indigo is a signature for septic fevers. The reddish tint towards the inside of the petal reminds one of "histaminic irritation." This indicates the application of Echinacea in inflammation, both in septic and irritated cases. It is an excellent topical remedy for bee stings, spider bites, and snakebite. Its cooling effect on the skin is quite pleasant in hot conditions.

Inside the petals we find the inflorescence, a black mound which has been likened to a boil or pimple. A constitutional tendency to the production of boils is a highly characteristic indication for this remedy. The black color also indicates the necrotic tendencies. The dark green leaves give way to the dark-reddish tint in the stems. This is often a signature for septic infection of the blood. Echinacea is well indicated when there are swollen veins in the arms or legs.

The black color of the root was taken as a signature for conditions where the tongue was black, according to homeopath J. H. Clarke. I have never seen a black tongue, but it is mentioned in eclectic practice as well. Felter mentions a "dirty-brownish" or "jet-black" tongue. Such cases would probably not occur outside a hospital today. I saw one patient who had a dark purple spot in the center of the tongue. Obviously there was local blood stasis—probably in the intestines. She was a teenage girl who had recently had her appendix removed, but still felt dull, tired, and fatigued; she was also plagued by acne. *Echinacea angustifolia* tincture in repeated, small doses, removed the symptoms in one month.

In summary, Echinacea is an excellent remedy for exhausted, prostrated, tired people who have been run down by too much work or study. I call it the "farmer remedy," because it is indicated for people who just can't take a rest, have to work hard, through a season, and then fall sick, prostrated, when they get a little vacation. It could just as well be called the "student's remedy," or even a medicine for poor work habits. My earliest cases were, however, farmers, and it was a pioneer farmer who first gave Echinacea one of its best names, "Prairie Doctor."

My first case was a young man, aged thirty, who came to me

because he was suffering from boils on his face, of which he was exceedingly self-conscious. I noticed that his facial skin had a dirty visage. I tried to treat him according to the standard homeopathic concept of a constitutional remedy and gave him Sulphur. This seemed to fit the important symptoms, but nothing happened. Next time I gave him a bottle of *Echinacea angustifolia* tincture to apply locally, taking a few drops internally, as he thought best. I thought it would probably fail and he and his friends would consider me an idiot. However, six months later he came back with a smooth, perfect complexion, a smile on his face, and an empty bottle of Echinacea. It was clear that the remedy had not only cleansed the local eruptions, but the entire economy. This taught me that Echinacea was a deep-acting remedy which affected the entire system in a searching and comprehensive manner. It was not just a local dressing for boils.

I happened to be talking with this patient sometime later, and he mentioned that he was raised on a farm. He complained about how his father delighted to make the boys work to the point of utter exhaustion. He rather resentfully referred to him as a "sadist." "He owned the last team of work horses in the county; he just liked to see them work." This meant nothing to me at the time, but it came back to me as I was talking with my next Echinacea patient.

A forty-year-old man came in from central Wisconsin, complaining of general lethargy. His skin had the same dirty, tired look. A thought quite naturally came to mind. "Are you a farmer?" I asked. "Or did you grow up on a farm?" Yes, he replied. His father was a cruel and vindictive man who worked him to the bone. A whole series of questions naturally framed themselves. "Do you have bad work habits? Do you work hard for a long time, then feel exhausted and sick for a few days? Do you have boils?" The answer was yes on every question. Indeed, his father also had boils. *Echinacea angustifolia* tincture had a profound, curative effect on the patient. The boils disappeared, the skin improved, and he changed his work habits.

Like Royal, I discovered that prostration, exhaustion, and tiredness are one of the most characteristic symptoms calling for Echinacea. I have also seen the dark, swollen veins he mentions. A man came to me suffering from a debilitating case of the flu. He had dull eyes, exhaustion, and purple veins running up the arms. A few drops of Echinacea, three times a day, and he was cured in three or four days.

Dr. J. H. Clarke gave a case history illustrating the complication from vaccination with an impure serum. A forty-seven-year-old man came down with septic deterioration. "The symptoms were: vitality ebbed; he became so weak he could not sit up; hair fell out; an eruption of psoriasis appeared on extremities extending to body. The disease advanced rapidly; the nails fell off. Left iritis supervened, and then keratitis of the right eye. Under Kali iod. [Potassium iodide] and phospho-albumen as a food, the hair ceased to fall off, but other symptoms became rapidly worse." *Echinacea purpurea* was now given, in twenty drop doses. "Slowly the disease was arrested, then gradual improvement and ultimate cure ensued."

Preparation and Dosage

The officinal preparation was made from the root of *Echinacea angustifolia.* However, many preparations currently on the market include all parts of several different Echinaceas. The thinking is that immune-stimulating compounds vary in different parts of the plant, and from species to species.

A good herbal tincture in full strength, or the first dilution (ten percent) should be used. Small doses (one to ten drops) act promptly when the remedy is well-indicated. Large doses (ten to sixty drops) are unnecessary when this plant is being used as a specific, and will tend to depress the system. I have definitely encountered people who had a variety of side-effects from repeatedly using large doses (sixty drops).

I try to use only the root of *Echinacea angustifolia,* as the Indians and the early doctors did. Unfortunately, the root takes about four years to mature and the plant is overpicked. I recommend that people using *Echinacea* as a general tonic in large doses use the *purpurea,* while people using it in small doses on specific and traditional indications use the *angustifolia.*

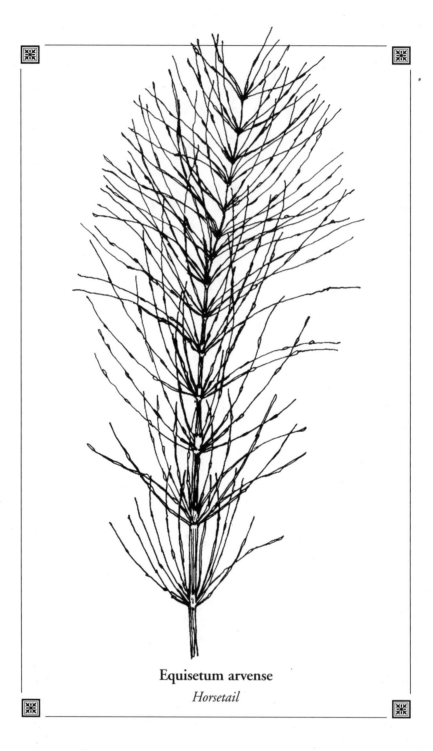

Equisetum arvense

Horsetail

Equisetum arvense
Horsetail

Horsetail is an ancient plant which dominated the forests of the dinosaur period. During that time, there were specimens that grew to be the size of giant pine trees. These giants were long believed to be extinct, but recently, several dozen plants were discovered living in a remote valley in Australia. Although the large kinds are virtually gone, Horsetail remains throughout the world as a small, distinctive plant. Because of the unique appearance and qualities, the Horsetails have long been utilized by indigenous cultures around the world and have found a niche in the herbal pharmacopoeia of many peoples.

Four species of Horsetail have been used in Western herbal medicine: *Equisetum arvense, E. fluviatile, E. hyemale* and *E. sylvaticum.* They are found in North America, Europe, and Asia. They grow in damp sands and soils at the margins of swamps, lakes, and streams. Field Horsetail (*E. arvense*) is the only kind with branches and is therefore easily distinguished. This and *E. hyemale* are the types preferred in herbal medicine. Culpeper writes, "the smoother rather than the rough, and the leaves rather than the bare, is most physical."

Equisetum arvense was introduced into homeopathy, basically on the traditional indications found in herbal medicine, which emphasize the kidney sphere. However, what is more important is that the narrow profile of this remedy can be enlarged to include almost the entire portrait of Silicea, one of the most important of the homeopathic remedies and one of Dr. William Schuessler's "twelve tissue salts." Horsetail, as we will see, is the "vegetable silica." This means that like Silicea it is a remedy for loss of nerve, nervousness to the point of fingernail chewing, hair-pulling, picking at the body or objects, a slightly chilly constitution, and a variety of problems with the hard sheaths and tissues of the body. I have used Horsetail for most of the common conditions for which Silicea is used in homeopathy, and I have not yet detected an important difference.

Herbal Flint

Horsetail stems are rigid, upright, hollow and very hard. The plant is more than thirty-five percent silica in content, so it is almost an "herbal sand" or "flint." The young shoots are edible, but not the mature, which are bound together and used as a scouring pad to wash pans. "Scouring Rush," as it is sometimes called, contains saponins which also help clean. However, it is the high silica content which seems to give Horsetail most of its properties. This gives it an affinity to hard structures throughout the body, strengthening the connective tissue, bones, cartilage, mucus membranes, arteries, skin and many other tissues.

A shortage of silica is not recognized by conventional science, because this mineral is found everywhere. Taking away the water, Earth and all her inhabitants are composed of ninety-seven percent alumino-silicates. However, there is a difference between minerals which have been absorbed into organic processes and those which remain in a mineral state. Horsetail provides a naturally occurring source of organic silica. It is therefore a remedy for conditions where there is an inability to absorb and retain silica. When this occurs there are weaknesses in the hard structures of the body. The hair becomes thin, fails to thrive, and fizzles away into split ends. The nails are often weak, breaking easily, with hangnails and lingering infections about the nail. Occasionally the personality suffers a similar weakness or "lack of flint." Such people have a lack of confidence, a lack of "flint" or "grit," as the homeopaths say about Silicea patients. They do not have the confidence to plunge into life, they remain behind, not safe, but picking at or chewing their fingernails, or picking out their hair, one by one.

These are the outward, observable indications of a system which is lacking in silica. There are also interior changes. The mucus membranes can be weak. They are easily irritated by foreign substances, so that allergies arise, especially in the sinuses. Horsetail is especially good when a person is allergic to all sorts of things, rather than one or a few. This is what I call "nonspecific hay fever."

If the lining of the bladder is weakened by silica depletion, the connective tissue can become inflamed and irritated. Chronic cystitis may result. No amount of antibiotic treatment will help because the tissues are innately susceptible. Horsetail is sometimes useful in nonspecific chronic bladder infections, where the condition results from weakness of the connective tissue of the bladder, rather than infection with bacteria.

The bones, cartilage, and muscles are likewise strengthened by Horsetail. It will sometimes do wonders rebuilding joints. In combination with Solomon's Seal I have repeatedly seen it make expensive, debilitating, complicated surgeries unnecessary. It strengthens the arteries and veins, eliminating varicosities—in people who need silica. Look to the hair, skin, and nails to determine whether the patient is one who would respond to Horsetail.

The older authors emphasized the capacity Horsetail had to prevent bleeding and cure wounds. Culpeper writes, "It is very powerful to staunch bleeding either inward or outward, the juice or the decoction thereof being drank, or the juice, decoction or distilled water applied outwardly. It also stays all sorts of lasks and fluxes in man or woman, and bloody urine; and heals also not only the inward ulcers, and the excoriation of the entrails, bladder, etc. but all other sorts of foul, moist and running ulcers, and soon solders together the tops of green wounds. It cures all ruptures [hernias] in children." However, remember that it is more specific to the silica person, than just anybody.

Horsetail also has an anti-inflammatory and antiseptic aspect, so that it is beneficial for old, inflamed, degenerated wounds. The warm distilled water is applied to "hot inflammations, pustules or red wheals, and other breakings-out in the skin," relates Culpeper.

In homeopathy, silica is known as the "homeopathic scalpel," because of its ability to act like a blade, like flint, to cut, to bring matters to the surface and to heal charitably. It cuts in, opens tissues, and releases pus and corrupted material, while cleansing and reincarnating flesh. It has a centripetal effect, removing heavy, unneeded materials to the surface and out. Sharp, hard Horsetail shares the same property.

The long, rigid tube-like stems also show an affinity to tubular structures in the body. Horsetail was particularly associated with kidney problems by the old authors. It "provokes urine, and helps the stone and strangury," writes Culpeper. Plants which grow in wet sands are particularly strong kidney medicines because both sand (like urinary gravel) and water are signatures pointing to this organ. Thus we have kidney medicines like *Eryngium yuccafolium* (grows on wet sands), *Eryngium maritima* (wet, salty sands), *Saxifraga* sp. (wet sands, peat and rocky ledges), *Eupatorium purpureum* (wet soils).

Cook comments on the influence *Equisetum* has upon the kidneys. "It possesses stimulating with astringing properties, and expends its power on the kidneys and urinary passages in a desirable manner. It increases the flow of urine moderately, aiding in the general elimination of the renal solids without exhausting the kidneys, but rather leaving behind a goodly tonic impression. Such qualities are desirable in many cases of dropsy, congestion of the kidneys with diminution of their function, hematuria, and similar troubles. In gleet [gonorrheal discharge] the article often answers a good purpose; and at times it has been spoken of for gravel, probably from its influence in increasing the renal glow. I have also used it in some cases of prolapsus [uteri] with leucorrhea and persistent headache." I use a combination of Agrimony, Horsetail and Gravel Root as a general remedy in kidney stones.

Horsetail also has a strong influence on the joints. The doctrine of signatures points us to the use of Horsetail in strengthening the cartilage. If you pick the young plant and break the seal between the joints, there is still an elastic material within the joint that holds it together. As you roll the joint between your fingers, you will notice that it flexes much like one would want the knee or any joint to flex when bending. The idea of cartilage is immediately presented to the mind.

Horsetail is an excellent remedy for the knees and other joints. It will rebuild damaged cartilage and structures. A woman in her fifties came in because she had "grinding" in the knees when she bent down, and pain and stiffness in these and other joints. An application of Horsetail to the knees took the grinding away in five minutes. "They feel less hot," she added. (Culpeper comments upon the ability of Horsetail to correct "swelling and heat and inflammation of the lower parts in men and women.") She went home with Horsetail and Calcium phosphate 30c.

The energy of Horsetail is centripetal, throwing the harder, solid substances to the surface, while maintaining the fluids in the center and depths of the organism. Thus it is in fact an old remedy for boils and abscesses, and can be called the "herbal scalpel." It also seems to gently support the upward movement of heat and refined materials and the downward descent of cold and coarser solids. It strengthens and hardens the protective membranes towards the exterior, while promoting the free flow of fluids in the interior. The gentle segregation of solids and fluids is found throughout the human body, but especially in the kidneys, which are responsible for keeping the balance between water and minerals. It also is seen in the blood vessels, where the blood has to flow and not get caught by "sticky spots" in the walls. The Chinese concept of the spleen also has a bearing here, since the spleen is said to raise the clear and descend the turbid through a gentle influx of heat. Finally, we see this influence in the nervous system, where the solids make a sheath around the fluids which coat the nerves. This extends up into the brain, and Horsetail also has an effect here as well.

The mature stem of Horsetail is topped off by a spore-carrying structure which looks like a head or alembic, a cap-like glassware used in alchemy and chemistry. Horsetail has an affinity to the "distilling" movement of cerebrospinal fluid through the brain, just as it does to the distilling tubules in the kidneys. On a more mundane level, Horsetail is indicated where there is a disturbance in the distillations, so that the little tubules which leave the brain through the ethmoid sieve are clogged, resulting in sinus congestion and dripping head colds. Thus it is, as Culpeper relates, "effectual against a cough that comes by distillations from the head."

Preparation and Dosage

Because Horsetail contains so much silica it cannot be eaten either fresh or cooked. In traditional herbalism, the tea is made by decoction. It also makes a nice tincture in alcohol. The dose need not be big: up to three drops is sufficient. The stems need to be crushed before drying, to remove the water in the joints. This can cause rotting of the material. According to William LeSassier, it is best when picked in a place which is shady, where the water is clean.

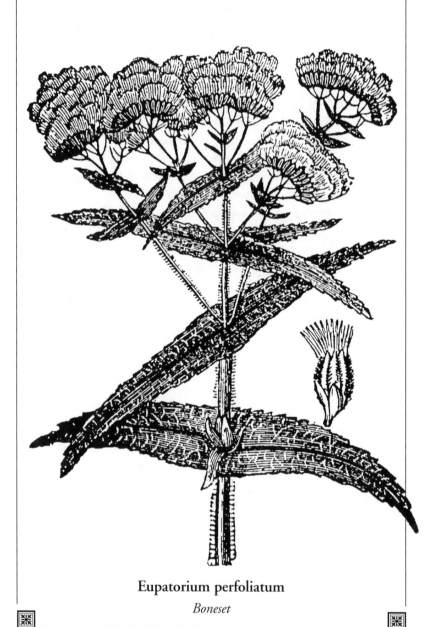

Eupatorium perfoliatum

Boneset

from an old American print

Eupatorium perfoliatum

Boneset

Boneset is a member of the Composite or Sunflower family. It is a common inhabitant along the margins of swamps and streams in the northern parts of eastern North America. There is a stand growing behind my barn at Sunnyfield Herb Farm, on the edge of the marsh. Boneset is easy to identify by the leaves (which are alternate and joined around the stems) and the flowers (which are bone white). When the stalks begin to get about four to five feet high towards the end of summer, the flower heads appear. They are often surrounded by honeybees.

When the European settlers first landed on American shores, they were faced with diseases peculiar to the new climate. Among these was an intermittent fever accompanied by strong chills and aching in the bones—the typical winter flu of the northern states. Boneset was universally used by the northern Indians in winter influenza, intermittent chill/fever, agues, and malarial conditions. According to Rafinesque, it bore an Indian name which translates as "ague-weed." (An "ague" was a fever characterized by intermitting chills and fever, and included both malaria and influenza.) The settlers quickly adopted this medicine into their pharmacopoeia. "There is probably no plant in American domestic practice that has more extensive or frequent use than this," wrote Charles Millspaugh in 1892. "The attic, or woodshed, of almost every country farm house has its bunch of dried herb hanging, tops downward from the rafters during the whole year, ready for immediate use should some member of the family, or that of a neighbor, be taken with a cold."

Eupatorium perfoliatum is most commonly called Boneset. The leaves merge together around the stalk; this is an old signature for bone setting in both Europe and North America. Despite the name, published literature denies the use of Boneset as an agent for bone healing. This is an unusual case where folk tradition maintains a use at variance with the conventional literature. I have repeatedly run across folk practitioners, mostly Indian and rural people, who consider this to be one of the primary uses of the plant.

The usual explanation for the name is that Boneset is used in the typical influenza of our northern climes, where the bones ache. All the old authors refer to this explanation. C. J. Hemple (1846) says that about 1800, "there prevailed throughout the United States, but particularly in the state of Pennsylvania, a peculiar epidemic, which, from the constancy of the attending symptom of pain in the bones, was called break bone fever." *Eupatorium perfoliatum* "so signally relieved the disease...that it was familiarly called bone-set."

There was much interest in the plant among professional physicians in our fledgling Republic after the experience with break-bone fever. In 1812, Dr. Anderson gave it a trial in the New York City Almshouse, in place of the more expensive Quinine bark. It proved to be quite successful in treating chill/fever, and from that time on it was used by many professional physicians as well as lay people. It was one of the few native herbs used by doctors of every school—allopathic, Thomsonian, eclectic, and homeopathic—representing one of the few therapeutic commonalities of the era. *Eupatorium perfoliatum* received a proving by Dr. Williamson about 1860, and was adopted by homeopaths on essentially the same symptoms for which it is traditionally prescribed.

Probably because it was reported as a remedy for malaria, Boneset has been ridiculed by some modern authors. Despite universal acclaim and the personal experience of myriads of people, I have seen modern books which report that Boneset has no value. Some people enjoy expressing opinions about things they know nothing about.

Boneset has three principal uses. It is used (1) to rid the system of intermittent chills, (2) as a bitter tonic for the mucosa, rebuilding the digestion and appetite after it has been destroyed by intermittent fever, and (3) as a bone healing medicine. It is traditionally used by hot infusion for the first purpose; as a cold tea for the second.

Intermittent Fever

Samuel Thomson gave the folk medical explanation for intermittent fevers. He explained that cold entered the system partway and got stuck. The body attempted to push it out, but since it was stuck there was an alternating chill and fever. The same explanation is used in traditional Chinese medicine. Intermittent fever is described as "halfway in, halfway out."

Intermittent fevers were traditionally associated with low, damp districts—even particular farms. We now know that this is because of the presence of malarial infestation in mosquitoes inhabiting swamps. This information, helpful from a public health standpoint, does not undermine the traditional concept of cold invading and getting stuck "halfway in." Some of the traditional remedies for intermittent fever—such as Boneset—were also used for malaria.

In severe, chronic intermittent fevers, there is a tendency to jaundice, bilious vomiting, and hepatic congestion. This probably occurs because tension in the circulation constricts the arteries around the gallbladder and liver. In both traditional Western and Chinese herbalism, intermittent fever is associated with the liver. Rademacher, for instance, catalogued intermittent fever under the liver. The botanical name *Eupatorium*, as we have seen, derives from the word hepatic.

Eupatorium grows in low damp areas where one is apt to get a chill. Although conjoined leaves are usually considered a signature for bonesetting, I find that they also indicate a relationship to chill/fever. Fever Root (*Triosteum perfoliatum*) also has this trait. It's as if the conjoined leaves represent an unnatural conjoining of hot and cold.

The chill associated with the *Eupatorium* condition may come on with much regularity: once a day, once a week, even once a month. It is accompanied by such symptoms as throbbing pain in the head, worse in the occiput, head cold with sneezing, bitter taste in the mouth, vomiting of bile, frequent green diarrhea, hoarseness and cough, soreness in the chest and liver region. Perspiration relieves all symptoms, except the headache. The chill and vomiting is preceded by thirst and great soreness and aching of bones.

Eupatorium perfoliatum was the first homeopathic remedy I ever used on myself. I had a slight chill one day and thought I might be sick.

The next day I felt better, but I never felt completely well. A month later I had another chill and wondered if I was sick, but it passed. Finally, another month went by, I felt a chill and I knew I was sick. I took *Eupatorium perfoliatum* 6x, a nice little sweat broke out that evening and the next day I felt well.

A much more serious case is described by Dr. Charles Millspaugh. "My friend, Dr. Henry S. Sloan, of [New York] city, relates his personal experience with this drug as follows: When a young man, living in the central part of [New York] State, he was attacked with intermittent fever, which lasted off and on for three years. Being of a bilious temperament, he grew at length sallow, emaciated, and hardly able to get about." During this time he was treated with cinchona bark and all its derivatives, cholagogues, and "every other substance then known to the regular practitioner," without any improvement. Finally the attacks came on twice a day. By this point he was unable to walk, except by supporting himself on rail fences and buildings along the side of the road. "As he sat one day, resting by the side of the road, an old lady of his acquaintance told him to go home and have some thoroughwort 'fixed,' and it would certainly cure him." On reaching home he received a tablespoonful of Boneset syrup, and immediately went to bed. "He had hardly lain down when insensibility and stupor came on, passing into deep sleep. On awaking in the morning, he felt decidedly better, and from that moment improved rapidly without farther medication, gaining flesh and strength daily." Soon he was completely and permanently cured. He only suffered a single recurrence, thirty years later, while lying in a swamp during a hunting trip.

Bone Setting

Conventional literature is quick to remark that Boneset is not actually used in bone-mending. However, acquaintance with folk practice shows that the reverse is the case. In some instances, the plant has probably been used in this fashion simply because of the name. "The lay practitioners didn't know that it wasn't supposed to be used for bone setting," was the comment of a sympathetic homeopath. However, there is a persistent, widespread use of the plant for this condition.

There can be little doubt that this tradition traces back to

American Indian experience. I have known a number of Native practitioners, uninfluenced by conventional literature, who use Boneset primarily for setting bones. We also meet with the tradition among rural people in Appalachia and the Ozarks. The late herbalist Tommie Bass, a resident of northern Alabama, specifically attributed this usage to the Indians, some of whom survived in unrecognized settlements in his area. Twylla Willis, proprietor of the Herb Bar, in Austin, Texas, remarked that her grandmother, who was raised in the Ozarks, used this remedy consistently for broken bones. "She had fifty six grandchildren," said Twylla. Folk medicine grants credentials from a different perspective than scientific medicine.

My own experience has settled my mind about this matter. I have used Boneset in simple and very serious breaks with repeated success. The healing always has gone better and faster than the doctors anticipated. I have also collected stories from other people. Homeopath Julian Winston of New Zealand collected several case histories of lay practitioners who used *Eupatorium perfoliatum* in homeopathic form, based on the common name.

In one instance I helped a woman who had a complete break through both the tibia and the fibula across the ankle-joint. While it is true that we used a variety of remedies, including the famous bone healer Comfrey, both of us thought the best curative influence came from the Boneset. The healing went so well that, after surgery to pin the bones together, the doctor decided not to cast the ankle. The words "amazing recovery" were used by her medical attendants several times.

One of my herb students told me her experience with Boneset. She has a nice sixty acre lot of woods out about ten miles past where I live. There are a lot of herbs out there. Several years before I met her, she had a serious auto accident. Two of her front teeth were knocked out and her right hand was crushed. They put the teeth back in her jaw and hoped they would grow. They didn't set the wrist, since the bones were crushed. There was some Boneset growing on my friend's land. She was attracted to the plant and liked the name, so she started drinking the tea. She craved it for about six months, before getting tired of the taste. Her teeth grew back and her wrist recovered without a problem. Boneset tea is very bitter and unpleasant, so evidently she needed the plant.

This case points out an interesting phenomena. Many people

who need Boneset find the taste attractive while other people find it horribly bitter. I have observed this several times, both in bone healing and influenza.

Perhaps the most charming story about healing bones with Boneset was related by a woman in Wisconsin. (The account is second hand, but precious nonetheless.) An elderly Indian lady of her acquaintance lived by herself in the woods in northern Michigan. She broke her ankle while in her boat, but cautiously made her way back to her cabin, where she had some Boneset tea. (Older Indian people sometimes keep the tea as a remedy for brittleness of the bones, or what we now call osteoporosis.) After three days she felt well enough to go to town and have the doctor check it. He was upset that she had not come in a month ago when he supposed it happened!

My friend Halsey Brandt of Bisbee, Arizona, speculated that Boneset cures both influenzal aching in the bones and broken bones because it stimulates circulation to the periosteum, the lining of the bones.

Bitter Tonic for the Mucosa

In addition to acting on the bones, *Eupatorium* is also a bitter tonic with a strong influence on the mucosa. It was commonly used to shore up people, like Dr. Henry Sloan, mentioned above, who had debilitated digestion from old intermittent fevers. It also acts on the mucosa of the lungs.

Dr. Frederick Locke describes the respiratory symptoms calling for Eupatorium perfoliatum in his *Syllabus of Eclectic Materia Medica* (1895.) "It relieves the cough of measles, asthma, and that cough so peculiar to old people. It is the remedy for colds, with pain in the chest, roughness of voice, and general muscular aching." I would also add that it is especially well indicated in cases where there is no cough, no attempt to bring up mucous, and when given, it renews the cough reflexes and starts bringing this old material up. This indicates, I think, an inactivity of the mucosa, an insensibility, so that the mucous remains "uncontested," so to speak, in the respiratory channels.

Herbalist Paul Bergner of Boulder, Colorado, gave an account of his personal experience with Boneset in a respiratory disease with flu-like symptoms. "After moving recently from Oregon to Colorado, the combination of the stress of the move, the climate change from wet to dry, and the weather extremes of the Colorado mountains, with wild swings from Spring-like to sub-zero weather, occasional 100 mph winds (!), and exposure to the new 'bugs' of the bioregion left me with a sick-week chronic viral bronchitis with periodic flu-like symptoms recurring every four or five days." After trying to doctor himself and working with a master of Traditional Chinese Medicine, Paul finally turned to Boneset. "I took three twelve-drop doses of a concentrated 1:1 boneset tincture over a period of eight hours. I felt the digestive stimulant and cholagogue effects immediately, as if something had become 'unplugged.'" He fell into a deep sleep and began to improve rapidly. Paul tells this story in his journal, *Medical Herbalism* (1995.)

As a tonic to the digestive mucosa, Boneset is most commonly used for debility from old intermittents which have damaged the tension on the gallbladder reflexes and caused problems due to wrongs of the bilious apparatus. Locke says it is an admirable tonic to restore the appetite, especially in alcoholics whose appetite has been ruined by drinking.

Ellingwood (1898 edition) gives two digestive cases quoted by Bergner. "In a case of neurasthenia (nervous exhaustion) of long standing, complicated by emphysema, the patient, an extremely nervous woman, regurgitated whatever food she ate. There was no nausea, the food simply came back up. Fifteen drops of the fluid extract of boneset every two hours cured the condition on the second day. It recurred several months later for a short time, but was promptly cured by a few more doses of boneset. Another case involved an elderly man who appeared ready to die from chronic incurable hiccoughs. Fifteen drops of boneset in an infusion of cayenne, once an hour, produced a permanent cure."

Preparation, Toxicity, and Dosage.

The traditional instructions call for the leaves. Pour a cup of hot water over about a tablespoon of the leaves and steep for fifteen minutes. The brew will be fairly bitter. The hot infusion promotes sweating, while the cold acts as a bitter tonic on the stomach, solar plexus, hepatic structures and respiratory mucosa. This is the method taught by Dr. William Cook (1869.)

The plant should be gathered at the beginning of flowering, towards the end of August. The flowers will continue to go to seed as the plant dries, if one picks it at the height of blooming—this is perhaps why the leaves alone are found in herb commerce. One does not have this problem if the tops are bottled fresh in alcohol. I prefer to use the flowers as well as the leaves, because the honeybees like them so much, and because they sweeten up the bitter taste a little. I make a tincture by macerating the tops in vodka or brandy. I use a dose of only one to three drops. The homeopathic potencies work about the same as the tincture. Many herbalists use much larger doses.

Eupatorium perfoliatum contains the pyrrolizidine alkaloids, which can be toxic under continuous use. No poisonings have been reported from the plant, which can hardly be taken in large doses, because of the nauseant bitter taste.

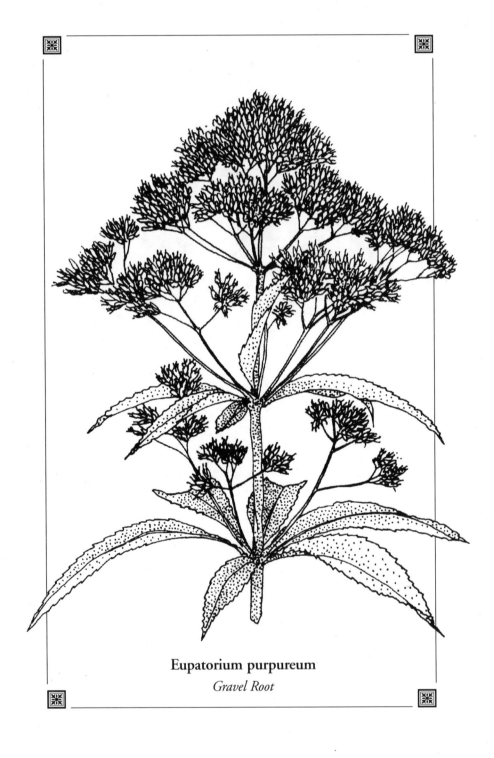

Eupatorium purpureum

Gravel Root

Eupatorium purpureum

Gravel Root

This plant does not look very similar to its cousin Boneset, though it also likes to grow along damp stream beds and in damp upland soils. Sometimes, however, we find it in the middle of the bog, where Boneset would never be found. The leaves are not joined round the stem and the flowers are pink-purple. When these come on in August, the plant suddenly appears in the swamp with a blaze, where before it went unnoticed.

Early in the settlement of the eastern seaboard, a medicine man by the name of Joe Pye became famous for treating a low form of typhus with this plant. In his honor, it was named "Joe Pye Weed." It is also known as "Gravel Root," referring to its excellent capacity to expel gravel and stone from the urinary tract. It is sometimes called "Queen of the Meadow," because of its beautiful appearance while in flower in the marshes of late summer.

Gravel Root was widely used by the Indians as a kidney medicine and just as widely adopted by the early settlers. "Probably no remedy is in such extensive use in domestic practice, for the relief of renal diseases, and those urinary symptoms which are commonly supposed to arise from calculi," wrote Dr. Edwin Hale. "Such an extensive foundation must rest upon some solid basis. In an extensive country practice of many years, I have usually found this sort of testimony to be worth as much as the dictum of some of our most learned medical men. It is from these popular uses that the Eclectic physicians have gained much of their knowledge concerning the use of indigenous plants." Gravel Root was adopted from folk practice by the professional physicians of the physio-medical and eclectic schools in the middle of the nineteenth century. It is still a common item in herbal commerce and practice at the present day.

After Hale introduced the homeopathic audience to *Eupatorium purpureum,* it was given a proving by the wife of a doctor. This produced extensive urinary tract symptoms. Hale had also seen these symptoms occur in people who had taken too much of the medicine during self-treatment. "When excessively taken, as it often is by the country people," Gravel Root has aggravated renal difficulties and even given rise to "the very symptoms for which it is so strongly recommended." It is used in homeopathy on pretty much the same indications as in herbal medicine. Some more detail has been added, but the genius of the remedy has not been brought out and it is seldom used today. Let us, however, remedy that situation.

Turtle Medicine

In order to get to the deeper reaches of this medicine plant, it would be helpful for the reader to have direct personal experience of the plant. Experience is the touchstone of reality, the philosopher's stone, the real McCoy. If that is impossible for the present, then follow what I have to say about Gravel Root.

Go out into the middle of a peat bog, where there is no mineral soil, only the organic deposit of dead plants. Pick some Gravel Root, take it home and clean it. While nibbling on the roots and rootlets, you will be surprised to find small mineral casts and stones. This cannot be the result of gravel found in the soil, since the plant was picked in a peat bog. This demonstrates that Gravel Root precipitates minerals out of solution around its roots.

This is an excellent signature, pointing to the use of Gravel Root for gravel and sand in the urine. *Eupatorium purpureum* works both ways, to bring minerals out of solution, or to bring them back in. It is a superlative kidney medicine, since the job of the kidneys is to maintain the balance of fluids and solids. This is also a signature showing that Gravel Root has a re-mineralizing capacity, and that it can be used, like its cousin Boneset, to heal broken bones and eroded tissue. It has also been used to dissolve deposits out of joints, like its cousin Water Agrimony. The motto of Queen of the Meadow is the motto of the old alchemists: dissolve and coagulate. It adjusts the balance between the fluids and solids.

There is an even deeper significance in this curious signature. In myths and legends from around the world, we learn how Grandfather Turtle rose out of the sea to become the nucleus for dry land. In just such a way, this plant precipitates mineral solids out of the waters. Legends also tell of how the earth is held upon the back of a giant turtle. Turtle is a symbol for the earth. It carries around upon its back a mineral shell like the hard places of the earth. In a sense, it is a piece of the earth itself.

Just as there is a soft, living body inside the hard mineral shell of the turtle, so is there a soft, living, conscious being inside the earth—Mother Earth. The living being inside the material world is what is also called in traditional lore, "the Underworld." It is to this place that the humble seekers-after-wisdom retreat, in order to learn of the hidden secrets of Mother Nature. Here, in the invisible Light of Nature, the essences of the creatures and medicines are made known, so that we can learn to work with Mother Nature, instead of carelessly rifling her treasures, as if we owned them.

Turtle is thus a symbol of the doorway to the Underworld. Actually, this is not a strong enough statement. *Turtle is the doorway to the Otherworld.* The dark eyes of Grandfather Turtle are filled with the wisdom of the ages. All things which have ever been true are registered in the soul of Grandfather Turtle, from the beginning of time down to the present. The impression of the eternal upon the temporal is also stored here, so that the interface of the Great Mystery with time and space is not forgotten, but recorded indelibly. Grandfather Turtle says, "Everything you always knew to be true, is true."

The dark eyes of the Indian people are conjunct the wisdom in Grandfather Turtle's eyes. The Indian people have an inalienable genetic access to the inner secrets of Mother Earth. They have long been famed and known as the bearers of some wonderful secret, from the time they were first "discovered" by outsiders. And yet, this depth of knowledge is for them a terrible burden to carry under the present regime. We live in an age when Mother Nature is ruthlessly exploited to yield her treasures. Just as the realm of Mother Earth is considered to be common or individual property rights without regard to Nature's agenda, the property rights (even basic human rights) of Native Americans are ignored and their possessions have been taken at will.

When a person is humble before the mystery of Mother Nature, and allows the living spirit of that realm, the "Spirit of the World," the *anima mundi,* to come within, then that person is initiated into the timeless mysteries of the hidden side of this world. This is what the turtle has to teach us. Grandfather Turtle is the root of wisdom, the philosopher's stone, in which the mysteries of Mother Nature are revealed. This is the First Earth, the *prima materia,* from which the world we live in is created, and to which it returns for renewal. We are able to understand the plants, minerals, and animals in their true nature from this source only. This is the true medical school where the true physician obtains his or her degree. With this knowledge it is possible to see the inner essence of the sick person, the disease, and the medicine. Nature is also the true pharmacy, from which we obtain our store of medicine.

Old Man Turtle teaches us to be patient, to wait for "the truth to out," as it always will. He rewards us for being subtle, so that we can penetrate through material obstruction to the core of true knowledge. Just as the mist rises from the sea to become the cloud and fall again to the earth, so do we learn to penetrate, like a cloud, through the barrier of this world, into the Next. This exchange, of water to mist, mist to water, is also associated with the precipitating mysteries of the turtle.

There is, however, a guardian at the doorway to the Underworld, who will test the will of any person who comes into that place without proper preparation. This can be represented by the wolf, the master of boundaries.

The second signature we turn to is the purple color in the flowers and stem of the plant. This is a signature pointing to low-grade, septic states, where the tissue is eroding and there is deteriorating protein in the blood stream. We often see the purple color around abscesses or veins when there is a putrid infection present, and the herbs which have this color—Wild Indigo, Echinacea, Dandelion, and Plantain, for example—are all powerful medicines for this condition.

The purple color has a deeper significance, however. It represents conditions of psychological morbidity and corruption, out of which the opportunity for spiritual rebirth arises. The flower rises from the rotting marsh like a Phoenix.

The Kidneys

In Traditional Chinese Medicine it is said that the kidneys "store the *jing*," the essence (see Teasel). This is the metaphorical *prima materia*, the ultimate source, of sexual and genetic material. It is the protoplasmic blob which is behind all of life, as well as the genetic articulation which gives rise to separate life forms. This blob is what the Western Alchemists called the *mercurius*. All sexual, genetic, and hormonal processes rise out of and reflect this primal essence. The most mundane definition of the word *jing* in Chinese is "sperm." The most material expression of the genetic configuration is the skeleton, the material shadow of the genetic blueprint. In Chinese medicine, the bones are considered to be an extrusion from the kidneys.

It is easy to see why the Chinese physicians call the kidneys the "source of life and death" and the "foundation of fire and water". The *jing* is considered to be the primordial origin from which arose both the *yin* and the *yang* of the body. Thus, the kidneys are also said to store the primordial *yin* and *yang*. Out of their combinations and changes, energy is created. This is the primal *chi* of the body, the "*chi* of the abyss," which is also said to be stored in the kidneys.

The entire urinary-sexual tract is seen as an articulation of the kidneys. The sexual tract covets, uses, and develops the sexual-genetic material, while the urinary tract expels that which is inessential, which is innately not part of the body.

The job of the kidneys, as a part of the urinary tract, is to adjust the balance of waters and solids. It does this by excreting the appropriate amount of fluids and minerals to keep the body in balance. The kidneys are thus the great balancing organ in the body.

Gravel Root acts on the primal level of kidney functioning, where the solids and fluids are kept in balance. It acts strongly throughout the entire urinary-sexual tract which develops out of the primal kidney energy. The folk doctors held that Gravel Root dissolved calculi, while the professional doctors claimed merely that it helped remove it. It promotes and strengthens kidney excretive power in small doses, but exhausts the kidneys in large ones. It also acts on the bladder, uterus, and prostate. Finally, it is held to strengthen and remineralize the bones, the "extrusion of the kidneys."

According to ancient and traditional Western medicine, the psychological function analogous to the kidneys is the ability to choose between truth and falsehood. These organs have long been associated with the scales of balance. In astrological medicine the kidneys are said to be ruled by Libra, the scales. Swedenborg, the great Swedish seer, describes how the prime function of the kidneys is to sort out the true from the false. He associated this organ system with judges, who are capable of listening carefully to the voice to determine innocence from guilt. This inference goes back to the Hebrew Bible, where the kidneys are associated with determining what is true or false. As it says in Psalms, "The Lord searches my reins," the kidneys, to determine what is true. As we have seen, the motto of the turtle is, "everything you always knew to be true, is true."

Gravel Root helps the faculty of imagination become subtle, so that we may pass to-and-fro, from this world to the next. It also helps the faculty of discernment, so that we may judge the truth in our seeing. It helps to establish or maintain the base or *prima materia,* the ground for psychological and spiritual judgment and integrity. If someone has not learned a lesson in life, they need to trace back to the beginning, run their mental fingers through their life experiences, and see where the problem lies. Gravel Root helps us get back to this base.

This influence upon the mind and psyche is demonstrated in the following case. One of my students gave Gravel Root in tincture to a friend of hers who was suffering from a bowel disease where the pores of the colon became enlarged and her entire system was poisoned. My friend thought she also suffered from a state of delusion about her life. After taking the medicine for a week the bowel condition aggravated. The woman stopped taking the Gravel Root, but got better. She then kicked out an abusive boyfriend and her thinking became more realistic. She still continued to blame the tincture for making her temporarily worse, so she still harbored that delusion!

Dr. William Cook gave specific indications for Gravel Root in the kidney sphere. "It promotes the flow of water, soothes irritation, and is especially beneficial in cases of reddish and reddish-brown urine, and where there is a deposit of reddish sand." He says it is specific for lithic acid gravel. "In oxalic and phosphatic gravel, it is of trifling service; and the same may be said of glutinous mucus deposits in the urine. In all febrile cases, when the urine is scanty and red, and the back painful, it is an excellent agent." He adds, "It has been used in dropsical affections, and is good so far as the kidneys are concerned; but in such cases it always needs to be combined with tonics and stimulants. By its relaxing property, it relieves irritability, and is not suited to conditions of extreme languor and depression; yet it leaves behind a very gentle tonic impression, and acts well when combined with such diffusives as zingiber and polemonium."

Scudder gives a survey of cases he treated with this medicine.

In one case of marked albuminuria, when other agents had failed to produce any relief, the continued use of this remedy for two weeks entirely relieved the patient. In two cases of diabetes insipidus, its use was attended with the same results. We have also employed it in incontinence of urine, especially in children, with good effects. It is of the most importance, however, in allaying irritation of the bladder. In many cases of this kind caused by displacement or chronic inflammation of the uterus, or arising during or after pregnancy, we have obtained more benefit from its use than from any other agent.

Hale comments, "It is in this class of diseases just named, that I know it to be most useful." He continues,

My experience with this variety of Eupatorium has been quite extensive, and my observations of its use are equally so," he writes. "I have cured with this remedy a severe case of strangury, in a female, due to uterine displacement; the usual remedies had been used without benefit. In a case of excessive irritation of the bladder, with large deposit of lithates in the urine, it removed all the symptoms in a week. Several minor cases might be mentioned. Next to Apocynum cann., I consider it the most powerful remedy we possess, for the alleviation, and even permanent cure of dropsy. It is even superior to that medicine, for its action on the kidneys is of a more pervading and profound character.

Hale then gives several case histories as illustrations. "One of the most intractable cases of dropsy, due apparently to renal disease, that ever came under my care, I believe to have been permanently cured by a tincture of the root." He then quotes a case from the practice of Dr. P. H. Hale. The whole body was swollen, extremities cold, the urine scanty and slightly albuminous, shortness of breath from water on the lungs, pulse feeble, with slight tendency to mental dullness. "Altogether the man was in a very critical condition." *Eupatorium purpureum,* eight to ten drops of the tincture, every three hours, cured in three days

Here is a case collected by Hale, showing a more decided action upon the bladder. Dr. B. L. Dresser, the homeopath whose wife proved the medicine, was consulted by a young man who had been mustered out of the Union Army during the Civil War. Almost immediately after joining his regiment he took a violent cold and began to experience an uneasiness in the region of the bladder which eventually became a serious cystitis. More than a year later he consulted Dresser, who recorded the following symptoms. "Smarting, burning in the bladder; soreness and pain in the bladder; severe, deep, dull aching in the bladder; smarting, burning in the urethra; most excruciating smarting upon passing urine; numbness of the legs; deep, dull, aching pain in the region of the kidneys; very much emaciated; hectic fever; night sweats; rheumatic pains shifting from place to place." *Eupatorium purpureum* diluted to about one part in a hundred (2x) cured in a few weeks.

The European species, Water Agrimony or *Eupatorium cannabinum,* has long been used as a "blood cleanser and purifier." The same idea became attached to the American species. "No remedy is better adapted to the relief of painful suppression of urine, either from inflammation or calcareous accumulations," wrote Dr. Hollembaek, a German-American eclectic quoted by Hale. It is suited to "cases when the kidneys fail to secrete a due amount of urine, allowing the uric acid and other component parts to be retained in the circulation." This may result in "erysipelas and other diseases of the skin … dropsy, rheumatism, gout and fever." Arthritic and gouty deposits were often seen as evidence of poor kidney function in European medicine and herbal tradition.

The Sexual System

Gravel Root also acts upon the sexual organs. "This remedy influences the reproductive organs of both male and female, more especially the latter," wrote Dr. Frederick Locke. "It is tonic to the uterus in atony or chronic irritability of this organ. It is of service given in four- or five-drop doses three times a day to prevent abortion due to debility in chronic metritis, prolapsus, retroversion and all troubles of the uterus of this nature." Cook adds, "It often answers a good purpose in [uterine] prolapsus, leucorrhea, and other female weaknesses, especially when the back is weak and painful."

A lengthy account of the action of *Eupatorium purpureum* upon the uterus was given by an eclectic, Dr. Paine, and quoted by Hale. Paine used the dried alcoholic extract, called "Eupurpurin." "There is, perhaps, no remedy of the materia medica that exerts a more powerful tonic impression upon the uterus," he asserts. "It has the effect to stimulate uterine contractions; and, in case of pregnancy, it has been known to produce abortion by producing premature labor. Hence it has great value in case of uterine inertia during labor, or where there is much debility and feeble uterine contractions." He recommended it in place of Ergot, the usual stimulant. "I have administered this in a large number of cases of complete uterine inertia, in combination with *Capsicum* and other stimulants, and have found most happy and immediate effects. In cases of debility of the uterus, it is a remedy of remarkable value. In the large number of cases of uterine leucorrhea, caused by exhaustion of the uterus and chronic metritis, the Eupurpurin... affords almost immediate relief. In cases of prolapsus uteri, and in retroversion of the uterus, and, in fact, all cases where there is debility of the uterus and its appendages, it can be relied on as a tonic and stimulant."

Dr. Paine then gives a case which shows that he used it as a uterine tonic, even during pregnancy, to improve uterine tone and insure a safe delivery. This shows a sort of "homeopathic" usage, since *Eupatorium purpureum* causes abortion. A woman who had suffered four or five miscarriages, and had never succeeded in bringing a pregnancy to full term. "She was in the third month of pregnancy, and within two or three weeks of her usual period to abort, when she came under my charge." He gave one grain of the "Eupurpurin," in combination with an iron tonic, three times a day. "This treatment I continued, with the addition of occasional light purges, for two or three months, when Iron was omitted." The "Eupurpurin" was continued with some kind of sitz bath and at nine months she delivered "a fine, healthy daughter."

Dr. Paine gives another case where the object was to insure conception. A woman who had been married fourteen years had never, to her knowledge, become pregnant. She suffered from amenorrhea, leucorrhea and dysmenorrhea. Dr. Paine used Eupurpurin and a host of other stimulants to the liver and mucosa (Leptandra, Euonymus, Cinchona, Hydrastis and Helonias). Her periods became healthy and regular, she got pregnant after seven months and delivered a healthy baby at full term. (Perhaps, indeed, *Eupatorium purpureum* helps precipitate the first matter out of the undifferentiated primal waters).

The action of Gravel Root upon the male sexual system is less well documented. The remedy has also been used for swollen, atonic prostate, impotence and night urination. Herbalist Tommie Bass uses the analogous southern plant, Queen of the Meadow (Eupatorium serotinum), as a regular remedy for prostate problems and diabetes. Although Gravel Root does not cure diabetes, it strengthens the kidneys which are weakened by the passage of sugar through them.

A diabetic man was suffering from kidney failure. He urinated every hour and a half at night and had considerable edema. He was scheduled to have a kidney and pancreas transplant. In the meantime I sent him Gravel Root. He took a few drops, several times a day. This cut the excess urination down to normal (once a night) and removed the edema. Eventually he had his kidney and pancreas transplant.

Deterioration, Death, and Ressurection

When we consider the importance of waste removal, we can see why Gravel Root should be associated with putrid phenomena and have a purple color. It is most beneficial in septic, putrid, eroding conditions where the tissue is not being incarnated, as in putrid ulcers. When properly indicated, it will stop the deteriorative process, cleanse the putridity, and lay down new tissue. It acts particularly on the large intestine, the focus for putrid waste removal, which is also a site where solids and fluids are balanced to promote proper disposal of waste.

I have several cases where Gravel Root helped deep, serious problems in the intestinal region. While working at Present Moment Herbs I helped a fellow employee, who was suffering from pain in the side associated with what the doctors had supposed was a tumor or cyst above the right ovary. The woman's family had a very bad history of ovarian cancer—four out of five sisters in her mother's generation died from the disease, the remaining one from an accident in her youth. The doctors scheduled her for a complete hysterectomy, no matter what the swelling was. While working together on a Sunday afternoon, my friend complained of a severe pain in the area—sharp enough to make her bend over and consider going home. I studied the symptoms carefully and came up with *Eupatorium purpureum* through a study of the homeopathic repertory. A dose of the 6x potency relieved the pain and continued to do so after she went home.

My friend went in for surgery as scheduled on Tuesday morning. The doctors then found that the "tumor" was actually a bag of pus fed by a fistula from the intestines: she had Crohn's disease and the abscess had ruptured. They completed the hysterectomy as planned, removed a foot of the small intestine and the fistula. They were surprised, they commented to her, that the peritoneal cavity was completely free of infection, since the abscess had already broken open. My friend and I felt pretty certain it was the Gravel Root that kept things clean. However, for years, I didn't know what to make of this odd case.

Finally, my friend Susan, "the near death expert," had a reoccurrence of her old Crohn's disease. I felt relatively helpless to do anything for the first six months of her deterioration. These things are expected of Crohn's cases, her doctor said. She was due for a relapse because it was nine years since her last surgery, "and all Crohn's patients relapse within ten years." All the old remedies we used the first time around worked temporarily or not at all. The doctor said a foot of intestine was narrowed and scarred. Any day he expected the formation of an abscess that would burst and surgery would be required to save her life. She had a "window of opportunity" for three weeks, he estimated. If she took prednisone and it could control the inflammation, she might not have to have a complete colostomy.

Susan tried the prednisone for a few days, then refused to take it. "It eats up my soul," she said. She'd rather die than surrender her spirit. Besides, she couldn't stand to go through any more major surgery and pain. Having been shot in the liver by an exploding bullet, stabbed, kidnapped, beaten, lost a third of her intestine in surgery, etc., in her forty-two years, she just couldn't do it. "That doctor just doesn't understand," she confided. He yelled at her. She went home to face the disease on her own, stopped all her herbal remedies and medical drugs (except potassium for the fluid loss from diarrhea) and thought about her life. If God wanted her to live, then he was going to have to save her, because she couldn't stand it anymore. In the depths of this state of mind, the telephone rang. The old case with Gravel Root and Crohn's had suddenly come into my mind. "Wait, wait, Susan," I said. "You've got to try this one last herb."

Gravel Root proved to be the right medicine. The next day we went out and collected some in a peat bog across the field from Sunnyfield Herb Farm. Susan enjoyed the walk in the fields. She took the root home and made a tea from it. The fever, hot flashes, and pain peaked the day after she started and then receded. She noticed that she craved the medicine and continued to take it. Month by month, she got better. It took about a year for her to completely recover from this extremis of life and death. She has been doing fine ever since.

Preparation, Toxicity, and Dosage

Eupatorium purpureum is supposed to have a cousin, *E. maculatum,* which is almost identical in range, appearance, and medicinal usage. The stem is more spotted and it is supposed to have a vanilla-like smell. There is some controversy over whether or not it should actually be regarded as a separate species in the first place. "Perhaps to be regarded as a race of *E. purpureum*" is the statement made by Brown and Britten (1913). My friend 7Song goes much further than this. "I have looked for the *purpureum* all over the country, looked up the specimens in herbariums and gone to the original sites where they were collected, only to find the *maculatum*." His conclusion? "*Eupatorium purpureum* is a botanical Holy Grail."

Eupatorium serotinum is a species found further to the south. It is used in some areas as a substitute for *E. purpureum.* Herbalist Tommie Bass calls it "Queen of the Meadow," in distinction to Gravel Root. He says it has similar properties, but is milder and prefers it over the other. "You use the roots to make a tea," he relates. "Take one to three cups a day for diabetes and prostate gland trouble. If it don't turn your stomach, it is simple and safe. It don't cure you but it gives you ease of diabetes." He gives some cases of apparent cure, however. His formula for diabetes mellitus is Queen of the Meadow root, Blueberry leaves, Red Root, and Goldenrod. "It's also good for rheumatism or gravel," Bright's disease, and swollen prostate.

Gravel Root is collected in August, when the plant is in flower and is easy to spot. Cook says, "any treatment by continued heat seems greatly to dissipate the good qualities of the agent, whence an infusion made at a low temperature gives the best results." He gave half a dram of the powdered root by warm infusion, three times a day. However, most doctors seemed to be satisfied with the preparations extracted and preserved in alcohol. Hale used "the mother tincture, or lower dilutions, a few drops at a dose every two or six hours."

Eupatorium purpureum contains pyrrolizidine alkaloids which possibly make it unsafe for chronic usage. Large doses can produce weakness of the sexual and urinary system, as mentioned by Hale. Paine considered it an abortifacient. It can be safely used for extended periods in small doses. The homeopathic potencies are also available.

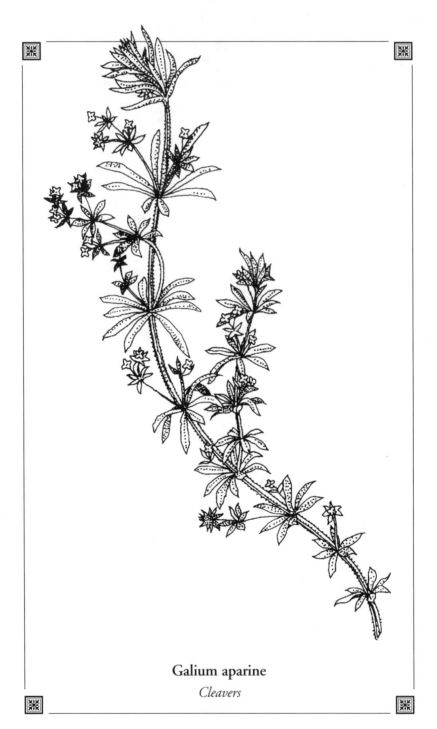

Galium aparine

Cleavers

Galium aparine

Cleavers

This dainty plant is native to Europe, but widely naturalized in temperate regions of the world. It grows in light woodlands and open fields, sometimes forming small luxurious beds. One of the common names for it is Bedstraw. The stems are lined with raspy little teeth which easily catch on the clothes. This, with the ease by which the stems detach themselves from the ground, cause them to easily cleave to the passerby. Cleavers is a member of the Rubiaceae or Madder family.

At an extremely early date, Cleavers proved itself of economic utility. A matted handful of the cleaving stems can be used as a simple sieve to strain hairs and dirt from milk. Dioscorides mentions this practice, as does Linnaeus. From early times it was also customary to prepare a bed for childbirth with Bedstraw. The idea got around that this is what Mary used when Jesus was born, so it was called Our Lady's Bedstraw.

The use of Cleavers to make a birthing bed was almost certainly picked up from the practice of our friends the Deer Nation. Many of us in the country have come across patches of Bedstraw with clear evidence that deer had made their bed there in the night. Two of my friends actually found newborn fawns lying in the groves of Bedstraw. The mothers evidently ran away at their approach.

Cleavers was used from an early date in medicine. Dioscorides gives a short account of it, but one which already points to the important affinities. He says it is a remedy for swellings and ear pain. (It is one of the most important remedies for swollen glands, especially around the

283

ears and down the neck.) He also says it is a good remedy for venomous bites. (This seems to have been a stock phrase in classical medicine.)

Knowledge of the plant continued to accrue through the centuries and it came to be widely used for glandular and renal difficulties. Culpeper says Cleavers is under the rulership of Venus, and so strengthens the parts she rules: the neck and reins (renal function). With the rejection of simple, nontoxic agents in the eighteenth century, Cleavers fell out of fashion but it continued to be used by folk healers, the Thomsonians, and the eclectics. Today it is still a favorite among herbalists throughout the world.

Dr. Frederick Locke (1895) gave a concise description of *Galium aparine* from the eclectic standpoint. "Galium is an excellent drug in active irritation or inflammation of any part of the urinary tract. It is a very good diuretic in fevers, lowering the temperature and helping the functions of the kidneys. The infusion stops the scalding of urine in gonorrhea when given in teaspoonful doses." So much for the acute conditions; Locke also gives chronic indications. "As an alterative it is used in scrofula and syphilis, and all cases in which we find bad blood."

Galium aparine is the preferred and officinal plant in Western herbal medicine, but many other varieties have been used indiscriminately, especially *Galium verum* (Yellow Bedstraw).

Indians also used a kind of Galium for bringing out the rash of measles. This is also an old European usage. Lincecum adds that they considered Bedstraw to be almost a specific to prevent miscarriage, and that in his experience it was virtually infallible. In Europe, Cleavers was used, as we have seen, to insure a safe delivery.

Dr. Edwin Hale introduced *Galium aparine* to the homeopathic audience. He was irritated by the use of different *Galium* plants on the same indications. "Such generalizations...will not be accepted by the Homeopathic school of medicine." He also noted the lack of specific facts in the tradition. Hale was careful to observe the folk use of Cleavers and in this he renders an important account:

> *While engaged in an extensive country practice, I often observed that the cold infusion was drank freely by fever patients, especially if any scalding or burning during micturation was complained of. At first, I disliked to have them use it in connection with homeopathic remedies, but I have found its use so general, and the idea of its mild curative powers so*

engrafted into the minds of the people, that it was a difficult matter to proscribe it. I have never noticed that its use interfered in any way with the action of homeopathic medicines.

In order to test Cleavers, Hale began to prescribe it in common with placebo pellets. In this way, he was able to build up a more exact knowledge of its properties.

It seemed to me particularly useful in the dysuria and suppression of urine in young children, from colds, or when it was attended with aphthae [canker sores], or what might be called a scorbutic state of the system; also in the strangury of women from uterine disease, hemorrhoids, or irritable bladder. It seemed to be useful in the strangury and scanty urine in rheumatic fever, and in the irritable bladder (from prostatic disease,) in old men.

Galium aparine has not been subjected to further scrutiny in homeopathy.

Cooling and Filtering the Inner Waters

Cleavers is a gentle, nontoxic medicine, which nevertheless possesses great curative powers. The cool, moisture-laden stems and the cool, moist ground upon which it thrives, indicate that it is a remedy which acts upon the water economy of the body, especially the kidneys and lymphatics. The sieve-like capacity is a nice signature pointing to the filtering element exerted on the waters by these organs. The long stems indicate an affinity to long vessels and passageways, including lymphatic ducts, blood vessels, renal tubules, the ureters, and urethra. *Galium* stimulates the water-bearing system from the distant ends of the lymphatics, under the skin, all the way through to the kidneys. It connects up the lymphatic system, from beginning to end, bringing all parts into communication. It removes fever, heat, swelling, or stagnation in the lymphatics, and burning from infection, heat, and dryness in the renal tract. It also acts on gravely problems from clogged filtering in the kidneys. In short, we may say that Cleavers cools, moistens, filters, detoxifies, and promotes transportation within the hidden waterways of the body.

By taking away toxins Cleavers gently opens the passageways leading to and from the liver, pancreas, and other internal organs, so that it has a general cleansing and decongesting capacity. Symptoms may include stitches in the side, indicating congestion of internal organs. It contributes to the general nutrition of the body by cleansing out the fluids surrounding the cells, making nutrition and waste removal easier. Thus, it has been used in anemia. By cleansing through the lymphatics under the skin and stimulating the kidneys to remove waste products, it has a notable action in chronic and acute skin disease. It is used internally and externally for scabs, eczema, psoriasis, wounds, burns, scalds, measles, and eruptions of various sorts. It is the "preferred diuretic for exanthemas," according to herbalists Priest and Priest (1982).

The Australian herbalist, Dorothy Hall, points out the connection between skin diseases and venereal infections. The theory, which ultimately comes down to us from homeopathy, says that venereal diseases in the parents will sometimes manifest as "taints" in the children. One of the most common expressions of this "taint" is skin disease. I have found similar indications of genetic "taints" in my own practice. I find Cleavers very useful for young children with swollen glands about the ears, from birth or early in life.

Hall says Galium is most specific for chronic, recurrent bouts of urethritis, especially when connected with grit, gravel, or calcium deposits, or a gonorrheal background. She also notes the traditional use of the plant for irritated and swollen prostate.

Hale gave several case histories for *Galium aparine* which illustrate its value in dysuria, or painful urination and infection.

> *A young child has been troubled with painful dysuria for several days. Every attempt at urination was accompanied with cries and screams. A weak infusion of Galium 3rd [one part in a thousand] was given, and in less than an hour the child urinated profusely and without pain.*

This was reported to him by Dr. Kendall, a homeopath, as was the following.

> *An old man had been troubled for months with intensely painful dysuria, frequent ineffectual urging, scanty discharge, etc. He was directed to drink a pint a day, of a cold infusion. In a few days he reported himself cured.*

Cleavers was also used by the Thomsonian or physio-medical doctors. William Cook (1869) comments, "It secures a goodly increase of the watery portion of the urine, thus rendering this secretion less irritating than it sometimes gets to be." Therefore, it "is among the truly valuable agents in all forms of scalding urine, as in oxalic acid gravel, irritation at the neck of the bladder, and the first stages of gonorrhea." Similar accolades are found in Beach, King, Scudder and a host of outstanding nineteenth century eclectic physicians.

When there is exhaustion of the kidneys there will often be tired feet (also see *Solidago.*) This symptom also is associated with Cleavers. Culpeper says a tea, oil, or ointment of Bedstraw "is good to bathe the feet of travelers and lacqueys [messengers], whose long running causeth weariness and stiffness in their sinews and joints." It is generally "very good for the sinews, arteries, and joints, to comfort and strengthen them after travel, cold and pains."

Galium also has a local affinity for the tongue, throat, and neck. It has been traditionally used for cancer of the tongue, goiter, and thyroid problems. It is routinely used by modern herbalists for swollen glands and sore throat in children. It helps clear away the debris in the lymphatics after a course of antibiotics. Cleavers is one of the few remedies indicated for infants and children with chronic swollen glands about the back of the head, around by the ears and under the chin. I have found in a number of cases that Cleavers is particularly effective for women suffering from cystic breasts, when there are numerous cysts (also see Easter Lily and Red Clover, which have few cysts).

Our lowly little Cleavers has long been used to cure cancer. Dr. F. A. Bailey, writing in the *British Journal of Homoeopathy* (1865) and quoted by Hale, gives a rather dramatic case history of apparent cancer quickly reversed with *Galium aparine.* The patient was a sixty-year-old woman who was admitted to the hospital, "on account of a hard, firm, somewhat circumscribed tumor of about the size of a boy's marble flattened, embedded in the substance of the tongue." It had gradually increased in size over the past five weeks, from the size of a hemp seed. "The upper surface was nodulated and uneven, and the swelling generally had the appearance and feel of a scirrhous formation." It was painful enough to keep her from eating and sleeping, and "exquisitely tender to the touch when handled." She had suffered from a general debility for some time, aggravated by lack of nutrition. Dr. Bailey recommended strong beef tea (for nutrition), a dark porter beer (those were the days!), and a strong dose of *Galium aparine* in extract, twice a day. She was also told to use the extract on the lump and hold it there for a while each day. In six weeks the tumor was gone, along with the pain, her complexion changed from sallow and pale to florid and healthy, and she had her original energy back.

Dr. Bailey readily admits this tumor could not be considered a cancer for certain (they had no biopsies then) but he felt confident from an extensive practice that this gentle herb did in fact cure cancer or delay it for long periods of time. He wrote:

> *I have for many years past been in the habit of employing this remedy in the treatment of cancerous affections of different kinds in my hospital practice, and have not failed to observe that in some cases it has seemed to favor the production of healthy granulations on the ulcerated surface, whilst in other complete cicatrisation has ensued.*

Locke also credits *Galium* with cancer-fighting properties. "It is a good alterative in cancerous diseases, some even claiming that it removes the constitutional tendency to the disease." A contemporary author reporting successful treatment of cancer with Cleavers is Maria Treben. She gives several case histories.

A Deer Medicine for the Nerves

The finely edged stems remind us of the nerves. Cleavers has a considerable action on the nervous system. It has been used for epilepsy, hysteria, spasms, and nervous complaints. I have used it for head, spinal, and nerve injuries. The mental state is one associated with an irritated nervous system.

One time I gave a few drops of Cleavers to a friend who was suffering from nerve pains and (according to medical tests) odd brain wave patterns associated with an old head injury; a television mounted on the wall of a bar had fallen on the back of her head. Within a few seconds after receiving the dose, she commented that she didn't like the remedy: it made her feel annoyed. Meanwhile, she was suddenly rolling her neck to break up stiffness. Sometimes it helps to know a person well—this was an old girlfriend. I was immediately reminded of little snitty moods she used to get into, so I knew the remedy was only bringing up a state she sometimes felt. This remedy helped her a great deal with the moods and nerve phenomenon. The specific physical symptom it removed was some edema around the eyelids. The specific thing I learned was that Cleavers helps people who are irritated by little things, rather than—or in addition—to big things. That is what we would expect for a remedy that helps to filter out little materials.

Shortly afterwards another woman came to see me. She had inflamed eyelids which had defied treatment for many years, though I often helped her with various other problems. She had a delicate nervous system and seemed to need a different nervine every year or so, depending on what problem was wearing her out. Now she was not suffering from exhaustion, but from a bored, fussy, displeased state of mind. She said she liked to roll her neck to get rid of the stiffness. She took Cleavers and the Bach flower essence Impatiens. Her mood improved quickly while the eyelids and the stiff neck improved over a longer period.

I remember another case where a woman in her late twenties was suffering from chronic acne. My usual remedies for this condition (*Lactuca, Arctium*) did not work, but when I gave her a few drops of Cleavers her eyes started to shine, so we tried this. Two months later she came back to show her fine complexion—and her eyes were shining!

All three of these women were fine-boned, delicate, and rather elegant if I may say so. I have used Cleavers for a variety of people of other makes and builds, but I do believe there is a Cleavers constitutional type.

Bedstraw is a Deer Medicine. These fine-boned, elegantly articulated, but somewhat nervous animals are associated with nerve medicines. The sharp edge of the stem seen in Cleavers (as well as various mints and other plants) is a signature pointing to the nerves, but it also reminds us of the fine, sharp-edged boney structure of the deer.

Preparation and Dosage

Cleavers loses its properties on drying and heating, so it can only be used by fresh infusion or preserved in alcohol or some other medium. I make a simple tincture by macerating the fresh herb in brandy. Because it is a strong diuretic, Galium is contraindicated in diabetics. Maria Treben makes a salve by stirring a sufficient amount of fresh juice of Cleavers into butter which she stored in a refrigerator.

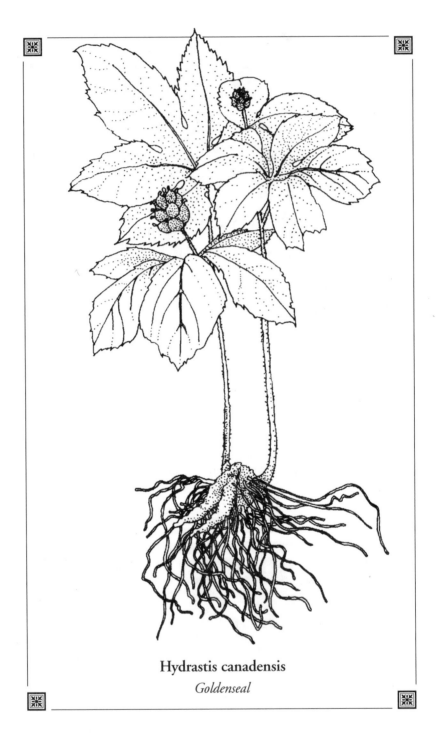

Hydrastis canadensis

Goldenseal

Hydrastis canadensis
Goldenseal

oldenseal is an old American Indian medicine plant. It was not well known to the white settlers until they crossed the Appalachians. Linnaeus was confused about its nomenclature and it was little known to the scientific world. Before 1800 its cousin Goldthread (*Coptis trifolia*) was widely used as a popular remedy, though mostly just for sores in the mouth and "webs in the eyes." As the Midwest opened up to settlement, Goldenseal quickly came to replace Goldthread. It also came to be seen as a more general tonic than Goldthread. In addition to curing sores, it was seen as a general tonic to the mucous membranes and digestive tract. Rafinesque first publicized it in 1828. From this time on Goldenseal was widely used by lay and professional practitioners. By 1910 *Hydrastis* was the most common item in American herbal commerce, and was being picked to extinction.

There is a major difference between the way Goldenseal was used in the nineteenth century and the way it is used today. The old lay and professional practitioners understood Goldenseal as a bitter tonic that would, in small doses, stimulate the mucous membranes of the digestive tract to greater activity, promoting tissue feeding and rebuilding while strengthening the heart and nervous system. It was therefore used principally as a digestive and nutritive tonic. This usage has been largely forgotten by herbalists today, although it is still used as a tonic by old folks in the south. It is commonly called "Yaller Root" down that way.

The discovery that berberine, the "active ingredient" in *Hydrastis,* is a "natural antibiotic," has led to its use in large doses to fight infection.

Today Goldenseal is one of the most popular (and overused) herbs in the marketplace.

As a native of heavily shaded woodlands in the Midwestern United States, Goldenseal has become increasingly rare in the wild. Overpicking and destruction of habitat endanger the wild population. There is some cultivation, but Goldenseal is already becoming rare in the wild. In an area which John Uri Lloyd mapped out as the center of the range of the plant at the turn of the century, I know a picker who says it is impossible to find Goldenseal in the wild unless one is a day's journey off the road.

Tonic for the Mucosa and Digestion

The nineteenth-century American doctors came to the conclusion that Goldenseal acted primarily upon the mucosa and the digestive tract, secondarily on the nervous system. Through these structures, through tissue feeding and nutrition as well as ennervation, it acted on the muscular element, the heart, and the general strength of the entire patient.

Here is a good summary of the old concepts from Dr. John William Fyfe (1909), an eclectic:

Hydrastis is an energetic tonic to the circulatory and mucous structures. It is especially valuable in diseases associated with irritation or debility of the gastric mucous surfaces. In acute indigestion due to sudden change of diet it constitutes a useful medicament, and in chronic inflammation of the glands, as well as of the mucous structures, it is employed with gratifying results. In hepatic torpor with constipation and chronic gastritis, small doses of Hydrastis exert a curative influence, and in hemorrhage from the uterus due to debility it is often useful. In fact, in all diseases characterized by sub-acute or chronic catarrhal conditions of the mucous membranes, whether of the stomach, intestines, bladder, vagina, urethra, uterus, bronchi or conjunctiva, the well-directed use of Hydrastis, both internally and locally, will always give good results. In convalescing it improves the appetite and nutrition, and acts as a good tonic when given in doses of from five to twenty drops, in water or milk, three times a day. When there is acute inflammation, with arrest of secretion, it is contraindicated.

Fyfe quotes an earlier eclectic, a Dr. French. He pin-points the mucosa as the central point upon which Goldenseal acts:

> *Hydrastis is primarily a remedy for relaxed and diseased conditions of mucous membranes. Its action is that of a tonic, promoting appetite and digestion, increasing the flow of bile and the normal secretions of the gastro-intestinal tract, while at the same time it lessens over-secretion, corrects unhealthy discharges, and restores the normal tone and function to the relaxed and diseased tissues.*

The eclectic authors often seem to have relied upon the appearance of the tongue in order to guide them to the right selection of the remedy. We have descriptions of the tongue calling for Goldenseal from a number of sources. Ellingwood gives a good description. In my own words, I would say that the atonic, somewhat pallid, slightly dry, enlarged, scalloped at the edges, with a slight yellow haze for a coating. In more advanced cases ulcerations appear, usually at the edges.

Hydrastis was proven by Dr. Edwin Hale, who brought so many native American plants into homeopathic use. Unfortunately, Hale emphasized the production of thick yellow mucus in the provings. This does not represent the true genius of the remedy. The herbal experience with Goldenseal teaches us that it is first a remedy for atonicity of the mucous membranes, resulting in poor nutrition and tissue-building. This process leads into ulceration of mucous membranes, then to the production of mucus, as the body tries to cover and protect the deteriorating membranes, and finally to the appearance of thick yellow mucus as bacteria settle into infected areas. The earlier stages in this chain of development are more important and commonplace than the latter. They have unfortunately been overlooked in homeopathy.

Homeopathic sources are generally not too illuminating about this remedy. However, a few of the authors give excellent accounts. One of these would be Dr. George Royal. He lists *Hydrastis* under a condition called "dilatation of the stomach" in his *Textbook of Homoeopathic Theory and Practice of Medicine* (1928). This refers to dilatation, thickening, ulceration and prolapse of the walls of the stomach. The constitution calling for *Hydrastis* is dyspeptic, debilitated and catarrhal. The characteristic symptoms are the following:

Frequent eructations of a sour fluid and occasional vomiting of all food. The tongue is thick, moist, coated, and shows imprint of teeth. The stools are lumpy and covered with mucus. Both fissures and hemorrhoids are found about the anus. The blood count is low. Anemia is marked. The skin is sallow. The subjective symptoms are a faint, all-gone feeling in the stomach, with constant, violent palpitation of the heart on exertion and after vomiting. In the abdomen we have heavy, sharp, cutting, dragging pains. There is a dull frontal headache, especially about the nasal sinuses. Use the 3rd [decimal dilution] and tincture.

Another of his homeopathic contemporaries, Dr. R. F. Rabe, gives a summary of the leading symptoms in *Medical Therapeutics* (1920):

Hydrastis affects the mucous membranes generally. Its first effect is to produce stimulation of the gastric functions, to which is added a general increased reflex excitability. This is followed by atonic, relaxed conditions of mucous surfaces, resulting in debility, general catarrhal discharges and a tendency to ulceration … In consequence, we have a remedy most valuable in catarrhal inflammations of the nasopharyngeal and gastrointestinal tracts. One strong, characteristic and guiding symptom is found in the tenacious, tough, yellowish nature of the discharges which are, in addition, sometimes bloody and usually thick.

Another point which makes the use of *Hydrastis* somewhat difficult for homeopaths is that it seems to work best in small material doses. Royal used the tincture and 3x potency. I have repeatedly seen that patients respond best to small amounts, usually about a drop a day is sufficient. Some people need slightly more, three to five drops, and some people less.

Because of its affinity for the mucous membranes and the solar plexus, Goldenseal is an important remedy in respiratory complaints. It deepens respiratory strength, improves tone and motility of the mucosa and removes infection and excessive build up of mucous. Once I used it to cure an infection of the ear which was causing a continuous discharge of clear yellow fluid from the ear (it looked just like Goldenseal tincture.) The man dabbed cotton to his ear continually, to soak up the discharge.

Hydrastis strengthens the solar plexus, toning up enervation of the stomach, gallbladder and intestines, stimulates the mucous membranes, promotes secretion, strengthens muscles and improves peristaltic action.

The atonic condition of the digestive tract is reflected in the appearance of the tongue.

The sensation of "all-goneness" in the stomach is a highly characteristic symptom produced in the homeopathic provings. It is felt by anyone who takes a strong sniff of Goldenseal powder. This symptom occassionally appears in the Hydrastis patient. It has been my experience that it corresponds with patients who have suffered an emotional loss. They feel like they have a "hemorrhage of emotional energy" from the solar plexus.

Weakness of nerve force in the gallbladder and gall ducts, or a mild prolapse due to poor nutrition and assimilation, probably account for the sallow complexion sometimes seen in the Goldenseal patient. *Hydrastis* is required in some cases of gallstone, inflammation of the gallbladder, and gallstone colic. It proves curative in these conditions by strengthening and toning, so that pathogenic waste and concretions are eliminated.

The intestines tend to become atonic in the person requiring Goldenseal, sometimes leading to constipation. This is one of the most important remedies for this condition when it is chronic, according to homeopathic authors such as Burt and Boericke. However, it will also be indicated for a few cases of diarrhea as well.

Here is a typical case illustrating the digestive problems associated with *Hydrastis*. A thirty-four year-old woman suffered from "candida" for many years. Her principal symptom was constipation. This diagnosis, vague as it is, was made both by alternative and conventional physicians, and satisfied the patient. She was able to control the symptoms through a special diet. Although she looked relaxed, she said she was tense. She did not look tired. The tongue body was broad, pallid, flabby, dry, scalloped on the edges, with a small ulcer at each side. The coating was slight, yellow and dry. The pulse was deficient in force and substance, but slightly tense. *Hydrastis* in tincture, one drop per dose, one to two drops a day, as needed, revitalized her entire system and removed the constipation. The patient reacted so strongly to her first dose that she asked whether it was an aphrodisiac. She responded promptly and the symptoms were largely removed, though she still had to watch her diet somewhat. Three years later she was still in good shape.

Because of its strong influence upon mucous membranes and nerve force, *Hydrastis* is indicated for atonic conditions of the female tract where there is a build up of thick, yellow mucus and ulceration of the cervix. Here it is traditionally given as a douche. It is also used to help strengthen labor at the end of pregnancy, but it is contraindicated (at least in substantial doses) during the earlier weeks, because of the jolting, possibly abortifacient properties.

Tonic for the Heart

Goldenseal is sometimes required for deficient action of the heart. Due to poor digestion and nutrition, the muscles and nerves become atonic. The heart may, under these circumstances, lack tone and strength. When *Hydrastis* is called for in cardiac conditions, the pulse will be weak and slightly tense, as mentioned above, but it will also be more irregular. Dr. Christopher used Cayenne Pepper and Goldenseal as one of his heart tonics. Ellingwood gives a detailed description of the effect of *Hydrastis* on the cardiovascular system:

> *It stimulates the respiration and circulation, imparting tone and increased power to the heart's action, increasing arterial tension and capillary blood pressure. The tone imparted to the muscular structure of the heart differs from that imparted by strychnine in being permanent and not spasmodic or intermittent in character. It influences muscular structure everywhere in the system in the same manner. It stimulates normal fibrillar contractility and increased tonus, encouraging the nutrition of muscular structure. It inhibits the development of superfluous muscular tissue and abnormal growth within that structure. It is thus most valuable in altered conditions of the heart muscle.*

Goldenseal is a topical remedy for herpes and various "damp heat" conditions where there is a red rash in moist places. It seldom cures herpes, but as an external salve in conjunction with a more specific remedy, like Ranunculus bulbosus or Prunus serotina it can be helpful.

An Important Remedy for Ulceration

Goldenseal is often beneficial for external ulcerations. It will often help diabetic ulceration because it improves nerve impulse, peripheral circulation and the health of the skin. The powder should be put on and in the ulcers.

Kathi Koville, author of several books on herbalism, related a story to me one time about a cure of diabetic ulceration which was undertaken by what sounds like Goldenseal, though the exact information was lost long ago. At any rate, it is a story that all herbalists should hear.

"About twenty years ago I was living on a hippie commune in the Sierra Nevadas," she explained. "We made some herbal remedies and put information on the labels." Every state and federal agency with any interest in regulations came down on them and they were faced with a trial for practicing medicine without a license. There was only one judge in the county, a seventy-six year-old man. When the state presented the case, he seem to be shocked by the fact that Yarrow and Plantain were in the remedies. "Why those grow in my back yard," he exclaimed. The defendants were surprised and relieved to find that he even knew what herbs were. He took them aside and said, "we don't want this to get down to the flatlands do we," referring to the state capital in Sacramento. "You just plead guilty and I'll take care of you." They followed his advice and were let off with a suspended sentence.

Later the judge explained his sympathy to the herbalists. "When I was six I used to ride the stage coach with my grandfather, who ran the stage coach line in this country. He had diabetes, his leg was ulcerous and scheduled for removal in two weeks. A man riding the stage asked, 'How'd ya' like to keep your leg?'" The old man replied why yes, he would. (I have known diabetics who preferred to lose a leg than try an innocuous herb.) The mysterious passenger opened up a traveling bag with numerous pouches. From one he extracted a golden powder. "Put this on the leg and drink it in a tea and it'll be all right." He kept that leg for twenty years, until he died. The little boy grew up to become a judge. He waited and waited for the opportunity to help an herbalist and return the favor, but none ever came along until he was very old and nearly ready for retirement.

The perfect commentary on this story was provided later that day at Brietenbush, by a woman who was a massage therapist, though she hadn't heard the story. "I like to give away a few massages, some for exchanges, some for free. If you do someone a favor you'll get something in return. The longer it takes, the better the gift."

The Remedy to Seal

Goldenseal is a specific remedy for gushing hemorrhages which are clean. It stops the bleeding and helps bring the edges of the cut together. Here the powder may be sprinkled directly on the cut. It possesses anti-bacterial properties. Any wound needing stitches, or having been stitched, suggests Goldenseal or Goldthread. It is absolutely contraindicated in dirty wounds, because it will seal in pus, dirt, and infection, causing a septicemia of the blood.

Thinking that Goldenseal will heal external hemorrhages, I started to use it to heal internal tears in tissues. In particular, I use it for torn disks in the spine, torn miniscus in the knee, torn bursa in the hip, etc. It is a superlative remedy in these problems. I simply have the person spread a few drops of the tincture on the area and it "seals up" quickly. The only thing that will hold it back is the presence of a lot of inflammation from irritation of the tissues.

I have seen this therapy perform miracles, restoring people to happiness and pain-free existence where before they were literally tormented by pain. Furthermore, it seems that the Goldenseal somehow nourishes and builds up the tissues of the disks, so that they are actually stronger. My good friend Susan was bucked off a difficult horse. She broke a few bones and dislocated her hips and suffered from excruciating pain down her left leg. I put her on Yarrow and Oak bark for the contusions and St. John's Wort for the pain. The bruises healed up quickly and the pain lessened somewhat. Then I had her take False Solomon's Seal, which corrected the dislocation. Her doctor and her chiropractor said she'd never be able to ride again due to the hip joint problems, but we straightened them out. This left the searing pain. The doctor was now able to perceive that it was a torn disk. In literally a week we completely eliminated the tear and the pain. The doctor by this time getting resigned to the remarkably quick curing going on. Then they discovered fractures up and down the spine. Well, we used Comfrey, Boneset and Solomon's Seal for that. And let's not forget Mullein at the end, to straighten the spine and get everything back in place.

And here are only a few of many more cases that bubble up in my memory. A woman down my way was writhing in agony from a torn disk in the neck. This had been going on for a year and a half. I gave her Prickly Ash for the pain. She had to take it constantly at first, but after a month she was only taking it a few times a day. About this time the inflammation in the neck began to settle down and the disk started to heal up. It took about three months and I had her on Goldenseal, Comfrey and Lady's Mantle, because the results were so slow and I wasn't sure if it was working. Eventually, however, she was completely restored to freedom from searing pain. Another time I used Goldenseal to cure a torn bursa. The woman felt "bubbles" of fluid rising up out of the tear in the hip. Goldenseal externally cured in less than a week! And once again, I helped a jogger who was unable to exercize because there was a tear in the miniscus of the knee. Total cure again in a short time.

An Energetic Understanding of Goldenseal

This is a medicine which really fits the Chinese way of looking at the organism and herbs. The intense yellow color of the root is a signature which points to the digestive and bilious functions. Yellow is said to strengthen "the center" (the digestive and assimilative processes, stomach and spleen) in Traditional Chinese Medicine. I suppose it is only a coincidence that Goldenseal flourishes in the central part of the United States—the earthy, nutritive Midwest. The rich, damp earth in which it grows is also a signature for nutritive enrichment. The single bright red berry, growing out from between the yellow-green leaves, always reminds me of the blood emerging from the nutritive process. This pictures the genius of Goldenseal.

More than anything, Goldenseal is a tonic for the center, the stomach and spleen, when there is a weakness or deficiency of chi. The spleen chi is responsible for assimilation and nutrition. It is also responsible for "holding up" the organs. The condition described by Dr. Royal, where the stomach was weak and prolapsed perfectly describes a condition where weakness of the spleen chi undermines the stomach. Goldenseal also acts on the stomach chi directly, for it has such a strong affinity to the solar plexus, the nerve and energy center for the stomach. And it is primarily through these organs that Goldenseal acts upon the rest of the organism including the mucosa and nervous system.

The flavor of Goldenseal is bitter, with a sweet aftertaste, the temperature is neutral, the impression jolting. Even a small sniff of the herb is felt as a jolt on the solar plexus. In large doses, Goldenseal weakens the solar plexus, and with it the entire digestive-assimilative complex, "the center," but in small doses it strengthens these functions. Although very bitter, there is a sweet undertone to Goldenseal. The bittersweet flavor usually works well on the digestive tract since it provokes secretion and activity.

Plants which create blood usually also control blood. Goldenseal has long been used to stop bleeding, especially from recent lacerations where the blood is flowing freely. Here the powder is sprinkled into the wound; coagulation follows and the edges of the wound seal quickly. However, Goldenseal is expressly contraindicated in infected, purulent, dirty wounds, because it will seal in infection, pus, dirt, splinters, etc. I remember one young woman in the country who was trying to treat herself with a burn. She used Goldenseal, but kept having a red inflammation set up where she applied it to the burn. I told her to stop, it was sealing up something that was trying to come out. The burn quickly healed.

Ben Charles Harris points out that the thread-like roots are a signature indicating the use of Goldenseal to stop bleeding in any wound that suggests stitches. It is especially indicated where stitches need help, as in a cut to the bottom of the foot, easily reopened by daily activity.

When we want to understand the essence of an herb we would like to understand the personality and some of the mental symptoms to which it is remedial. I am afraid that here my knowledge falls short. There has been little discovered so far about the mental symptoms calling for Goldenseal. Boericke has the most to say: "Cerebral effects pronounced: wits sharpened, head cleared, facile expression." This is, however, more of a physiological statement than a psychological one.

If I had to characterize the typical Goldenseal patient, I would say that he or she is sort of ponderous, lacking in the ability to go with the flow, and stiffly out of touch. However, all of this is rather subtle and difficult to pick up. I usually look to the tongue, rather than the mind, to led me to Goldenseal. The pale, atonic, somewhat apathetic, slightly coated, scalloped tongue reveals to me a person who has been hit by strong experiences that wear down their energy, but these may be physical rather than psychological.

There is, however, one emotional condition which I think calls for Goldenseal. Patients who have lost a strong emotional connection, suffering a shock over the loss, will sometimes feel an "emotional hemorrhage" from the stomach. This results in the "all-gone sensation" mentioned in homeopathic literature. This, however, is not a symptom that I commonly find in cases requiring Goldenseal.

Preparation, Toxicity, and Dosage

Goldenseal works best as a digestive tonic in small material doses. I prefer single drops of the mother tincture, or a few drops of the 1x dilution. The few homeopaths who used Hydrastis usually used the low potencies like Royal. The powder or the tincture are also beneficial. Remember to be careful with this remedy during pregnancy and to avoid excessive and prolonged use.

Analogs

Recently there has been talk of using substitutes for Goldenseal. It is closely allied with Goldthread (*Coptis trifolia*), a native of the northern states and the Canadian shield. In southern Appalachia, Yellow Root (*Xanthorhiza simplicissima*) is used on pretty much the same indications as a tonic. There is also a Chinese Goldthread (*Coptis chinensis.*) All of them are in the Buttercup (Ranunculaceae) family. They have fine, thread-like yellow roots which are bitter because of the presence of an alkaloid, berberine. Other plants containing berberine are Barberry Root (*Berberis vulgaris*) and Oregon Grape Root (*Berberis aquifolium.*)

Any berberine-containing plant can be used as a substitute for another, if we are looking for the crude effects of the plant as a "natural antibiotic." However, when we speak of specific indications and symptoms reflecting the essence, we cannot be so cavalier. On this level there are considerable differences between these plants. Yellow Root has long been used as a substitute for Goldenseal as a stomach tonic. Because it contains less berberine, it is not as successful as a "natural antibiotic." Barberry Root can also be used for fever, but it is associated with more dampness and has an affinity to the liver and kidneys. Its cousin Oregon Grape Root also has an affinity to the liver, but for heat or fever with dry tendencies. Goldenseal seems to have the most affinity with the mucosa, the stomach, solar plexus, and through the nerve reflexes to the gallbladder. It is less active on the kidneys than Barberry.

There are, however, some interesting analogies between Chinese

Coptis and Goldenseal. *Coptis* is also used as an infection fightening medicine. It is one of the few remedies for the condition called "heat crushing the pericardium," where fever causes unconsciousness and delirium. In the days before antibiotics, the berberine-containing herbs were one of the few medicines strong enough to combat dangerous fever and infection.

The Chinese herbalists consider *Coptis* to be contraindicated in "deficiency of the spleen *chi*," meaning the nutritive and assimilative functions going on in the center of the body. This is exactly where Goldenseal has its greatest affinities as a tonic. In fact, it would be indicated in "spleen *chi* deficiency." It is probable that *Coptis* would also have this property, if used in small doses, as the Indians and the early doctors did. It is also clear that this small contraindication would apply to Goldenseal; in large doses it would weaken "deficient spleen *chi*. " Here is another demonstration of the homeopathic law that what a medicine causes, it will cure.

Western herbalists should take a lesson from these facts. Goldenseal is useful as a "natural anti-biotic." It does fight bacterial infections with fever and inflammation. However, the use of large doses can be deleterious. I have sometimes seen patients weakened by the overuse of Hydrastis. The tongue becomes pale and atonic, the mucus membranes lose their tone—in fact, we have exactly the conditions which call for Goldenseal.

I do not have a very high opinion of the use of Hydrastis as a "natural antibiotic." I always tell my students, "why not just use regular antibiotics, it's the same idea and they're more effective."

Here is a case history demonstrating the fallacies of large and inappropriate doses of Goldenseal. The patient was a thirty-seven year old woman. She had been suffering from a sore throat and swollen glands, for the past three weeks. These appeared concurrently with an herpetic lesion, but that had already disappeared. The tongue was large, pallid, flabby and slightly dry. Pulse weak, especially deficient on the left wrist. She had taken an Echinacea-Goldenseal formula in large doses, which did nothing. I recommended Goldenseal in single drop doses, up to 3 per day. After a short time she was completely healed. I advised her never to take Goldenseal in large doses.

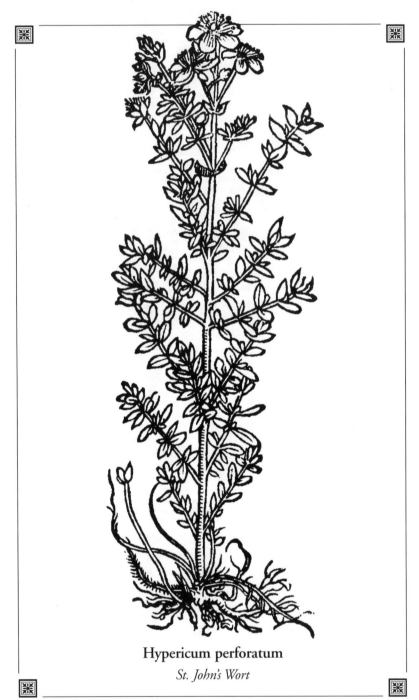

Hypericum perforatum

St. John's Wort

from *Herbarium Imagines Vivae,* published by Christianus Egenolphus, 1535

Hypericum perforatum
St. John's Wort

St. John's Wort is native to Europe, but widely naturalized throughout North America. There are several native American members of the family, but none of them have the exceptional healing properties of this particular species. They are in the Hyperaceae family.

Dr. Charles Millspaugh noted in 1892, "this European immigrant has become so thoroughly naturalized with us as to become a very troublesome weed upon our farm-lands." It indicates poor soils, so most of these fields have been fertilized, abandoned, or turned into pasture. It is for the stockman that St. John's Wort has proved most troublesome. Cattle grazed on land infested with it can become photo-sensitive and die of sunburn. However, this pest for the farmer is a healing balm in the hand of the herbalist.

The Greek name for this plant was *hypericon*. This seems to indicate that it was placed "above the icon," or possibly that it had power "over the image," or specter. Such ideas only gained momentum with the centuries. During the Middle Ages, St. John's Wort was used to protect people against demons, witchcraft, and lightning. "Among the more superstitious peasantry of Middle Europe the most astonishing virtues were assigned to the herb," adds Millspaugh.

The name St. John's Wort refers to the fact that the plant begins flowering on St. John's Day, just before the summer solstice. This is considered the best day to pick it—though fortunately for us lazy, ill-timed people, St. John's Wort remains in flower until the end of summer. The fact that it flowered at such an auspicious time was not lost on medieval

Catholic peasants. They also noticed that the branches, when viewed from above (not from the side) fall perfectly into the shape of a cross. This must have furthered the idea that it was a holy herb which would protect them. This might also suggest protection from above, from lightning, a piece of lore distinctive to this plant.

These are not, however, the most important signatures presented by the St. John's Wort. The leaves, when held up to the sunlight, seem to have little perforations in them—hence the name *perforatum*. These are actually little glands, so these little "holes" are actually windows. This suggested the use of St. John's Wort in wounds, or perforations of the skin. It also added to the magical associations. The use of pins to poke holes in dolls representing victims is an ancient practice, and it was thought that St. John's Wort would protect against insidious occult invasion of people. The bright yellow flowers, when placed in water, oil, or alcohol, give up a dark, red, somber tincture which looks like blood. This also indicated the use of St. John's Wort in wounds as well as some special connection to that most magical of substances, the blood. *Hypericum* has been used since the most ancient times as a wound medicine.

Paracelsus drew on these traditions for his understanding of the properties of St. John's Wort. "The hypericum is almost a universal medicine," he says. "The veins upon its leaves are a signatum, and being perforated they signify that this plant drives away all phantasmata existing in the sphere of man. The phantasmata produce spectra, in consequence of which a man may see and hear ghosts and spooks, and from these are induced disease by which men are induced to kill themselves, or to fall into epilepsy, madness, insanity, etc." This is quoted by Dr. Franz Hartman, who adds the comment: "Have those who ridicule this statement ever employed the hypericum in cases of hallucination?"

Samuel Hahnemann applied the law of similars in a different fashion. He gave *Hypericum* a homeopathic proving and introduced it into his materia medica. He fine tuned the traditional use of the plant as a woundwort. Homeopathy has shown that *Hypericum* is specific for wounds to parts rich in nerves, attended with sharp, shooting pains, inflammation along the course of a nerve, pinched nerves, injuries from sharp, penetrating instruments, etc. These experiences actually confirm the ancient association with needles in a strange way.

Hypericum was largely ignored by the eclectic and physio-medical doctors of nineteenth-century America. They seem to have identified it closely with "the enemy," i.e., homeopathy. However, it slowly crept into American usage, probably from European immigrants. It is often used in homeopathy in the mother tincture, salve, cream or oil, so the jump to herbalism may easily have come from this direction as well.

It is hard to imagine that this herb could ever have been abandoned by herbalists. It has the most beautiful, warm, balsamic, healing taste. I sometimes think of it as the archetypal medicinal herb. Father Sebastian Kneipp called it the "perfume of God" and the "flower of the Fairies."

Despite such precious traditions, the FDA has toyed with the idea of outlawing the sale of *Hypericum* because of the problem with sunburn in cattle. There are no well-documented cases of this difficulty in people, who consume minute quantities, by comparison to cattle. However, as we know, the motto of the FDA is: "This motto has not been approved for medical use!" But more about those Fairies.

St. John's Wort and the Little People

This is one of those plants about which the mantle of European folk culture hangs heavy with curious lore. *Hypericum* blooms around the Feast Day of St. John the Baptist. Just as Christmas Day is the official church holiday associated with the winter solstice, St. John's Day is the holiday near the summer solstice. In the Biblical account, St. John the Baptist was Jesus' cousin, born six months before him, so naturally his feast day fell at the summer solstice. Just as Jesus took over the functions of the dying and resurrecting pagan god of winter, St. John was associated with the pagan god of summer vegetation and life. The Bible recounts that St. John went off to live by himself in the wilderness, dressed like a "wild man," feeding on wild plants. The medieval Catholics recognized a resemblance to the "Wild Man" or "Green Man" associated with the blooming fertility of summer.

These associations transferred to St. John's plant, which not only blooms at Midsummer, but had long been used as a fumigant to remove diabolic and dangerous influences from the home. The little holes in the leaves suggested protection against "spectra" or "phantasms" which might penetrate the psyche or body. And not to forget, St. John's Wort looks like a cross when the branches are viewed from above. The moral wing of the church deduced that St. John's Wort must protect one against the dangerous witchcraft and pagan influences which flourished at the Midsummer festivals. At any rate, there was a time when almost every door and window was crowned with St. John's Wort on St. John's Eve.

One of the most charming stories I have heard about St. John's Wort is that it is the plant of the "Little People." In ancient tradition, the Little People were acknowledged to be very powerful beings (not necessarily little) who exist in the Underworld. They sometimes kidnap mortals and take them to their kingdom. They teach them secrets, sometimes releasing them after a period, but other times holding them captive forever. There are certain "holes" in the countryside, where it is easier to pass over into their world, intentionally or unintentionally. Often these places are situated where water and stone are found in proximity, or where the Elder or the Hawthorn grow.

The medieval Catholic church understood that the Fairy Folk were not the same as the Fallen Angels, or demons, but a different kind of people. Because of this, the church adopted a doctrine which agreed with the traditional admonitions of folk lore. People were warned not to dance with the Little People because, although immortal while this world lasts, the Fair Folk have no souls. On the Judgment Day they will cease to exist, along with their guests. Their fabulous celebrations therefore have a sad, hollow quality beneath the surface. Their home is not the true abode of the human race.

Despite such dangers, we can learn from the Little People about the secrets of the natural world, dreamtime, and seership. They speak to people through dreams and visions, and in some measure even direct these activities. Unlike the demons, whose main interest is to turn people onto a crooked path, the Little People are interested in human companionship. They are willing to trade this for knowledge, but they can become terribly possessive. They sometimes act as companions for children who live and play by themselves in the woods, but they also can steal people away.

The Indian people noticed this other race as well. In the Great Lakes region they are called the *maemaegewaehnssiwuk*. One of my friends showed me a rock by the edge of a lake in central Minnesota. "That's the rock where the Little People used to come out and play, before the white man came." There are Little People who are native, and ones that came over from Europe. The former have long black hair down to their toes and live in the forest. The latter dress in clothing and live more in the fields. The way I heard it, the European Little People taught the Native American Little People about St. John's Wort and they taught the Indian people about it.

Stories about the Little People are always colorful. Like St. John's Wort, they can help heal people who have "holes" in them. One of my close friends was dying from a serious disease. A "New Age shaman" who knew a thing or two "stuck a patch" on her side and "had the Little People hold it on." She felt them jump up on the her bed that night and come over to her side. A year later, when she was well, she saw them leave. During that time she went to a sweat lodge with some Indian people on a sacred mountain. "The Little People are here," one of the spiritual leaders commented. "I've never seen them on the mountain before." I know all the parties involved in this case and can attest what happened.

Herbalists need to know that the Little People can cause them to get lost in the woods. If a person is out in a familiar place in the woods and suddenly he or she gets turned around and lost, the Little People are trying to get some attention. Put out an offering and things will straighten out. This happened to one of my friends. She was out in a field picking St. John's Wort. She put the flowers in a wide mouth bottle as she went along. After an hour she put the bottle down by a tree and wandered off to look for other plants. When she came back she couldn't find it. She circled the tree three times, then circled all the trees in the field and finally walked around the perimeter of the whole area. Then she thought about the Little People. She walked to a nearby truck stop and bought a bag of jelly beans. "I figured an hour's worth of work was worth a $1.39." She put some out, but she was pretty mad at the Little People. She threatened, "If you want the rest of these you'll have to show me that bottle or I'll eat them all." Just then she looked at the tree: from a hundred feet away she could see the bottle. When she got to it she found it between two trails where she had trampled down the grass. She couldn't imagine how she avoided kicking it as she walked by!

Wounds to the Nerves

Hypericum is widely used in homeopathy for nerve-trauma. It is especially beneficial when there is inflammation irritating the nerves, so that there are sharp-shooting pains along the course of the nerves. It is also beneficial for injuries to places rich in nerves, where the pains are considerable. It is used for blows to the coccyx, from falling on the ice, down stairs, or delivering a baby. It is especially indicated for pinched nerves or injuries which occur as a result of sudden movements, as when people catch at something to stop themselves from falling. Boericke comments that the judicious use of *Hypericum* in surgery can make morphine unnecessary. I have talked to homeopathic patients who testified that this level of pain-control is possible. "Every homoeopathic physician of at least three month's practice can attest to its merits," writes Millspaugh.

Back there in my early days of practice I saw the following case. A young woman stuck an awl up under her finger-nail, resulting in great pain. Within twenty-four hours, a red streak was shooting up the arm. She asked what she should do. I said, "Why don't you go to the emergency room?" She said she wasn't going to do that and I knew she wouldn't. I thought about it a little while and realized she and her husband had a homeopathic home remedy kit. *Hypericum* 30x had the streak and the pain diminished greatly by morning and she recovered without difficulty.

Many of the old homeopaths said that St. John's Wort will prevent or cure tetanus, even after it has set in. Dr. Guernsey gave a dramatic history about a young boy who was cured after the tetanus had locked his jaw and neck entirely. Dorothy Shepherd also attests to this, pointing out that she dressed wounds of children and adults injured during the bombing of London with *Hypericum* and never once had tetanus set in, although many cases were admitted in the conventional hospitals nearby.

Dr. Shepherd gives a good account of the wound-healing properties of *Hypericum* in *A Physician's Posy* (1969), including many case histories. The one I like the best, however, is her own. While in an isolated resort in the mountains of Switzerland she was bitten by a horsefly. The wound turned septic very quickly, with a rapidly spreading cellulitis of the foot and leg and swollen lymphatics further up the leg. "Septicemia sprang to mind. I remembered seeing cases dying within two or three days of neglected sepsis of the foot." A friend went out to collect a local variety of St. John's Wort (*Hypericum androsaemum*). They made a decoction of the whole plant, soaked a clean handkerchief and dressed the wound with it. In twenty-four hours she was able to put her foot to the ground again and walk about.

Hypericum has been used in homeopathy and herbalism externally as a soothing anti-inflammatory for fresh, bleeding wounds, sores, burns (in all degrees), bed-sores, chaps, folliculitis, abrasions and injuries from work or cleaning agents, bumps, boils, furuncles, dry and wet eczemas and insect-stings. It is also useful as a cosmetic skin-care cream for scaly, dry, or unclean skin and very effective as a massage oil for muscle spasm (remember the tetanus), cramps, stiffness, ache, overuse, sprains, bruises, articular ache and back ache, rheumatism, gout, sciatica, neuralgia, and poor circulation to the extremities. The oil can also be massaged into the gums for inflammation and atrophy.

Very often, when we have a medicine which acts this strongly on nerve trauma, we find that it will also act on the nervous system. St. John's Wort has a particular affinity to the solar plexus and the nerves of digestion. It has been especially popular among the herbalists of central Europe, and it is to them that we turn for the best accounts of its use in internal conditions affecting the organs and viscera of the body.

Soothes the Solar Plexus, Stomach, and Digestion

A Greek herbalist, Stefan Doll, gives several specific indications. He says St. John's Wort is beneficial during developmental periods in youth and aging. This includes bed-wetting in the young, menstrual problems (cramping, irregularities, and pain), and menopause. He also notes that it is good for people who are sensitive to changes in the weather. He uses it for "recuperation and invigoration after long diseases and operations."

Another source on the Middle European tradition is my friend Fred Siciliano, an herbalist in Ventura, California. He learned about St. John's Wort from his teacher, Sidney Yudin, who studied herbal medicine in the Soviet Union. Fred says that St. John's Wort helps co-ordinate the functions of the different organs of digestion. (In otherwords, it strengthens the action of the solar plexus, which oversees these functions.) "St. John's Wort gets people on the high road to health by improving assimilation of food, and this promotes tissue cleansing. It is more a tonic than a cleanser, but it is the appropriate cleanser when the patient is too weak to bear stronger medicines. It decongests the liver and removes mild tension that accompanies this. It harmonizes the stomach, spleen, pancreas, liver, and gallbladder, so that weak digestive organs are not pushed over by a too-strong action of the liver."

St. John's Wort is indicated in chronic illness associated with chronic pain, nervous exhaustion, emotional depression, mental and physical weakness. It can be used when there is anxiety, stress, or fear. It is used as a subtle strengthening agent for the nervous system, especially through the solar plexus, so that the stomach is soothed and healed, improving the digestive function. Dr. Yudin used it for both hypo- and hyperacidity of the stomach—for ulcers, heartburn, and bloating. It goes further into the system, helping the small intestine to absorb food better, bringing nutriment to the lymphatics for distribution in the interior of the organism. It is also beneficial for intestinal inflammation, cramps, and colic. It promotes increased cleansing from the lymphatics and tissues generally. By removing catarrh from the stomach and small intestine, digestion and assimilation are improved. The gallbladder is mildly influenced and strengthened through the nerve reflexes from the solar plexus, gently decongesting the liver as well.

Hypericum relieves tension in various parts of the body by relieving liver tension and improving blood circulation and cardiovascular tone. It has also been used to treat kidney and sacral pain, kidneystones, bed-wetting, urinary incontinence and irritation, irregular and variable menstruation, pre-menstrual depression, catarrhal bronchitis, and intermittent fever or influenza.

Flower Essence practitioner Yolanda LaCombe of Los Angeles wrote to me, "St. John's Wort has a strong relationship to the solar plexus and aids in digestion. I use it to bring emotions and thoughts into synchronicity. It is a good remedy for overload and for processing information. It is also an excellent protective remedy. The golden-yellow color of the flowers indicates that it has great applications for most forms of depression and Seasonal Affective Disorder in particular."

One of my students had a good experience with *Hypericum* which illustrates the affinities to the digestive tract. Her father had cancer of the intestine, parts of which were surgically removed. At the same time, chemotherapy had been given. After a time he became exhausted from the nausea and pains in the guts and depressed from the whole affair. His daughter came over with the bottle of St. John's Wort tincture. After the first dose he broke out with a rash over his body. Fortunately, he understood that this was a good sign. The next day the rash passed and from that time on his strength and spirits improved. He took the medicine for several months—one drop, one to three times a day. He still takes it from time to time, when he feels the need.

Within the last decade, research on animals showed that

Hypericum possesses anti-retro-viral properties. It was introduced to HIV+ patients with good result. The first HIV positive person I talked to who got good results from St. John's Wort was a man who was infected through intravenous drug use. Now there's a literal application of the pin-prick signature!

Remedies which act on the solar plexus are often psychological in their influence because they improve the gut level instincts, and this helps people to deal with unconscious phenomena in their lives. Thus, we come back to St. John's Wort as a remedy for demons, witchcraft, hallucination, and insanity. But the Little People may have something to say about this as well.

Preparation, Toxicity, and Dosage

In herbal medicine the bulk herb is used as a tea or tincture. The oil does not catch the best ingredients, and is not always as effective as a remedy—though it is well-suited to external application. I prefer to use the tincture. In homeopathy, the potencies are used. I often have better success with the tincture and this should never be overlooked, even by the most inveterate high potency homeopathic prescribers.

In its internal and external applications, *Hypericum* is similar to *Xanthoxylum*. The former works better when the person feels worse from moving, due to the inflamed, swollen tissue around the nerves, and the resulting nerve irritation. The latter works best when a person is writhing in agony; one cannot sit still from the pain.

Hypericum causes serious sunburn in animals grazing on pastures over-run with the plant. White animals are more sensitive to its effects. Animals have even been killed from the burns. Cases of serious burn caused by St. John's Wort in human beings are not well documented, but people who are photo-sensitive should use this medicine with care.

315

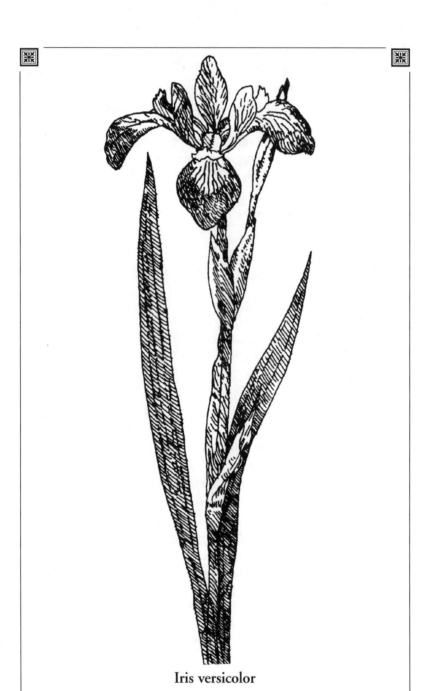

Iris versicolor

Blue Flag

Iris versicolor
Blue Flag

Various representatives of this family are scattered throughout the Northern hemisphere, and have entered into the indigenous medicine of Europe, Asia and North America. *Iris versicolor*, the Blue Flag native to the Eastern Woodland forest, is the officinal plant in botanical and homeopathic medicine. It was used by the Indians for many purposes.

William Bartram, the early American botanist, noticed that the Creek Indians planted Iris near their villages. "They hold this root in high estimation, every town cultivates a little plantation of it, having a large artificial pond just without the town planted and almost overgrown with it." Bartram did not speculate as to the meaning of this plantation, but it is probable that Iris indicates clean water or helps keep it clean. A woodsman from up in northern Wisconsin told a friend of mine that, "there are some plants in the bog which keep the water clean. One of these is Iris." The Indians used the root as a cathartic and bowel remedy.

Because it was a reliable cathartic, this remedy was adopted by the colonial settlers and doctors, who knew of similar properties in the European Iris. It was not used in a very subtle fashion until the last years of nineteenth century, when its affinities to the liver and pancreas became evident. It was then utilized as an "alterative," or "blood cleaner," which basically means that it cleaned up metabolic waste products. It is still used in herbalism today, usually in combination with other such "blood cleaners" as Burdock, Yellow Root, etc. The indications are not very specific.

Iris fared somewhat better among the homeopaths. It was proven by the low-potency wing of the school. The indications generated were limited, but useful. "Iris acts powerfully upon the gastrointestinal tract, the liver, and especially the pancreas; causing burning sensations and a high state of congestion," writes Millspaugh. "Upon the nervous system, its action is marked . . . by the severe toxic neuralgia of the head, face and limbs." Among the more characteristic symptoms are the migraine, starting with a blur before the eyes, concomitant with nausea, worse after relaxation from strain, and better by slowly moving about. This is a common enough pattern, so that Iris has come to occupy a specific niche in homeopathic materia medica, as a "migraine remedy."

The deeper affinities of this remedy had to await developments in the twentieth century. The concept of "low blood sugar" appeared only in the 1920s, and I do not believe that this remedy could have been entirely understood before that pathological entity had been recognized. Iris is nearly a specific for this condition. This was first brought out in my earlier book, *Seven Herbs, Plants as Teachers* (1987). Since that time I have had so many confirmations—as have several of my friends—that any question about this affinity is moot. I think we have helped over a hundred cases with Iris. It is perfectly suited to all the main symptoms associated with that complaint. The following description is based primarily on my experiences with the remedy, interspersed with a few characteristic symptoms gleaned from homeopathic literature.

The Hypoglycemia Remedy

The typical Iris patient suffers from the characteristic symptoms of low blood sugar. If he or she goes for more than a few hours without food, she becomes tired, faint, dizzy, lightheaded; which is relieved immediately after eating, especially something sweet. If, however, the person has too much sugar, he or she runs the risk of getting hyper; this is followed by exhaustion. These ups and downs are accompanied by characteristic symptoms such as migraine headache, starting with a blur before the eyes, accompanied by nausea. A peculiarity of this headache is that it occurs while the person is relaxing, after stress, and is ameliorated by moderate movement about the house. (This is unlike *Chelidonium* and *Sanguinaria,* which seek bed rest.) A characteristic symptom is the sensation of a weight on the neck, which occurs in conjunction with a deep depression. The interesting thing about this depression is that it is not especially associated with personal issues, but is a sort of "generalized nonspecific depression." The patient feels like he or she is "carrying the weight of the world" on his or her shoulders. The Iris patient usually has an "addictive personality"—not to the serious narcotics, or even alcohol or tobacco—but to sugar, chocolate, junk food, or TV.

I have never had any success using Iris for the treatment of diabetes, and I believe that the limit of its action is hypoglycemia. It does, however, have a history of use in pancreatitis. Dr. William Burt, who first proved Iris in 1880, noticed that it caused a burning sensation in the pancreas, and recommened it as a remedy for this condition. This has been clinicially verified since then; Iris is an important remedy for this condition.

The poor management of sugars in the body causes the deposition of glycogen in the liver. This results in inflammation of that organ, but not congestion. Therefore, there is no build up of bile resulting in a yellow complexion. At least, I have never been able to get Iris to work when there was any jaundice. Instead there seems to be a liquification of the bile, so that it flows freely from the hepatic structures. This produces the yellow to orange diarrhea with itching of the anus, characteristic of Iris in the homeopathic provings. The buildup of sugar in the liver results in the inability to digest sugars, which results in hypoglycemia. When this occurs, the sugars start to be stored in tissues throughout the body. We see them building up in the skin, resulting in a "sugary red glaze" on the cheeks that is highly characteristic.

Inflammatory conditions of the liver usually result in a reddened tongue and wiry or tense pulse. We observe these in moderation in the Iris patient. The characteristic pulse feels like there is a "glaze" through the middle of the artery. I know this sounds a little far-fetched, and it is subtle, but I have been surprised again and again to find this particular feeling in the pulse requiring Iris. This "glaze" is like a plane of wiriness parallel to the surface of the skin, bisecting through the middle of the artery. The tongue often has red edges, but not the heavy, dark red we often see when the liver is seriously aflame. The tongue has more brightness. Sometimes the edges are swollen.

Here's an example illustrating the use of Iris in hypoglycemia. Woman, aged thirty-three, has a breakout between the fingers and elsewhere, that looks like poison ivy. She and her mother have little tiny cysts

319

under the skin, and she bruises easily. Face reddish, looks sunburned. Seven years ago she was treated by a holistic M.D. for "candidiasis." Symptoms were flushes of heat after eating sugar or barbecued food. Treatment was Niastatin and diet. Relief until about a year ago, since then the flushing has been increasing. Present symptoms: flushing, more often when relaxed, feeling of uneasiness, can't completely focus on what's going on. This happens a few times a day, more in the late afternoon. No problems if she is exercising. She does not notice reactions to eating sugar, but has typical symptoms of low blood sugar: dizziness, faint-feeling, headache (pounding, front and back), a little nausea, blurring before the eyes, relieved by eating sugar. Tongue red in the middle, swollen along the edges. Pulse has the typical "glaze" through the middle. Iris 12x, once a day, or less, as needed. Quickly removed all low blood sugar symptoms, as well as the skin irritation.

The red, glazed complexion of the typical Iris patient looks a lot like sunburn. This prompted me to try it as a remedy for this condition, in which capacity it has proved quite successful. I recommend the Iris Face Oil, made by Weleda. The following case history illustrates its value. A young man asked me for a good remedy to combat sunburn. He was in a National Guard unit that was scheduled to go to Panama for one month, on "maneuvers"—this was before the Noriega debacle—and wanted something that would really do the trick. He was thinking of Aloe vera, but I recommended Iris Face Oil. I saw him several months later, and asked how it went. "Great, at first," he replied. "All my buddies wanted some: they only had Aloe vera." What was the hitch? "It worked great until my Sergeant took it away so he could use it himself."

Preparation, Toxicity, and Dosage

Dr. Fredrick Locke wrote, "All that has been said of Stillingia applies to this preparation. If preparations of Iris are in the least representative they are liable to decomposition and gelatinization. They change to a brown magma and then become worthless. Specific Iris is made of Ohio-grown Iris. The root found in the South is of little value, the oleoresin being as found by Prof. Lloyd, practically replaced with red tannates." It yields its properties partly to water and completely to alcohol. In large doses Iris is a cathartic with toxic side-effects. In small doses (one to ten drops of the tincture) it flushes sugar from the liver. However, most cases that I have treated have responded to the homeopathic 12x potency or a flower essence. Patients with the red, sugar-glaze on the face should definitely use Iris soap, face lotion or moisturizing cream.

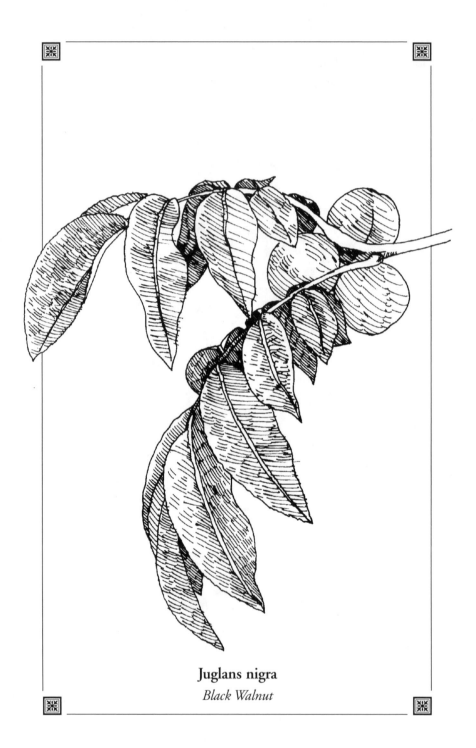

Juglans nigra

Black Walnut

Juglans nigra
Black Walnut

Black Walnut has long been famous for its wood and nuts. The herbalists considers it just as important as a source of medicine. The inner bark and the hulls of the nuts have long been used as a mild laxative and intestinal tonic. Although ruthlessly harvested for its wood, Black Walnut is widely distributed in North America; it is found from the Atlantic to the Pacific, as far north as Minnesota and south to central Mexico.

Black Walnut has a cousin, Butternut (*Juglans cinerea*), which inhabits about the region (further north and not as far west.) The wood is not as desirable and the nuts—though tastier—do not store well. However, Butternut bark is used interchangeably with Walnut bark. There does not seem to be any significant difference in the properties. Butternut bark is usually just used locally, where Walnut is not available. I live about ten miles north of the natural range of the Black Walnut, so I use Butternut.

These two trees have yet another cousin, *Juglans regia,* usually called "English Walnut" in America, but native from Scandinavia to the Hindu Kush. This tree is not a gentle laxative, but a harsh cathartive, so it was not as popular in the medical traditions of the Old World. The early settler learned about Black Walnut and Butternut primarily from the Indian people, not their own traditions. The two native American trees were widely employed by lay practitioners, not professional doctors. Their use has been maintained in the twentieth-century by herbalists.

Dr. John Christopher used and promoted Black Walnut hulls, so they are widely known at the present time.

English Walnut more recently gained popularity as one of Dr. Bach's thirty-eight flower essences. The psychological profile worked out by Dr. Bach for the English Walnut applies well to the American cousins, as we will see, and enriches our understanding of all these trees.

Despite differences, there are important similarities between all of these trees. Although we may, in time, be able to mark subtle differences between the three, at the present we have more to gain from a comparison.

English Walnut

When I was a freshman at the University of Minnesota, one of my botany professors brought up the doctrine of signatures as an instance of scientific fallacy. As an example, he cited the Walnut. "The nut inside the shell looks like the brain inside the skull, therefore they thought it was a remedy for the brain," he said. He laughed almost uncontrollably, but to me it made total sense. I was thinking, "I actually learned something valuable in college. Who would have predicted this!"

I saw this example of the doctrine of signatures referred to elsewhere and wondered where it came from and why it had been chosen as an illustration. Eventually I found that it was mentioned in William Coles's *Adam in Eden* (1657). When I finally tracked that book down at the Lloyd Library in Cincinnati, I found that Walnut was on the opening page. Evidently it was selected because no modern scientist wanted to read the rest of the book. This is what Coles actually says:

> *Wall-nuts have the perfect Signature of the Head: The outer husk or green Covering, represent the Pericranium or outward skin of the Skull, whereon the hair groweth, and therefore, a salt made of those husks is exceedingly good for wounds in the head. The inner woody shell hath the Signature of the Skull and the little yellow Skin that covereth the Kernal is like the hard Meninges and Pia Mater, which are the thin skarves that envelop the Brain. The Kernal hath the very figure of the Brain, and therefore it is very profitable for the Brain and resists poysons, for if the Kernal be bruised and moystened with wine and laid upon the crown of the head it comforts the brain and head mightily.*

Coles also mentioned the well known action on the intestines. The husks are loosening to the belly, cure colic and wind, and "kill the board Worms."

The association between walnuts and the head is very ancient. Plinius says that the Greek name means "heavyness of the head." He also says that the nut of the walnut prepared in oil or wine "serveth to anoint the heads of young babes for to make the hair grow thick." Likewise, "it is used to bring the hair again of elder folk, when through some infirmity it is shed."

Although I had learned something valuable in college, it was many years before I was able to make any use of this signature. Then I ran across Dr. Bach's work. The picture of a protective covering over the brain was strangely relevant. "The remedy gives constancy and protection from outside influences," Bach wrote. It is "for those who have definite ideals and ambitions in life and are fulfilling them, but on rare occasions are tempted to be led away... by the enthusiasm, convictions or strong opinions of others." He called it the "link-breaker."

However, Walnut is especially associated with the intestines, so this simile still does not exactly explain the properties of the plant. However, the old Greek physicians saw a connection. They believed that some mental illnesses could be cured by "purging the humors off the brain" through the intestines. For this purpose they gave laxatives. When there is heat in the viscera it rises and agitates the mind.

Returning to the head, we note that Walnut has long been used for the hair. Black Walnut is found in "natural" shampoos. Coles also refers to this: "The leaves with Boars grease, stayeth the hair from falling, and maketh it fair: the like also will the green husks do." Walnut prevents loss of hair from active scalp disease (not male pattern baldness), and darkens the color.

Butternut

Hopping across the ocean, in the tracks of the European settlers, we come to the American representatives of this genus, Black Walnut and Butternut. These beautiful trees are native to the Big Woods of eastern North America. They were widely used by the Indians for food and medicine, and later by the settlers. Both these cultures put a high value on purgatives and cathartics. Even in the best of times, meats were poorly preserved and the water supply was often contaminated. Of all the available purgatives, the Indians and pioneers liked Black Walnut and Butternut the best. They used the bark and the hulls. During the Revolutionary War, when colonial physicians could not obtain foreign drugs and camp fever was widespread, they began to use Black Walnut and Butternut. In this way, these trees entered popular medicine. From this time onwards they were widely used in folk practice and for a time in professional medicine.

Peter Smith gives a frontiersman's view of Butternut in *The Indian Doctor's Dispensary; being Father Smith's Advice Respecting Diseases and Their Cure* (1812):

> *This differs from all other purges that I know of in this—that your doses may be less and less, but other physic must have more and more, or it will not purge. Other purges generally leave the body in a worse habit but this in a better. Its general ease and safety, and its answering in almost every disease, so that I venture to say the trial of it will never be wrong, make it a far preferable medicine to salts or any other purge, where repeated applications are wanted.*

Smith recommended it "in a weak and debilitated state of the bowels." It is good for "pain in the stomach, worms, colds, consumptive coughs, costiveness, laxes, hemorrhage, or what you will, all is safe." Butternut (and Black Walnut) are indicated in constipation, because they purge out impacted bowels; in diarrhea, because they purge out heat and infection; in parasitic and amebic infections, because they kill low forms of life.

Father Smith's advice on dosage is quite helpful. The bark "may be taken in as small quantities as you please," he says. If it does not immediately purge, it acts "as a stimulus and tonic to the system." By repeating a small dose every night (a pill or two), for up to a month, "a good habit of body" will be produced and constipation or irregularity will be removed. "The doses may be increased a little every night till they purge; then take less and less till the patient is quite well." This is still the standard way to use Butternut and Black Walnut.

John Monroe (1824), who studied under an Indian doctor in northern Vermont, writes that Butternut bark is "one of the best and safest physics ever known. It is a great cleanser of the lungs; good in phthisis, and all other disorders of the like nature. The oil of the nuts is an excellent application for sore nipples of women."

Dr. William Cook (1869), whose father-in-law was a "root doctor" very much like the preceding two, gives a similar but more sophisticated account of Butternut bark:

It is among the moderately slow but very reliable cathartics, relaxing and stimulating, influencing the gall-ducts and gall-cyst, and the muscular fibers and mucous membranes of the bowels. It secures the ejection of bile, and the dislodgment of all hepatic and alvine accumulations; but does not excite watery stools, and always leaves behind a desirable tonic (but not astringent) impression on the alvine canal. In sensitive persons, and those of the nervous temperament, it often causes sharp griping—an effect more common to the recent than the long-dried root. Bilious and bilious lymphatic temperaments rarely feel any griping.

J. I. Lighthall (1876), "the great Indian medicine man," pronounced Butternut the "king of constipation." More specifically, "Where piles are produced by constipation it is almost a certain cure."

In addition to acting on the bowel, Butternut acts strongly on the skin. It is often indicated when dermal problems are connected to bowel problems. This is remarked upon by one of the eclectic writers, Dr. John William Fyfe (1909):

Butternut exerts a marked influence upon the skin, and may be employed in either acute or chronic skin diseases. It also allays irritation of the mucous membranes, and promotes their normal function. In dysentery and diarrhea it is a frequently indicated remedy, and in some cases of intestinal dyspepsia it gives much better results than the bitter tonics.

Here is a nice case history from my own records, illustrating the positive action of Butternut bark on the intestines and the skin. A little boy had pinworm and impetigo. Butternut bark tincture, a few drops three times a day, removed the problem in three days. This case also demonstrated the relationship of Walnut to "breaking the link." The boy's mother died of cancer when he was three and a good friend of hers was appointed legal guardian. For him, the link had been broken too precipitously.

Black Walnut

Although Butternut seems to have been the more popular member of the family in the nineteenth-century, in our own century Black Walnut has taken up the torch. This may be due to the influence of Samuel Thomson and his followers. One of these was Dr. Christopher, who preferred Black Walnut hulls.

Dr. Christopher tells a particularly famous story about Black Walnut in *The School of Natural Healing* (1976, 1996). When he was serving in the army during World War II, he was assigned to run a pharmaceutical warehouse. At one of the weekly meetings with the medical department a man was brought in who had a half inch crust of impetigo on his head. The doctors had tried everything. Even the best physicians in New York City had been called in, to no avail. They were going to send him home, but he objected. He came into the army a clean man, he said, now they were sending him home with a disgusting disease. At that point corporal Christopher chimed in. He said he could work a cure in a week. The major and the other doctors laughed and worried about their liability, but the man insisted that the corporal be given a try. Christopher sent home for some Walnut hulls. When they arrived he made up a bandage over the head and soaked it continually with Black Walnut tea. When the week was over, the man was brought into the weekly meeting. The cap was peeled back and the scalp was healthy! After that, the army doctors respected corporal Christopher's talents and let him practice herbalism.

A backwoods cure was told to me by a fellow at a workshop in Ohio. He was living on a little farm in Arkansas that had terrible water. They called it "Black Sulfur Water." The septic system ran down into the well. One day when he was away his wife and son decided to give the water a try. They came down with dysentery. "I didn't really keep herbs on hand, you know, just used whatever was around. I knew there was Black Walnut in the woods, so could I use the bark and added a little Cayenne. That cured them in no time."

The combination of Black Walnut with a pinch of Cayenne is an old Thomsonian standby. Cayenne is used as a dispersive to stimulate circulation in the deep interior of the body. It is antibacterial and widely used in tropical countries in food, to prevent infection with bacteria and parasites.

Dr. Shook, who was one of Dr. Christopher's teachers, offers a short synopsis of the uses of Black Walnut:

Internal ulcerations, inflammations, mucous and hemorrhagic discharges, bleeding piles, leucorrhea, diarrhea, dysentery, relaxed and ballooned intestines; outwardly, for ulcers, tumors, cancers, abscesses, boils, acne, eczema, itch, shingles, and so forth. It is also used for sore throat, tonsillitis, aphthous sore mouth, relaxed uvula, epistaxis, nasal catarrh, falling hair, ringworms, hoarseness of the voice.

The Parental Tree

We learn something very interesting if we study the natural history of the Walnut clan. The roots of all trees in this family secrete substances which inhibit other forms of life from developing, including their own offspring. Thus, the ground under a large Walnut becomes denuded. This is how the tree protects itself from competition.

The question naturally presents itself as to how the nuts are able to germinate if they cannot do so under the parental tree. If you have ever seen a walnut fall off a tree you would know the answer. The hulls are about the size of a baseball and the consistency of a softball. When they fall off they tend to bounce a distance before coming to rest. This is especially true for nuts growing on high branches. The ones that bounce towards the tree will not get a chance to grow, but those that bounce away may one day become tall, majestic trees. The thick hulls do not provide protection for the nut as much as a life-giving bounce.

The Walnut tree is like a parent that encourages the child to break the link and get a clean start on their own. At the same time, they provide that extra padding and bounce that helps when the child leaves the nest. These properties correspond to the psychological state to which Walnut is remedial.

Preparation, Toxicity, and Dosage

Traditionally, the dried hulls of the nut have been used in American herbalism. This still is the practice among Indian herb doctors. Recently, however, Dr. Huldah Clark introduced the idea of using the green hulls instead. She has used them to treat a wide range of serious conditions, from cancer to AIDS. Many people have jumped on the "green hull" bandwagon and there is now a major movement behind this form of the preparation. Personally, I am satisfied with the traditional method of making a preparation from the dried, darkened hulls. It is certainly much easier to make!

It should be noted that it is customary to use the inner bark after it has dried for a year: the fresh bark tends to cause griping and cramping in the intestines. Fresh bark can be used to make a tincture, but the dose has to be much smaller. Either method will produce a rich, oily, sweet product, not unlike the nuts themselves. Dose of the tincture is from one to twenty drops, three or four times a day, according to the condition. Start small and build up, increasing the dose drop by drop until it starts to purge, then cut back, as described by Smith and Lighthall.

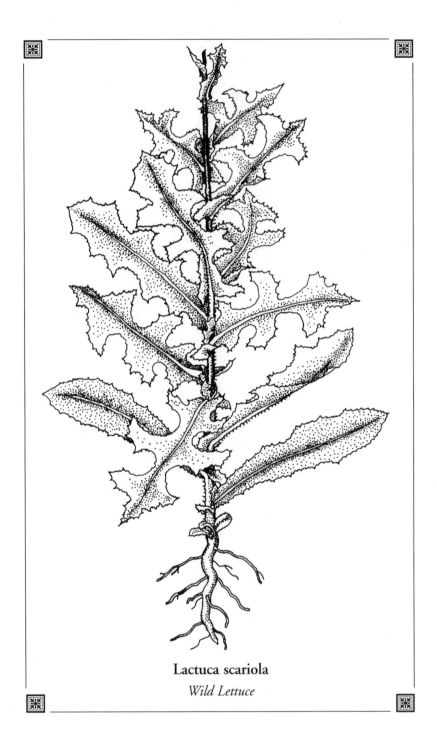

Lactuca scariola

Wild Lettuce

Lactuca scariola

Wild Lettuce

When garden lettuce "bolts" or grows past its prime, the stalk gets tall, the leaves become long and slender, and the sap gets bitter and white. Little yellow flowers that resemble Dandelions top the stem. At this point, garden lettuce closely resembles Wild Lettuce.

There are many species and varieties in the genus. *Lactuca virosa* (Wild Lettuce) is considered the officinal plant in Western herbalism and homeopathy. It is native to Europe but naturalized elsewhere. *L. scariola* (often called "Prickly Lettuce") is also native to Europe and widely naturalized in North America. We also have a native Wild Lettuce, *L. canadensis*. All seem to have about the same properties.

Dioscorides was familiar with a kind of Wild Lettuce (*Lactuca scariola*). He says that "it is similar in virtue to the Poppy," since it is suporific and painkilling. The sap has long been used as a sort of mild substitute for opium. He also used it for burning heat in the eyes and to purge "watery matter through the belly." The seed of wild and domestic lettuce also averts "wanton dreams and venery."

This may be a suppressant effect. In the Galenic system, Wild Lettuce was classified as cold in the fourth degree, the class for medicines which diminish consciousness, like Opium. At the present time Wild Lettuce is used in herbalism as a "nerve sedative." There is hardly any further explanation in the literature.

Lactuca virosa received a homeopathic proving on fifteen subjects in 1846, but this did not result in widespread usage. Hughes (1880) wrote that "very little is known about this drug." Cowperthwaite added (1916) that very few of the symptoms "have been verified by practice." Timothy Field Allen (1893) gave only one symptom as "often" verified by clinical experience. There was, however, one homeopathic author who seems to have had an intimate knowledge of *Lactuca*. In the *Text Book of Materia Medica* (1865) Adolph Lippe gives many useful symptoms. Most especially, he gives the distinctive pulse indication, "slow and hard."

This is an extremely important symptom. Whenever I run across a slow, hard pulse, I immediately think of *Lactuca,* and it virtually never fails. If it does not help, I usually get results from *Artemisia absinthium* (hard, but more so in the middle pulses) or *A. vulgaris* (suited to female problems). This pulse indication is also important because it points to the core problem in the *Lactuca* profile. A slow, hard pulse is a classic indication for "internal cold" in Traditional Chinese Medicine. It corresponds to a person who is cold, stiff, deadened, hardened. If there is, more specifically, infertility, impotence or stiffness in the lower back and loins, we have what is called "cold in the liver meridian."

The symptoms of "internal cold" are essentially the ones which *Lactuca* produced in the homeopathic provings, and which it will, as a result, positively cure. The homeopathic provings show muscular tightness, deep-seated tension, suppression of function from tightness and tension, emotional coldness and deadness. The *Lactuca* patient suffers from a general sense of tightness and coldness affecting the whole body, but especially the chest, groin and extremities. At the same time, however, a suppressed sort of heat shows itself here and there, especially in the eyelids, as Dioscorides mentioned.

Cold Suppressing Heat

Plants with a white sap are usually cold in nature. Most people who have consumed lettuce in salad would agree that it is a cold plant. The homeopathic provings bring out a great deal of coldness. At the same time, the bitter taste is considered to indicate an affinity for inflammatory conditions. *Lactuca* is suited to conditions where cold has supervened over the normal body-heat. This results in a cold, tight state, with tight sinews and muscles, rheumatic aching the joints, but with evidence of heat still showing through at the corners. When the heat has been completely extinguished, we need Wormwood or one of its cousins, Mugwort or Sagebrush.

Internal cold is not caused by a lack of heat in the system, but by external cold which has invaded, and become locked in. When cold results from a lack of internal heat it is called "yang deficiency" in Chinese medicine. Because of the deficiency of yang (fire) the patient is not only cold but weak and relaxed. Internal cold, on the other hand, is associated with tension because the cold has forced its way in.

The homeopathic provings show that *Lactuca* has a sedative effect on the brain and nervous system, reducing the frequency of the pulse. The sensations are predominately those of tightness and coldness. After an initial sensation of heat, there is a prolonged feeling of cold. Icy coldness in the throat, chest and stomach. Contraction at the pit of the stomach. The thorax feels compressed and narrowed, especially while sitting with the body bent. One prover felt a desire to breathe deeply, an ardent longing for the open air, and yawned frequently. Constant sighing. Mucus with a painful cough. The tightness of the chest usually remained with the provers for several days, while a slight pressure in the abdomen was relieved by the passage of gas.

I have many times used *Lactuca virosa* 6x or *L. scariola* ø for asthma associated with tightness in the chest (but no active infection or phlegm production) and often for pain and stiffness in the lower back and extremities. This is the one symptom often verified according to Timothy Field Allen. It is significant in and of itself, but it also points to the deeper Lactuca problem of generalized stiffness.

"The Herbal Street Person"

The wild varieties of lettuce are somewhat rough looking. They assume an appearance opposite to edible lettuce, looking unkempt and uncultivated. *Lactuca scariola* particularly likes to hang around in the cracks in the sidewalks along the side of a building or the street. They are much more common in the city than in the country. If they appear in the countryside, it is usually around houses and barns. I always say to my students that Wild Lettuce "looks like a street person."

This picture corresponds well to the mental state calling for the plant—though most people who need it are not homeless. Wild Lettuce is the remedy for people who have been through adversity and harshness. Internal cold can result from the invasion of cold from the environment. However, it usually results from prolonged emotional suffering, resulting in emotional deadness or coldness. The *Lactuca* patient has been through rough, de-humanizing, deadening experiences. They are not, however, completely deadened—that would call for Wormwood or Sagebrush.

Hughes generalized about the mental state produced in the provings. "The disposition manifested itself in sadness, anxiety, and causeless chagrin." Thought processes terminate in negative and disagreeable ideas—what we would nowadays call "negative thinking." This is really a great remedy for negative thinking in general, people who say, "Oh, but that would never work."

I asked one young man I was working with if he suffered from this kind of thing. He commented, "Well, I always worry that someone will be murdered and I will be charged and sentenced for the crime, even though I didn't commit it. Is that what you mean?" *Lactuca* cured him of this "causeless chagrin," along with emotional deadness and muscular tension. One of my students mentioned this story to a woman she was helping with Wild Lettuce. She had the same fantasy!

In another case, a 13 year-old boy was brought to me by his aunt on the chance that I could help with his emotional problems. His mother was dead, his father was a heroin addict and a pimp. His grandparents had just shipped him off to the aunt, who had only met him once. In addition, his girlfriend had just committed suicide. The only physical symptoms he cared to mention were sharp, biting pains in the eyes (a pathogenetic symptom under *Lactuca*). The margins had a slight redness, but a sharp look. The pulse was slow, hard and superficial. Usually the *Lactuca* pulse is deep, so I judged this to be a rather recent entrance of cold into the system, probably quite treatable. *Lactuca virosa* 6x cured the physical symptoms in less than a day and made a notable difference in the mental state as well.

One of my friends in Madison, David Millbrandt, phoned to share a case which was, he said, "so Matt Woodish I had to call." Several years ago he picked up a hitch-hiker in the Dakotas and brought him back home. "I owed my wife some work around the farm and our friend could help us out," he commented. The man was a Vietnam Vet whose wife had joined a religious cult and absconded with their son. He was now a homeless wanderer. He helped around the farm and stayed in the garage. He complained of insomnia. He sought help at the Vet Hospital for paranoid delusions, got a job at a filling station and moved out—for a while. Later he was back in the garage.

David wanted to help him with herbs, but the man's attitude put that out of the question. One day he had a toothache, so David had a chance. "I walked out to the street—that seemed appropriate—picked some *Lactuca,* threw it into the blender and added some brandy. After one dose the man fell into a deep sleep for the first time in a long while. The toothache disappeared. A week later he was back on the road to Wyoming, but he settled down, got a job and now leads a happier life. "Maybe it was just a coincidence," commented David. "Maybe he was getting his life together slowly all along, or maybe it just came at the right time, but after that Wild Lettuce, his life turned around."

Cold in the Liver Meridian

The liver is particularly affected by invasion of cold into the interior. At first, cold invasion causes tension and restriction in the circulation, resulting in alternating fever and chills. In traditional medicine (both east and west), this is associated with the liver. As the cold takes a grip on the organism and the heat is extinguished, pain, chill and tightness affect the extremities. The liver is associated with "the tendons" in Traditional Chinese Medicine. This is called "cold in the liver meridian."

Since the liver meridian runs from the foot, inside the legs, twinning up about the loins and sexual organs and then across the abdomen to the liver, this kind of blockage results in cold, pain, stiffness and aching in the lower extremities and loins, pain and distention in the abdomen, impotence, blockage of sexual energy, hernia, sterility and infertility. A "cold uterus" prevents successful pregnancy. The pulse is slow and hard, the tongue pale or coated white. *Lactuca virosa* (or *L. scariola* for do-it-yourself wild crafters) is perfectly suited to this condition.

Here's a case illustrating the value of *Lactuca* in this syndrome from the male side of the aisle. A 39 year-old man was suffering from chills and achiness, "like a flu." Muscles were tight, breathing constricted, he felt depressed. Two days before the symptoms came on he had been

337

struck on the testicle very hard by an electric plug that he yanked out of a socket. He suffered excruciating pain at the time. *Lactuca* 6x quickly removed the symptoms.

And here's a case from the female side. A thirty-six year old woman, six months pregnant, came to see me at Crescenterra chiropractic clinic on a "return visit." We meet on the front steps on a fine autumn day. "Oh yes, I remember you," I said. "What was the problem and what did I give you and what happened?" She smiled. "Well, you can see the result," she said, pointing to her round belly. I had given her *Lactuca scariola* ø for a tendency to miscarry at the twelfth week. She had lost six pregnancies. *Lactuca* fit this case because she suffered from cold and stiffness in the lower back and extremities generally and some considerable hardships. It helped her go full term.

Preparation and Dosage

I prepare a tincture from the leaves of *Lactuca scariola*. I would have thought that the plant was most powerful when gathered at flowering, after it has thoroughly "bolted," to use the gardening phrase. This is when the white sap is most bitter and when the wild specimens are most dissimilar to the garden varieties. However, experience has taught me that the plant is most medicinal when gathered in the spring or early summer, before it goes to flower. *Lactuca* can be dried, but I fancy that the white sap is better preserved fresh in alcohol. The doses commonly used in herbalism are sizable (30-60 drops). However, when the plant is indicated as a specific, we can use small doses (1-3 drops) and we still see a strong sedative effect. I have to warn people not to take it before driving—it is best taken at night. I have also used homeopathic potencies of *Lactuca virosa* from 3x to 200c.

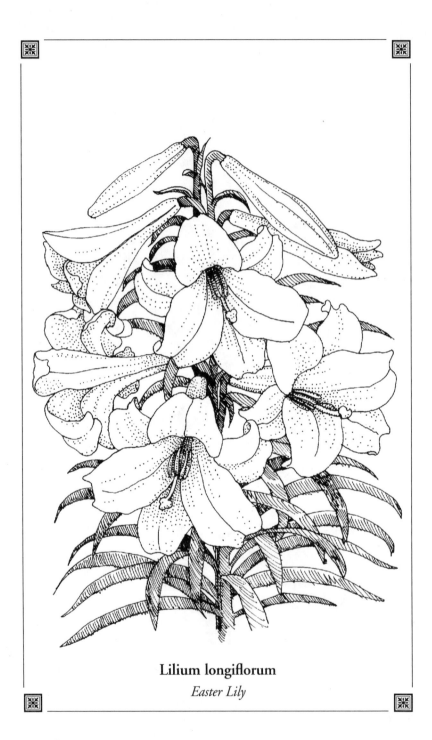

Lilium longiflorum

Easter Lily

Lilium longiflorum
Easter Lily

The European tradition has long used White Lily (*Lilium candidum*), a native of the eastern Mediterranean. It can be cultivated and is sometimes naturalized in temperate regions. It is also called Madonna Lily, and is associated with purity (*candidum*) and Mother Mary.

Easter Lily (*Lilium longiflorum*) is native to China and Japan. It was introduced into Europe in 1817, as an ornamental, and is now widely propagated. In my area it is easier to grow than White Lily, though it needs to be planted next to the foundation of the house to provide warmth in the winter. Easter Lily has long been used in Traditional Chinese Medicine.

The properties of the White and Easter Lily are similar or nearly identical.

Stagnant Mucus

In my book *Seven Herbs, Plants as Teachers* I included an account of Easter Lily as a remedy for fibro-cystic disease of the breasts, cysts in the ovaries and under the skin, and menstrual problems. It is particularly indicated in women who are having troubles with sexual issues, like purity versus impurity, or personal desires versus higher, spiritual aspirations. Since that time, my friends, colleagues, and students, as well as myself, have used this remedy with success in literally hundreds of cases. It has turned out to be a virtual specific for cysts.

341

A short time later I had a case that showed that Easter Lily was also valuable for respiratory infections. A twenty-two-year-old woman had been afflicted with a bronchial infection for three weeks. She had recently quit her job as a stripper! The cough was deep and brassy. It gave the impression that there was implated mucus in the farther reaches of the bronchial tree. She had a clear, luminous, pale skin, which at the present time was generally reddened and slightly full looking. It seemed as if there was a sort of "stuckedness" quality to both the fever and the mucus. My choice of remedy was based on the complexion and the recent occupation. I did not think of Easter Lily as a respiratory remedy at that time, but it worked fine. The flower essence tincture cured in thirty-six hours.

Within three months I had a similar case. A thirty-eight-year-old woman was diagnosed with bronchitis. One week previously she came down with a fever which settled into the lungs and dried up the mucus. The intensity of the fever had subsided but she was left with a deep, brassy cough, slight fever, and dried up mucus in the lungs. Easter Lily flower tincture cured within twenty-four hours. She long remembered this illness, and the remedy, because it came at a time when she was breaking up with her boyfriend, and decided not to sleep with him.

From this time on I began to use Easter Lily as a remedy for "stagnant mucus in the periphery of the respiratory tree." Later I read that soft, moveable tumors or cysts are often classified as "stagnant mucus" in Traditional Chinese Medicine. This tied my experiences with Easter Lily together. However, the textbooks on Chinese herbal medicine described Easter Lily as a remedy for "lung *yin* deficiency." That would describe conditions where there is hectic fever, the fluids of the lungs start to dry out, the membranes loose lubrication and become irritated. This did not jibe with my experience. I mentioned this to Mitch Stargrove, N.D. He remembered that his teacher on Chinese materia medica in naturopathic school said that Easter Lily was "not really for lung *yin* deficiency" but for "stagnant mucus" in the lungs. "Stagnant mucus" is associated with a drying out of the phlegm so that it becomes lumpy. "Yin deficiency" dries out the membranes and makes the mucus secretions scanty. "Stagnant mucus" is considered a less important category and is sometimes included in the other.

In short, Easter Lily is nearly a specific medicine for "stagnant mucus," whether in the lungs or in the form of "soft, moveable tumors."

Here we have another almost cartoonlike confirmation of the doctrine of signatures, because the dried pieces of bulb that come to market from China look hilariously like dried chunks of mucus.

Although I do not use Easter Lily very much for respiratory conditions, some of my friends do. A few years ago I made a business arrangement with some of my neighbors who sell herbs by mail order. I gave one of them a taste of my Easter Lily by way of introduction. Almost immediately, he started to discharge mucus from the sinuses. This is David Eide, of Natural Health Products, in Mound, Minnesota. He now uses Easter Lily on a regular basis for removing mucus. He even had one case where it helped with mental illness in a teenage girl. It cleared the mind (fine, phlegmatous particles are thought to obstruct consciousness in Chinese and other systems of folk medicine). It also helped her deal with her emerging sexuality. My friend, David Milgram, D.C., of Flagstaff, Arizona, has also used Easter Lily for respiratory conditions. He found that internal doses of the flower essence cured conjunctivitis in several patients when indicated by broader symptoms.

Madonna Lily is used for about the same purposes as Easter Lily. Culpeper notes that it treats "swellings in the privities." It is also a respiratory and skin remedy. In addition, it was used as a salve to break "plague sores" and cleanse dirty wounds.

A Woman's Remedy

Lilium longiflorum is a superlative remedy for the removal of cysts from the breasts and ovaries, and has generally a purifying action on the female organs. It has a special affinity for the cervix and appears to remove dysplasic cells, if not neoplastic ones. It is not an appropriate remedy for fibroids, which would not usually be classified under stagnant mucus.

The symptoms of the mind and senses lead especially to the selection of Easter Lily. I mention in my book *Seven Herbs* a general correlation between purity/impurity issues in the Easter Lily patient.

Cases confirming the use of *Lilium longiflorum* as a remedy in cysts have come in from many of my peers, students, and friends. David Milgram had a particularly dramatic case. The patient was a woman in her mid-thirties who had been diagnosed in her late teens as suffering from "poly-cystic disease." She was told she would never be able to bear children. While seeing Dr. Milgram for chiropractic work, she asked if he "had anything for cysts." Maybe, he replied. He gave her *Lilium longiflorum* flower essence tincture. Three months later she reported that the cysts were gone and she was two months pregnant. She was rather mad about it for a while, but got used to the idea in time for the arrival of a healthy babe six months later.

In addition to promoting fertility by removing cysts (and perhaps by removing impurities from the female tract), Lily has been used to facilitate labor. Gerard (1597) quotes from "Iulius Alexandrinus the Emperors Physitian." He reported, "That the water thereof distilled and drunk causeth easie and speedy deliuerance, and expelleth the secondine or after burthen in most speedy manner."

Here is a little case which may confirm this observation. Down in St. Peter, Minnesota (where the herbalist Jethro Kloss had his clinic around the turn of the century), I met a woman who had used Easter Lily for this purpose. Her niece was a mere slip of a girl, aged twenty-one, carrying her first child. The doctors were fairly certain she was not big enough to have an ordinary birth. The aunt gave Easter Lily flower essence tincture (because it was Easter), and the baby was delivered without incident the next day. When asked about the pain of labor, the new mother replied, "Oh, it was about like an ordinary period. What's the big deal about labor?"

We should not think of Easter Lily exclusively as a remedy for women, as the following case shows. A twenty-three-year-old man, father of an expected child, had "lumps in the skin" at the neck. They were broad, shallow and moveable. *Lilium longiflorum* flower essence tincture cured completely in short order. He took it externally and internally.

I am often asked if I have a remedy for lipomas or fatty tumors. I do not believe that Easter Lily will work with this condition. It has no affinities to fat production and storage. Chickweed, which is used to "dissolve fat," has proved beneficial in some hands. I should also mention that Cleavers is an excellent remedy for cysts, especially when there are many and the breasts are fibrous. Red Clover is good for a single, hard encysted gland. These are my stalwarts in fibro-cystic disease.

Preparation and Dosage

The bulb is the officinal part in Chinese herbalism. A decoction is made by simmering an ounce of the pieces in a quart of water. However, I use a flower essence or herbal tincture made from the flowers of *Lilium longiflorum*. Three drops of the flower essence dosage tincture, one to three times a day, as needed, is usually sufficient. Response is usually prompt. Women with menstrual problems should take it for seven to ten days before the period, for three periods. It usually takes a few days, or three periods, to complete its cleansing action on the organism.

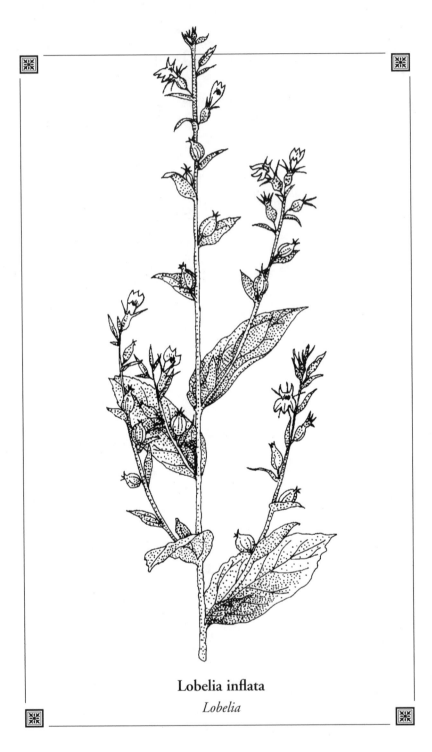

Lobelia inflata

Lobelia

Lobelia inflata
Lobelia

How can we explain Lobelia? To what can it be compared? Dr. Christopher said it had brains. Let's agree with that and add: it is smarter than any human being. The brains of Lobelia are the intelligence of the life force itself. As Dr. Christopher said, Lobelia knows where to go in the organism and it goes there. When it arrives, it can produce opposite kinds of reactions—arousing or sedating—depending on what is needed. It is an important and powerful remedy, but one whose actions can never be predicted. When correctly indicated, Lobelia does things that nothing else can do. In completing its work it will sometimes produce bizarre side effects and aggravations. Like the life force itself, Lobelia must really be witnessed to be understood. It is the wildest and craziest article in the herbal materia medica, one that every herbalist must strive to understand, yet one that can never be mastered.

These difficulties are further aggravated by the controversies surrounding the introduction of the plant into herbal medicine. Its use by the Indians is not well documented, though it was and is certainly used by some Native American practitioners. The ethnobotany of Lobelia took a wild gyration from obscurity to infamy about 1800, when Samuel Thomson, an uneducated "root doctor" from New Hampshire, introduced it into practice as a powerful antispasmodic and general panacea. By 1809 he had attracted notoriety and condemnation from the medical establishment for his cures of asthma and other serious complaints by the use of this powerful agent. In that year he was imprisoned on the charge of murder by the use of Lobelia. After languishing in an unheated, urine-soaked cell with a child molester, the case was brought to court, the charges were shown to be fabricated, and he was released without being allowed to stage a defense. Despite these facts, the charge that Thomson killed a man with Lobelia was repeated for the next hundred years by almost every allopathic author on materia medica and many of the homeopaths as well. At the same time, the use of Lobelia as an antispasmodic for the paroxysm of asthma was adopted by the allopathic profession, without giving Thomson credit for the discovery. The misunderstandings and literary free-for-all which resulted have never been resolved, and even today Lobelia is a poorly understand medicine in the literature of all schools, except among Thomson's own followers. The late Dr. Christopher was a member of that school, and his writings preserve the traditional Thomsonian view.

The Archetypal Diffusive

Thomson conceived of the vital force as an actual substance spread out evenly throughout the healthy organism, circulating from the center to the circumference. Disease resulted from a shortage or blockage in this continuous flow of substance. From experience, Thomson learned that some herbs act primarily through what we would call the nervous system, making a strong impression noticed by the senses, while other herbs act slowly and imperceptibly through the tissues. The former agents were called "diffusives" by Thomson's followers—he did not really have an adequate vocabulary here. These diffusives cleared blockages in the flow of the life force, the nerve force, or the blood. If there was inactivity, they stimulated, if there was tension, they relaxed. Over all, they equalized conditions and brought the organism back into a homeostatic balance.

Chief among the diffusives was Lobelia. Thomson saw it as the great equalizer for disturbances in the hegemony and homeostasis of the life force. "It clears all obstructions to the extremities, without regard to the names of disease," he wrote in *The Thomsonian Materia Medica* (1841). "It produces an equilibrium in the system, and will be felt in the fingers and toes, producing a prickling feeling like that caused by a knock on the elbow."

Thomson visualized the life force as residing in the stomach, from here radiating to the extremities. Although he was not particularly interested in the doctrine of signatures, Thomson did notice a resemblance

348

between the seedpod of Lobelia and the stomach. "This pod exactly resembles the human stomach," he wrote in his first book. And he preferred to pick Lobelia after it had gone to seed, unlike most other plants, which are selected during or before flowering.

Thomson's followers were more erudite than he, and the description of the action of Lobelia slowly evolve through the century. The term "diffusive" was introduced by Dr. John Thatcher, an allopathic author, about 1812. This term was picked up by his followers. These included the "Thomsonians," who were lay practitioners, and the "physio-medicalists," who were professional doctors. Lobelia was eventually adopted by the eclectics as well, although they did not like to credit Thomson.

I think it is Ellingwood, one of the eclectic authors, writing almost a century after Thomson introduced Lobelia, who is finally able to put the peculiar action of Lobelia into words. He writes:

> *From my own personal observations and from the conclusions I have drawn from the observations of others, I would say that lobelia seems at once to supply a subtle but wholly sufficient force, power, or renewed vital influence, by which the nervous system and the essential vital force within the system again reassert themselves and obtain complete control of the functional action of every organ. From this influence, in a natural and sufficient manner, a complete harmonious operation of the whole combined forces is at once resumed, in some cases in an almost startling manner. Other agents stimulate, prop up, whip up or temporarily increase the force and power of one or another function, while this remedy with this peculiar power at once assumes control of the whole, and succeeds against all the opposing influences.*

Lobelia was adopted into conventional medicine as an antispasmodic to break the paroxysm of asthmatic attack. Later, the alkaloid lobeline was isolated and used for this purpose. It fell out of favor. Wilson and Gisvold, in their allopathic *Textbook of Organic Medical and Pharmaceutical Chemisty* (1954) give the explanation: "Because its action is somewhat capricious and fleeting, it has not been well received." The eclectics were somewhat more tolerant of its idiosyncrasies. Dr. George Hite (1890) wrote, "Lobelia inflata is a remedy whose excellency is equal to its nastiness."

Turning now to our own senses, we observe that Lobelia makes an impression on the tongue and nervous system which is sharp, shocking, and highly diffusive. A drop of a strong preparation, placed on the wrist, will shortly be felt as a sharpness at the back of the throat, or vice versa. Lobelia seems to travel the nerves as fast as possible. Because it is both a stimulant and a relaxant, the therapeutic potential of the plant is extensive, but contradictory and complex. "Excellent but nasty, capricious, and fleeting" would be a good summary of Lobelia.

Taking Hold of the Organism

In order to offer the best possible overview of this remedy, I have divided the conditions for which it is remedial into six basic groups. This may not cover all the expressions of disturbance to which Lobelia is suited, but it helps to gain initial insight into this highly complex medicinal agent. These are: (1) Clearly observable spasmodic conditions, where the pulse is tense, wiry, and spasmodic. (2) Oversecreting, hyper-relaxed, and collapsed patients, where the pulse is feeble, and the secretions are free-flowing from the body. (3) People with suppressed secretions. The skin feels doughy and the pulse feels doughy. (4) People with a wiry and fast pulse, a red tongue, fever, spasm, collapse, sweating, and loss of secretions. (Prolonged heat and loss of fluids can result in spasm, inflammation, and dryness.) (5) Affections related to the vagus nerve; usually spasmodic. Bronchial spasm, hiatal hernia, nausea, vomiting, heartburn. (6) Conditions caused or aggravated by tobacco. These six conditions intermix, and more than one may be found in a single person. Let's take a look at each one separately.

Spasm. There are different kinds of spasms. The spasm suited to Lobelia is extremely intense—even life threatening if the throat, heart, or lungs are involved. What is characteristic about it is that the muscles tend to "torque up." The torsion in one muscle spreads to another, and on throughout the whole system, until the entire body is bent out of shape. As a diffusive, Lobelia "equalizes the charge on the muscles." It relaxes the entire edifice of torqued muscles so that the whole organism can resolve itself back into place. In severe cases of some duration, it will be necessary to give the remedy for a while until the entire frame gets relaxed. This produces an overall feeling of prostration, which, however, is followed by unkinking and unwinding.

Some of the most dramatic case histories result from the use of Lobelia to cure spasm. In one of my classes I was talking about Lobelia.

One of the students was a massage therapist. The next day she was work-ing on a regular client. At the end of the session the woman wanted to talk. Her husband was in great pain from what sounded like a spasm. They called him up. The pain was so great he was literally crying on the telephone. They rushed to the house and found him writhing in agony. "It was like he was giving birth to himself," commented his wife. "I've had six children and I know what childbirth feels like." She thought there was a spasm in the latissimus dorsa. "I knew he needed Lobelia," said my friend. She tracked some down and gave him two drops on the tongue and a few rubbed into the back. He experienced temporary relief, then the agony returned. She gave another dose which resulted in slight amelioration, then aggravation. The writhing agony seemed to be even worse and after a half hour he begged to be taken to the emergency room. My friend went home and called me, worried that she had made things worse. It certainly sounded like a Lobelia case to me—maybe a kidney stone. I tried to reassure her, but what could I say? Lobelia has a mind of its own. She hung up the phone. A minute later the wife was at the door. "We got five blocks from the house and the whole thing blew over," she said. "Come see him now." He was sitting out in the car "like a newborn or a Buddha, just beaming energy…" "He looked wonder-ful," commented the massage therapist. "We felt giddy; it was just like after a birth, when everybody's gathered around that new born child… The whole thing did seem crazy."

My friend was quick to see that Lobelia would make a useful rem-edy in spasmodic labor. Scudder comments on this fact. "Lobelia is specific in difficult labor from rigid os, vagina, or perineum. It also stim-ulates the contractile function of the uterus, and thus strengthens the pains. This use of Lobelia will be greatly prized when known." However, the potential surprises from the exhibition of Lobelia are enough to make the obstetric practitioner wary.

Here's another case from my own practice. A thirty-two-year-old married woman, who appeared to be robust and strong, had been nau-seated from the moment of conception so severely that she was forced to lay down all day long. After two months she and her husband decided on an abortion, but the nausea continued without reprise. After anoth-er month she felt severe abdominal cramping and thought her period might be suppressed. The nurse practitioner suggested that there were still clots in the uterus and wanted her back for another surgery. The pulse felt like the end of the beat was chopped off, so I concluded that it probably was a spasm and gave one dose of the Lobelia 6x homeopathic—all I had on hand. The period came so quickly that she bled right on the chair. She was perfectly well within a day and never needed another dose.

I might point out here an additional lesson which is often seen. People who attempt to plan for or treat the "worse case scenario," as this nurse practitioner was trying to do, and which is commonly done in conventional medicine, will usually miss the cure completely. One can sense intuitively what "feels right," and it usually is right. Attention should be made to the "worse case scenario," but also to the "best explanation."

Suppressed secretions. To judge from the literature, this seems to be a much rarer condition. The usual symptoms are a slight edema and doughy skin, from suppression of the perspiration. There may be internal symptoms as well. Scudder mentions the "doughy" pulse as indicating Lobelia, and it is suited to just these cases, not to all situations calling for the medicine.

Here is the single case history I have on this pattern. A twenty-seven-year-old man was retaining a great deal of water. He was of a robust and large build. Normally he had an outgoing nature, but at the present time he was dragged down. This condition had been going on for several months. The skin and the pulse felt doughy. Single drop doses of Lobelia in tincture cured him in three days.

Hyper-secretion. This is a less common condition as well. Lobelia is suited to conditions where the "periphery collapses" and there is profuse, continuous sweating, with or without fever.

Here is a case history. A middle aged woman of thin physique, yielding personality and physical weakness, suffered from watering eyes and copious, uncontrollable perspiration. She was addicted to smoking cigarettes. Lobelia 3x potency controlled the sweating and cut the dependence on cigarettes dramatically. She did not quit, but she was more healthy and smoked much less.

Severe inflammation and dehydration. Lobelia is a remarkable agent in severe fever, where the fluids are drying up, the muscles are affected due to lack of lubrication, and there is tension and heat. Characteristically, the tongue is bright red and dry, sometimes cracked. In all conditions, the tongue suited to Lobelia tends to display an unequal distribution of coating and color. This is a good, characteristic symptom.

I have had some trouble finding good case histories in the literature, though the condition has been described often enough. Fortunately, I have several from my own experience. A fifty-three-year-old woman was suffering from relapsing bronchitis. She had been treated unsuccessfully by regular physicians with several courses of antibiotics over the last several months. Dark around the eyes, chalky, sallow complexion, tongue bright red and dry (as if she had been sucking on a cherry cough drop—which she had not), thirsty, dry skin, wheezing, much phlegm difficult to raise, hot flashes (menopausal), edema in the ankles and waist. She was an addicted smoker. A sorry case. I tried Calcium carbonate 6x, which cleared up the hot flashes, then Calamus, which cleared up the edema. Both temporarily helped the bronchial infection, but it still was not cured—but was in fact progressing. The tongue was still red and dry which indicated that the infection was deep, and I was inclined to have her start up on the antibiotics again. She went back to a conventional physician who diagnosed pneumonia and prescribed antibiotics and prednisone. After two weeks on the last drug, she could not stand any more and begged for some alternative. The wheezing was quite bad. I said, "Well, I'll give you the remedy that would have been official in the regular pharmacopoeia long before prednisone." I was thinking rather allopathically of trying to suppress the bronchial spasms with Lobelia, but this turned out to be the correct remedy. She took Lobelia tincture as needed, up to three times a day, sometimes not at all. Stopped the antibiotics and prednisone. She slowly, *but naturally,* got better. After six weeks the tongue was of normal color and moisture, the complexion was much better, the eyes were not dark, the wheezing slight. She still had not quit smoking. She occasionally noticed nausea from a dose of the tincture, after which she would wait for a while before taking a dose. I lost track of her after this.

Action on the vagus nerve. Due to this affinity, Lobelia has a relationship to conditions of spasm in the bronchial tubes, diaphragm, and stomach. It is remedial for some forms of bronchial asthma, bronchitis with wheezing, heartburn, nausea, spasm in the stomach and esophagus, and hiatal hernia.

A number of the physio-medicalists, from Thomson down to Dr. Christopher, give case histories of spasmodic asthma cured by Lobelia.

Thomson mentions a woman in Newington, Massachusetts, who had been unable to sleep lying down for over five years, without being attacked by an asthmatic paroxysm. She was cured after a few table-spoons of the tincture. In *The School of Natural Healing,* Dr. Christopher describes an asthmatic who was unable to lie down to sleep for over twenty years; he had to sleep sitting in a chair. One day his doctor was out of town and the patient was out of his prescription. In desperation he was brought to Dr. Christopher. After one tablespoon of the tincture he coughed up a big chunk of mucus and was completely cured.

Dr. Jeanes, our lone homeopathic authority on Lobelia, gives a good case illustrating the use of this medicine when there is spasmodic contracture of the stomach. A thirty-eight-year-old married woman had chronic dyspnea. This was accompanied by the following symptoms. "Sensation of weakness and oppression at the epigastrium, and extend-ing from thence into the chest. Burning in the stomach, and a sensation as if there was a burning lump in the pit of the throat, which appeared to impede swallowing and respiration. In swallowing, it seemed as if at this point something rose up to meet the food and obstruct its decent into the stomach. Frequent eructation of acid fluid with sensation of burning. Frequent vomiting of the food after meals, especially after eat-ing warm food." She "had not known what it was to be without heart-burn for one hour for the last year." The urine was high-colored, and deposited a copious red sediment. Pain in the left lumbar region of the abdomen. Lobelia in low potency produced a gradual but complete removal of the dyspeptic symptoms.

Antidote to tobacco. Lobelia has been used as an antidote to the tobacco habit in herbalism. I have known dozens of people who have used Lobelia to help them quit smoking. It seems to be an antidote to both the craving and the withdrawal symptoms. It does not work in all cases and causes unpleasant symptoms in some. The active ingredient is lobeline. Wilson and Gisvold explain: "A curious cross-tolerance exists between nicotine and lobeline, in which animals tolerant to the former also exhibit tolerance to the later. Based on this phenomenon, a suggest-ed use for lobeline is as an aid in breaking the tobacco habit." Lobeline is not approved by the FDA. Indeed, Lobelia is rightly considered a sus-pect herb by them.

Homeopathy did not adopt Lobelia as an antidote to cigarette smoking, but it was noticed that the Lobelia patient is aggravated by exposure to tobacco smoke. I would like to enlarge upon this observation from personal experience. The patients are especially sensitive to the kind of stale, stagnant smoke found in a bar or place where people smoke habitually. Also, some people are never healthy after quitting smoking. Lobelia probably assists these patients by restoring the proper internal secretions and relaxing the muscles of the thorax.

Lobelia may also be an antidote to other substances. Thomson wrote, "In cases where they have taken considerable opium, and this medicine is administered, it will in its operation produce the same appearances and symptoms that are produced by opium when first given, which, having laid dormant, is roused into action."

This brings up an important point. Lobelia tends to heighten the effects of other medicines and substances. Thomson used Lobelia in compounds with other herbs, in order to bring out the effects of the more dormant remedies. Dr. Christopher used to say Lobelia "has brains," and directs the other remedies to where they have to go in the body. This is a quaint way of stating Thomson's basic theory.

Not only does Lobelia help other herbs find their appropriate points of application throughout the organism, but it seems to work better when used in combination with other agents. Compounding seems to take the edge off this unpredictable plant. I always feel more secure using it if I can add Lobelia in with other herbs. It seems as if the Lobelia likes to have other remedies to boss around and is more fully engaged in a compound.

Despite my best efforts at classification, here is a case history which does not neatly fit any of the above categories. This again demonstrates the wide range and peculiarities of this medicine. A sixty-year-old woman had been suffering from despair, fatigue and various digestive problems for many years. She was currently under the care of a chiropractor, who was working out kinks in the musculature of her neck, following a whiplash, which had been painful for many years. He also had her off amine-containing foods to reduce inflammation. Whenever she ate them her pain got worse, but when she didn't she felt like she was suffering from the shakes. She felt angry over restrictive diet, very hyped, but agitated and very fatigued at the same time. Unstrung, jittery. Would be constipated but she takes a mild herbal laxative. Pulse fine, thin and wiry. Tongue: some coating at the back, swollen edges, one very red spot towards the front, off to the side. The spot on the tongue was about the only symptom that seemed really distinctive—Lobelia is the only remedy I know of which has "lopsided" tongue variations. The fatigue combined with the jitters was also a possible symptom for this remedy, and the food withdrawal reminded me of tobacco withdrawal. Lobelia 6x, significantly improved the ability to cope, the neck pain and tension, and the shakes. The fatigue was improved, but not removed.

How the Homeopaths Repeated the Mistakes of the Allopaths

Here is a case where the homeopaths botched the opportunity to acquire a good remedy. Lobelia was proven in 1836 by Dr. Jeanes of Philadelphia, and latter by Noack and Trinks in Germany. Jeanes did some good work with Lobelia, but it was quickly forgotten. Being school-bred doctors, the homeopaths rejected the testimony of Thomson and copied the theories of the allopaths. These early experimenters latched onto the idea that Lobelia acted on the vagus nerve (or "pneumo-gastric," as it was then called) and missed the real insight which Thomson had into the "diffusive" properties of the medicine. As a consequence, homeopathy—just like allopathy—missed the fundamental understanding of the remedy. It is sometimes still used for asthma in homeopathy, but this represents only a fraction of its properties, as Thomson said. This is the only remedy I am acquainted with, which I think Boericke (1927), in his important little *Pocket Manual of Homoeopathic Materia Medica,* completely misunderstands and misrepresents.

Boericke's description of Lobelia is misleading. "Languor, relaxation of muscles, *nausea, vomiting and dyspepsia* are the general indications that point to the use of this remedy, in asthma and gastric affections," he writes. These are mostly the crude symptoms produced by massive dosing. Such a symptom picture is rarely encountered. I have used Lobelia scores of times, but only had one patient who fit this description.

The only sound account of Lobelia I have been able to find in nineteenth century homeopathic literature is that of Dr. Jeanes. (I am working from his work as quoted in C. J. Hemple's 1848 translation of Jahr's *Symptomen-Codex.*) This contains many good observations, characteristic symptoms, and case histories. Jeanes stuck to the allopathic concept that the vagus nerve was the center of action for Lobelia.

However, he still had a working knowledge of Lobelia.

The list of characteristic symptoms given by Jeanes are quite useful, whether one is a homeopath or an herbalist:

Constant dyspnea, which is increased by slight exertion, and aggravated so much by slight exposure to cold, as to form a kind of asthmatic paroxysm. A sensation of oppression and weakness at the epigastrium, extending upwards from thence into the breast, with or without pyrosis and cardialgia. A sensation of a lump or quantity of mucus, or of pressure, in the pit of the throat. A pain extending around the forehead from one temple to the other. Pain in the back about the lowest dorsal vertebra. Pain in the left side of the abdomen, immediately below the short ribs. High-colored urine depositing a copious red sediment.

Lobelia as an Activator or Accelerator

Samuel Thomson often used the diffusive herbs as activators, to stir up the other herbs in a formula and direct them to the desired tissue or organ needing therapy. Lobelia was especially used in this manner. Dr. Christopher said that it had the brains to tell the other herbs where to go. Lobelia is used especially as an activator for problems involving the musculature and respiration. Cayenne is used to stir and direct the blood, Bayberry for its actions on the lymphatics, and Prickly Ash bark for its action on the mucosa.

The use of activators or accelerators is an old American Indian tradition which seems to be unknown in European herbalism. It is still used today by Indian practitioners with traditional training, such as Cherokee herbalist David Winston. It is possible that Thomson adopted this technique from Indian medicine, but it is also possible that he came to the idea through his acquaintance with Lobelia. His reliance on this plant as one of his mainstays could have led him to this discovery.

The activators used by Thomson generally have a strong effect on the nerves. In addition to Lobelia, he used Prickly Ash, Bayberry Bark, Goldenseal, and Cayenne Pepper, all of which show their strong affinity to the nerves by causing tingling or burning. Each has its own sphere of influence. Lobelia acts especially on the nerves of the muscular system, Prickly Ash on the nerves of the mucosa and the nervous system generally, Goldenseal on the nerves of the mucosa, Bayberry Bark on lymphatic tissues and boggy membranes, and Cayenne on the vasculature. To this group could also be added Echinacea, which was little known in Thomson's era. It also causes the same tingling reaction on the tongue, acting as an accelerator for the lymphatics and venous side of the circulation.

Not all activators have to have cause tingling, however. We should recall, from an earlier chapter, how one ancient herbalist commented that every formula directed towards the stomach should contain Wood Betony. This remedy has such a general, stimulating effect on the stomach, through the solar plexus. It probably activates other herbs directed to the stomach.

Some plants just work together well, like Lobelia and Black Cohosh, or Agrimony and Solomon's Seal, or Burdock, Dandelion and Yellow Dock.

It took me a very long time to come to an appreciation of Lobelia as an accelerator, because I am such a homeopath at heart. I tend to like to use herbs as simples—by themselves—rather than in formulas. Lobelia is, however, an herb which actually seems to work best when it is used in combination, in small quantities, with another or other herbs. It really seems to like having other herbs to boss around! Lobelia causes less trouble when it is combined with another agent.

Herbs are so darn peculiar! I have long enjoyed the homeopathic model. By placing the emphasis on the single remedy, it helps us to get exact, concrete information about the materia medica. However, the homeopathic concept of provings, case-taking, and use of the single remedy in single doses is also wooden and stiff compared to the wild, strange world of the herbs themselves. They like to do all sorts of things. They really do have a magical level of action and this goes far beyond the artificial constructs of the human mind. They are multidimensional.

Preparation, Toxicity and Dosage

Lobelia is currently on the list of "suspect" herbs maintained by the FDA. It can be used in a homeopathic dilution, if one wants to avoid using such a plant, but it is difficult to say whether it is as effective.

The seedpods are the most potent part of Lobelia. These and the stems are considered the officinal parts in herbalism and homeopathy. Thomson speaks of great fluctuation in the size of the crop from year to year. The quality and properties of the crop also vary greatly so that it is difficult to find any two batches which have the same intensity. Some are relatively inert. This is just the sort of uncertainty we would expect from Lobelia, but it makes it hard to use. The bulk herb should be so active that it causes irritation at the back of the throat when the container is opened. The tincture should also convey this prickly sensation when dropped on the tongue. Thomson prepared his tinctures with either vinegar or alcohol. I prefer the latter, though the acetate was often considered to be more potent by the Thomsonians.

Lobelia is a very tricky remedy when the question of dosage is raised. Thomson and his followers used the famous "emetic" dose, but it is not necessary to produce vomiting to get the curative effects of Lobelia. Even if it is used as an emetic, the dose should still be moderate. Scudder writes, "To obtain the curative effects of a Lobelia emetic, the remedy should be given in small quantities frequently repeated, as it can be absorbed from the stomach, so that emesis, when it does occur, shall be from the general influence of the remedy in the blood, and not from its local irritant influence upon the stomach. Many physicians fail to obtain the benefit they have reason to expect because of its improper administration; it is not absorbed, but simply irritates the stomach." Scudder used "one drop or less" as a stimulant dose. "In some cases where there is necessity for a speedy action, as in cases of angina pectoris or neuralgia of the heart, I give one to two full doses of twenty drops."

I have used the tincture in single drop doses, no more than once a day. If the person is suffering from a severe condition of spasm or fever, they may need a greater dose and repetition. Sometimes I have used the 3x, 6x, 12x or 30x homeopathic potencies, and I know of people who have used the 200c with success. It is virtually impossible to know in advance how a given person will react to Lobelia, and what dosage will be appropriate. Lobelia works best if the patient can figure out the dosage for him- or herself. Using one to two drops per dose will seldom bring on nausea or emesis, and is to be preferred when an emetic is not desired.

Excessive doses of Lobelia can cause salivation, nausea, and temporary spasm. I have seen two drops, taken fifteen minutes apart, provoke vomiting. "I needed that," said the person I gave it to. Perhaps more dangerous is the capacity Lobelia occasionally shows to change blood volume rapidly. I know of a case where somebody got dizzy and feared she might black out and fall down. I would sit quietly for ten or fifteen minutes after the first dose of Lobelia.

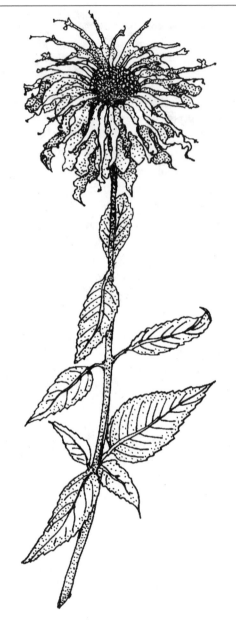

Monarda fistulosa

Sweet Leaf

Monarda fistulosa
Sweet Leaf

It has been the custom of authors writing on the botanical medicine and anthropology of the American Indians to discuss their use of medicinal herbs in the past tense, as if these practices were long gone. This is a good technique for suppressing the magical feeling which is associated with this marvelous tradition, to which many people still look with nostalgia. However, it gives an entirely false view of the situation. By no means is Indian medicine dead. After the anthropologists with their fixed opinions left, the Indians went back to helping themselves, their friends, and their families as they always had. The Indian Medicine Society still exists. Here and there, the knowledge of herbal medicine remains, from one end of the country to another. I have again and again met Indian people who unobtrusively proved this point in their humble use of the healing herbs. I have long been amused by accounts of medical anthropologists running off to the Amazon to discover new drugs, when I have learned so much from Indians right here in North America.

Even if there were no surviving practitioners, Indian herbalism would never die, because the Indian ancestors remain in the psychic ethers of the woods and prairies of our continent. They will always be here to help their faithful children, whatever their color or origin. However, there still are many Indian practitioners. I was reminded of this recently. A woman I know was trying to contend with breast cancer, without the help of conventional medicine. She had been calling a clinic in Sioux Falls for most of the day, trying to get through, but "there was something wrong with the phones." When she finally gave up, there was a knock on the door. An Indian man she had never met before was standing there with some herbs. He said, "These medicines will cure you." And he has been helping her ever since!

Monarda fistulosa is an example of a plant which is still widely used by American Indian healers, from one end of the continent to the other, but which is hardly known to non-Indian practitioners. It proves the point that Indian herbal medicine is still alive, still operating in a parallel reality distinct from the dominant culture, still full of rich discoveries that the medical anthropologists have never dreamed of. I was fortunate enough to learn about this magical plant from an Indian practitioner; it has been one of the most valuable plants in my herbal cupboard ever since.

This is also a medicine plant which Cherokee herbalist David Winston has shared with the herbal community. He uses the red species *(Monarda didyma.)* I originally thought, based on the accounts of Midwestern and Plains Indian people, that only the purple variety *(M. fistulosa)* was used in medicine. He corrected me, noting that the red species is preferred in Cherokee medicine.

Indian, pioneer and early medical practitioners also used the closely related Horse Mint *(Monarda punctata.)* This seems to have similar but not identical properties.

Getting the Name Right

I had never been able to resonate with the names for *Monarda fistulosa* found in the literature. "Wild Bergamot" was derived from a vague resemblance to the European Bergamot—a small unrelated citrus. "Bee Balm" seemed nice enough, but there are a half dozen "Balms" in herbaldom. "Oswego Tea" reflected local events in western New York, not the essence of the plant. *"Monarda"* was pretty enough, but it was derived from the name of a botanist. To make things even more confusing, all these names are also applied to a cousin, *Monarda didyma.* This plant looks almost identical, but has crimson to burgundy red flowers. It has similar volatile oils and properties, but is not the preferred plant in the area where I live. According to David Winston, it is a very valuable plant with similar properties.

The first thing I learned from Indian practitioners was the name

"Sweet Leaf." It was so beautiful and appropriate. I knew instantly that I would be able to understand this medicine.

In Indian herb training, the apprentice is often taught the "true name" of the plant. This name reflects in some way the essential nature of the medicine and gives insight into its personality and application. Sweet Leaf is the perfect name. In half a dozen Indian tongues the word "sweet" indicates something fragrant, tasty or beautiful, somewhat like the English word "fair." There is also an added inference in the word, as if there is an offering of bounteous richness from Mother Nature. These associations capture the essence of this plant so clearly. It is also known by Indian people as "Perfume" or "Indian Perfume." This reflects the same root word.

Sweet Medicine

Sweet Leaf is a member of the Mint family. It grows in open fields and meadows which have not been cultivated for some time, near the edges of forests across much of North America. It is cultivated in gardens as an ornamental. The pale violet, purple, lavender or white flowers mature in a circle around the globular head so that the flower top looks like a little crown. All parts of the plant are high in essential oils, giving it a rich, buttery taste and a magnificent smell. In Europe thirty-five tons a year are grown as a crop for the volatile oils. It is often cultivated as a culinary herb, having properties similar to Oregano. It combines well with Lavender in perfumes and with Sweet Marjoram in cooking.

Monarda fistulosa is one of a half dozen of the most important herbs used by the Indians of North America. It is considered to be a powerful medicine, a natural perfume, and a general "good sort of thing to have around." It even has a place in ceremony, including the Sun Dance. Despite this background, Sweet Leaf was little appreciated by white settlers and failed to find a place in the domestic or professional medicine of the dominant culture. This may have been because Europeans had many of their own mints transported from across the ocean, but Sweet Leaf is still irreplaceable, if not simply the best of the bunch.

Not only is Sweet Leaf largely unappreciated as a medicine, it is not correctly classified according to the Indian standard. The classification of plants by Indians and white botanists often differ. For instance, the old

Indian doctors considered *Trillium erectum* (white, upright flower) and *T. pendulatum* (red, pendulous flower) to be the male and female representatives of the same species. The same idea applies to the White and Red Cohosh. In the case of *Monarda fistulosa*, the Indians recognize many different types where the white botanists see only one. (Of course, no one should ever think of botanical nomenclature as a fixed or permanent part of reality!)

Melvin Gilmore addresses this problem in his *Uses of Plants by Indians of the Missouri River Region* (1919). He says that the Pawnee differentiated four types of *Monarda fistulosa*, based on their fragrance, appearance, and use. They classified the best as *parakaha* (fragrant, sweet) and the least choice as *'tsusahtu* (ill-smelling). The first species has stems "as weak as straw," the second has weak stems, the third has somewhat weak stems and small leaves, and the fourth has stiff, strong stems and larger leaves.

Gilmore comments, "The differences noted by the Indians among these varieties, if we may be allowed to call them varieties, are fixed and hereditary and not accidental or dependent on season or situation. Of this I am assured by my own experience with living specimens." He transplanted representatives of the third and fourth kinds into his garden and observed them for five years, at all seasons. They continued to breed true and preserve their distinctive properties. "I give this extended discussion because I have found taxonomists reluctant to admit the possibility of the distinction; at the same time they did not put it to the proof." The distinctions between the four races of Sweet Leaf are still observed by Plains people today. In South Dakota it is customary to prefer the soft-stemmed sweet variety. There are, however, other ideas about which plants to pick.

Perhaps each batch should be assessed individually. The taste, smell, and properties of *Monarda fistulosa* vary greatly, according to the location, season, and variety. The taste differs from extremely hot and pungent to rather sweet. The content and quality of the volatile oils will change quickly. Some samples taste buttery, because of the high oil content. Others pick up flavors like asphalt or petroleum from exposure to chemicals. These factors modify or destroy the medicinal properties.

Here are the indications I look for in Sweet Leaf. The stems should be somewhat flexible and soft, as Gilmore remarks. One should be able to feel the volatile oils on the stalk, leaves, and flowers. The taste should be sweet, pungent, peppery, hot, and (most important) "buttery." There need to be enough volatile oils to cause this "buttery" sensation in the mouth.

Generally, it is best to find a patch and keep picking from that spot year after year to get the same results. You can hang the herbs in bundles in the kitchen all winter. There is such an abundance of volatile oils that the properties are not greatly diminished by storage in the open air. The plant will last at least two years even left in the open air.

Draws Fire from the Skin

The right name leads to an appreciation of the essence of a medicine; so does knowledge of the characteristic action of that plant. If we can summarize the properties in a brief sentence that "says it all," we are well on the way to having a new herbal friend. The person who taught me about Sweet Leaf understood this very well. The basic definition of the action of the plant was very simple: it "draws out fire."

In the American Indian medical tradition burns are usually treated by applying hot to hot. This approach is sometimes found in European and American folk-lore, though more often the contrary idea (cold to hot) holds sway.

In her excellent book *Country Folk Medicine* (1995), Elisabeth Janos alludes to the Native American perspective on the treatment of burns. She interviewed an Indian healer who sometimes gave lectures on Indian medicine. He explained the basic concept. A burn should not be placed under cold water, but instead it should be warmed. He used the proper treatment of frostbite as an analogy. If a person's extremities are warmed up too quickly, the pain will be more severe and the tissue may mortify. Likewise with the burn. If it is cooled too quickly, the healing process will be hindered.

In addition to the idea of treatment by warm to warm, there is also a folk-medical concept that fire is a substance and can be "drawn out" of the body. It will flow into something similar (hot) but not something opposite (cold).

In short, Sweet Leaf is a plant which will draw out the fire. It is warm or even hot to the tongue, and it acts as a drawing agent for the particular substance of fire. As we will observe below, it is specific where the surface is cool but the depths are hot. When Sweet Leaf used as a burn medicine, the flowers are chewed up and the saliva placed on the area. Saliva contains an enzyme which activates the Sweet Leaf for this use. It may be necessary to clean off the area every few minutes if it is a bad burn.

My friends and I have verified this application many times. Cynthia, down the road, uses it for sunburn. "My son was burned on his neck. I went over and got some Sweet Leaf from the garden, chewed it up, and started to put it on him. 'Yuck,' he said. 'I don't want spit on me.' The next day he said, 'Mom, ya missed part.'"

Another time, I was visiting some friends in Chicago. One of them burned her finger at the stove. She complained in a loud, plaintive voice, "You're the homeopath, do something." I gave Cantharis, a homeopathic burn medicine, but nothing happened, so I had her put some spit on her finger and added some Sweet Leaf tincture. The pain disappeared immediately and the blister was gone in fifteen minutes. I was surprised.

Sweet Leaf does not work on every burn and it does not always relieve pain, but it is important for many. It probably works best in those cases where there is a cold sweat accompanying the burn. My favorite burn medicine is Agrimony (or its cousin Cinquefoil.) Here the characteristic is that the pain causes the person to catch the breath. Nettles is also an important burn medicine but I don't know the individualizing characteristics.

Draws Fire from the Internal Organs

Once we understand the characteristic nature of a medicine plant we can expand upon its uses because we comprehend its underlying "logic." I was not told that Sweet Leaf was a fever remedy (though it is listed as such in the books), but I figured that it would "draw out fever" the way it would draw fire out of a burn. When I mentioned this to the person who frist taught me about using it in burns, it was clear that he was fully aware of this usage as well.

What Sweet Leaf does for a burn it will also do for heat in the interior organs of the body. It draws fire out of the stomach, intestines, lungs, kidneys and deeper circulation. I have seen it settle hyperacidity, bronchial infection, diarrhea and constipation, and especially inflammation of the bladder. It is so highly diffusive and diaphoretic that it opens the pores of the internal organs as well as the skin, to remove heat. At the same time, it helps to retain the cooling fluids in the interior so that they are not lost through the skin.

I find that Sweet Leaf is particularly effective when there is fever with a cool, clammy skin. When it is given in an appropriate case, the skin will change from feeling clammy to having a warm, oily sensation. The fever is coming out and the cooling waters remain in the interior.

One time I was shopping at Present Moment Herbs in Minneapolis. A woman brought in her sixteen-year-old daughter for bronchial asthma. The shop clerks were harried and overworked so I was drafted to help out. She was a beautiful girl, a student of ballet, a bit noble in appearance, with a straight back. I thought of Sweet Leaf right away. The skin was clammy and cool. I didn't have any Sweet Leaf with me and the store didn't have any on hand either, but the family lived right down by the park where we had first seen the Sweet Leaf. I met them down there and we picked some Sweet Leaf. I saw the mother a year later. "Oh yes, my daughter is completely cured."

Sweet Leaf has been at my side when I really needed it. An eighteen-year-old boy from a town just south of my farm, came to the doctor with a severe pain in the lower right abdomen with swelling and tightness. It felt "constricted, like a pulled muscle, tensed up." The doctor thought it was probably appendicitis and sent him to the Emergency Room. The doctors down there thought the same thing. "It's probably appendicitis, but we won't know until we cut you open." That didn't sit right with the young man, so he refused surgery. The parents supported his decision. "We trust in the Lord," they explained. The surgeon was flabbergasted. "Lots of people are praying for him," his mother added as they left.

They gave him Echinacea without much success. If things turned bad his mother was going to make sure that he went to the hospital. While they were praying that evening, my "name came up." These were people who really knew how to pray and listen for an answer. They had trusted their lives to God years ago.

I got home late that night and was too lazy to run the messages off the machine. Imagine my surprise when I got to their message the next morning: "Our son has appendicitis and we heard you were an herbalist from so and so…" I called them right back and told them I'd be there as soon as possible. I wasn't worried about whether the boy would die from appendicitis and I would get in trouble. This family had faith in God, in me, and in the herbs, and I wasn't going to disappoint them. If I was afraid to do the right thing, my life would be worth nothing when it came time for me to face my Maker.

In twenty minutes I was at the bedside. The temperature was hovering at 100, the skin was very clammy, perspiration filled the room with a rank odor, the pulse was weak, slow, and lethargic, the tongue slightly swollen with adhesive coating, malar flush, eyes dull, pain in lower right abdomen unmitigated, has not been able to eat for two days, last bowel movement two days ago. He felt totally "worn out," but incapable of sleep or eating. I put some *Echinacea angustifolia* on his wrist, but it only produced a faint change. Then I put on a few drops of Sweet Leaf. The eyes and the skin dried off rapidly. I had the mother place a warm, moist cloth saturated with a half a dropper of Sweet Leaf tincture on the appendix area. Within a minute he said, "my right leg is cold…now it's cold and sweaty." Indeed, it was. I was a little unnerved to see such a prompt reaction. The father asked, "So how long have you been doing this work?" We soon realized it was a detoxification. I had him sip Sweet Leaf in water every ten minutes for the next day.

Within four hours the leg stopped sweating. He slept well. Twenty-four hours later the temperature was normal. Forty-eight hours later he ate a little gruel. I saw him three months later and he was in the bloom of health. Not only had he saved the expense of an operation (the family was uninsured), but the slow recovery that occurs after surgery. Furthermore, he had removed the stagnation or toxins that produced the problem, and which would probably have caused other difficulties later on.

What was most important, however, is that this young man had gained what the Indians call "medicine power." That's a special power, a confidence we gain when we put our life is God's hands. He had literally faced the prospect of death, and his parents had faced the prospect of losing him, but their courage, conviction and connection brought them through.

I was impressed, not only with the action of Sweet Leaf, but with the courage of the family, the exactitude and power of their prayers, and the healing power of God. They were true Christians. They could stand up and testify to the healing power of God.

The doctor this family first saw at the clinic was a friend of mine. Tom had been the teaching assistant when I was in a field botany class twenty years before. He was sympathetic to alternative medicine and loved plants, as I did. He added an additional piece of the story. "I sent them to the Emergency Room instead of a surgeon, so that they would have more time to think about what they were going to do." And indeed, they used that time to make a spiritually wise decision. Tom likes to pun, so he also quipped, "It must be the right herb, the appendix is like a fistula—*Monarda fistulosa.*"

Tom commented to the patient when we all met long after the incident: "The Lakota have a saying, 'Now is a good time to die.' " The young man understood exactly. If we stand on our principles, our life will have meaning and power. That is medicine. If we simply take the easy route, the obvious fork in the road, the statistically correct and conventional avenue, our life will not possess that spiritual power and testimony. It will be worth that much less. This, unfortunately, is the path of conventional medicine. Save the body at any cost but ignore the spirit. Treat the patient like a statistic, not an exceptional person.

In a sense, the word medicine has exactly opposite connotations in conventional Western and American Indian practice. For the doctors it means saving the body at any cost, including the loss of spirit, character and self-regulation. For the Indian people, it means connecting with something that comes from the Great Mystery, causes a change that the person by him- or herself could not manage, and leaves the healed person with a little piece of acquired "spirit power." Sometimes I think the differences between the two cultures are summed up in the contrast to the way the word medicine is used. Modern society is not geared to bring out the spirit, but ignore or even destroy it.

Another dramatic story was related to me by one of my friends. Wendy and her friend Maryann were invited to attend a Sun Dance on the Rosebud Reservation, just this side of the Black Hills. They were going to be staying with friends.

There was a white family who had been living with an Indian family out there for five years. The Indians lived in a shack, the whites in a tent behind it. The white woman had been bitten by a rattlesnake. She was just leaving the gate at a sacred spot where the Sun Dance grounds were being set up when the snake struck. One fang sank into her calf, the other grazed the skin. "It could have killed me," she said later. "But it didn't. It only sank in one fang." She was sure there was a lesson in it for her.

The Book of Herbal Wisdom

The people took her to the Indian Health Board hospital. The doctors considered her outside their jurisdiction since she wasn't a tribal member, but they couldn't turn down an emergency patient. They determined that she was allergic to the rattlesnake antidote and sent her home. Then the medicine men came and doctored her. They said, "We will try to keep the swelling away from the heart." The leg was swollen to twice its size and the swelling extended up to the diaphragm but stopped just short of the heart. If the swelling got to the heart, they said it would kill her. In addition, there was a purple-black streak running through the swelling up to the hip. The woman was wracked with pain and unable to sleep. This was the condition Wendy found her in when she arrived a week later.

The woman was resting with her head and chest elevated slightly to keep the venom in the leg. She was so tense and out of it, that it was hard for her to talk. At this point there was no guarantee that she would actually survive. The skin was cool and clammy, but she said she felt like she was burning up inside the swollen areas, "Like there's sunburn all over inside." She couldn't stand to be touched there, like someone with sunburn. Wendy, Maryann, and the woman's daughter chewed Sweet Leaf flowers and put them over the legs and abdomen. They changed the medicine every few minutes. Within minutes the heat started coming out, the swelling started to subside, and within an hour they could touch the area. That night she slept for the first time. The next day, Wendy noticed the purple-black color was not going down, so she put some Elderberry tincture on it and it started to break up. That evening the woman went to dinner at a friend's house. On the second day the swelling was almost gone and the purple streaks were turning red. She was able to take up her duties at the Sun Dance on the third day.

Draws Fire from the Urinary Tract

Sweet Leaf settles the nerves as well as fighting fire. As a remedy for nervous tension and burning pain, I thought it would be a great medicine for bladder infections. With experience, I found out that Sweet Leaf is unsurpassed in this complaint. It works in probably nine out of ten bladder infections—not only in people, but for cats. I have seen it work in chronic and acute conditions when there is a wide variety of symptoms and differences between cases. Sometimes it helps when there is lingering infection in the kidneys, but I would not necessarily rely upon it for acute kidney infections, which are very rapid and dangerous in progression. These generally demand medical advice or faith in God.

After hearing about this medicine, my good friend Margi Flint, herbalist (AHG) and "earth goddess" in Marblehead, Massachusetts, adopted this remedy into her armamentum. She had such success with it as a remedy for cystitis of unknown origin that the doctors at the hospital where she worked became very interested and started sending her patients. It has seldom failed her in this complaint. Some people get bladder infections from an unknown internal predisposition, rather than a bacterial infection. There is no known cause, it is very painful, and not easily treated. Margi's experience suggests a possible new remedy in this complaint. Sweet Leaf apparently works whether there is a bacterial infection or not.

Anything which is good for the urinary tract and removes heat and pain is also likely to help arthritic inflammation. In the folk-medical model, the condition of the kidneys is directly related to the joints, because the balance of fluids and solids influences whether or not minerals fall out of circulation, resulting in arthritis. I have not seen Sweet Leaf work in such conditions, but I have heard from reputable sources that it does.

Sweet Leaf is also beneficial for skin problems where there is pain imitating a burn. I once used it successfully for eczema on the scalp and eyelids. The skin of the forehead and forearms was clammy. Even a single dose noticeably relaxed the nerves and pulse.

An Excellent Remedy for Yeast Infection

I reported back to the person who first taught me about Sweet Leaf, noting how good it was for bladder infections. He didn't stop to boast, he just added the next piece of information. It was a very important remedy for yeast infections. Such conditions are often associated with infections of the bladder.

After learning this I gave *Monarda* for a vaginal yeast infection and it worked. I was grateful to be able to have another remedy in my arsenal for this difficult-to-treat condition. There are so few. (Barberry Root deserves notice here.) I told Pam Montgomery of Green Terrestrials in Milton, New York, about using Sweet Leaf for yeast infections. A year later she told me that she had used it three times for systemic yeast and it worked every time. In the last few years my friends and I have had quite a few successes with it in chronic candidiasis.

Recently, Oregano oil has appeared on the market as a remedy for yeast infection, vaginitis, and candida. Some of my friends say it works. I believe it would, since it is a native European plant very similar to Sweet Leaf in culinary and medicinal effect.

Chronic yeast infection is usually associated with what is called "leaky gut syndrome," where the pores of the intestines are too open and too much of the toxic contents of the bowels spills into the bloodstream, causing a burden on the liver and a generalized increase in toxic material in the body. It is believed that the yeast cells send down roots into the pores, which then keep them stuck open. It is my belief that Sweet Leaf works so well in many cases of chronic candida because it "tones the pores" of the intestine, just as it seems to "tone the pores" of the skin. It is for relaxed, open, perspiring skin pores, and it is likewise probably active on the pores of the bowels and other tissues throughout the body.

Calms and Tones the Nerves

Like many members of the mint family, Sweet Leaf is a sedative acting on the nervous system. The square stem of the mints, or the ridged stem of other plants (such as Cleavers), are a signature pointing to the nerves, both in American Indian and European herbal tradition.

As we shall see below, Sweet Leaf acts strongly on the brain, mind, and senses. It also acts on the solar plexus and the organs supplied by nerves from this center: stomach, liver, gallbladder, and intestines. It is a good remedy for digestive complaints, where it is soothing, calming, and cooling. By stimulating the nerve reflexes it helps the liver detoxify the blood and it releases the bile from the gallbladder. It also livens up the intestines, improving the tone of the nerves and tissues of the tract. Thus, it is beneficial in complaints such as constipation, gall stone colic, and hang-over. It helps clear the senses when the body is preoccupied with digesting a big meal or the liver is working on some alcohol, drugs or poisons.

I helped one woman who had constipation at an herbal conference. Her forearms were clammy and I figured she had a nervous stomach from being in a different place. Probably the gallbladder reflexes were tensed up. The next day she was regular. A few days later I was at an astrological conference. One of the presenters was suffering from diarrhea. He was sweaty and probably nervous. I thought, if Sweet Leaf works for constipation with nervousness and clammy sweat, it will probably work here. Sure enough, the cure was quick and effective.

Sweet Leaf is used as a tea before the sweat lodge ceremony in some Indian communities. It promotes perspiration, relaxes the nerves, reduces tension, and brings harmony and beauty to the participants. It is also used to calm babies when they are crying or upset.

This hints at an even deeper action of this powerful medicine plant on the nervous system. It only not calms and tones the nerves, but it acts very deeply to restore and improve the nerves of sense and thought. I learned this unexpectedly, from experience. I have never seen another remedy which acts so deeply on the nerves.

Deep Nerve Problems

I was helping a woman named "Carrie," who had been diagnosed with "atypical Meniere's disease" by doctors at the Mayo Clinic. I figured that meant she had some anomalous nerve disease. I had her on homeopathic *Lycopodium* for about a year. It stopped the dizziness and mental confusion and calmed down the ringing in the ears somewhat. I tried *Lycopodium* in lower and higher potencies like a good homeopath, but it just wouldn't hold. Sometimes I had to insert an "intercurrent" remedy when some symptom or other flared up. Her life was kept livable, but she wasn't getting cured.

Carrie had a friend who was a classical homeopath. "Well, I think I could do better," she said. "You should have just a single dose, taken once." This woman had no respect for the difficulty of the case. Carrie said, "I almost lost respect for her right there." Like so many classical homeopaths this practitioner was a fanatic rather than a seasoned observer who understood the limits of our art. Eventually Carrie felt obligated to give her friend a chance. The woman gave *Lycopodium* in a high potency. All it did was make the low potencies I had been giving not work anymore.

I had been helping Carrie for a year and a half and I had been using Sweet Leaf for a few months when they collided in my mind. I didn't know why, but I had to try it. The effect was immediate and powerful.

The dizziness, confusion, and buzzing were all dramatically improved. I only had a little bit of my preparation left and I was going out of town, so I told her to call a certain little Indian craft store and get some from the proprietor, "Gina."

Meanwhile, Gina was having a serious set of symptoms. She was suffering from dizziness, confusion, and buzzing in the ears. I was out of town and so was another herbalist she relied upon. "Where are my medicine men when I need them!" she complained. She was even ready to go to a medical doctor. Just then Carrie called her up. Gina was busy and wanted to get her off the line, but when Carrie mentioned her symptoms, Gina recognized them as her own. She got some Sweet Leaf for Carrie and took it for herself and was cured.

When I got back Gina said, "Matt, you're a real medicine man. You healed me even when you were away." Since then she has used it to cure or palliate Meniere's disease in other people.

I told this story to a class out in Buffalo, Minnesota, west of my place. A woman got really interested in Sweet Leaf and wanted some of it for her tinnitis (ringing in the ear.) I noticed that she had a bloated, yellowish complexion and thought, "She ought to make an appointment and see me, she needs to get that gallbladder cleared out. Probably constipated too." I thought her interest in Sweet Leaf was ridiculous. The story about Carrie and Gina was so crazy, even I didn't believe it would work again. Furthermore, this woman only had tinnitis, not Meniere's. Still, at her request I got her some Sweet Leaf tincture. That was on a Saturday.

On Wednesday she called. "Well, I haven't given up hope, but it hasn't worked yet." (Of course not, I thought to myself, she ought to make an appointment to see me. I was just humoring her until she saw the light.) She rambled on. "I used three dropperfuls, three times a day." That stopped me. "What?" I asked. "The directions on the label say three drops, three times a day." I suggested she try the lesser dose (though I was still humoring her.) If it didn't work at three dropperfuls a dose, it probably wasn't going to work at three drops.

I got a call the next morning. The very next dose of three drops gave our enthusiast diarrhea. It turned out that, yes, she had been constipated for twenty years. She woke up the next morning and the tinnitis was half gone. The ringing did not get better but it didn't worse after the initial improvement, but she was very grateful. "I can hardly remember what it used to be like; it drove me crazy." Only then did I remember that Sweet Leaf was a remedy to open the gallbladder and stimulate the intestines.

Years later I ran into this woman at a health food store. I didn't even recognize her because the swollen, bloated yellow complexion was gone. I commented, "I see the gallbladder is better." Hunh, was about the limit of her reply. The ringing had eventually subsided, now she had hypersensitive hearing.

One of my students gave some Sweet Leaf to a man who was suffering from some nervous complaint. He immediately got a bit dizzy after taking the first dose. Within the next few days his senses improved. He claimed he could see and hear better. My friend commented that he seemed more grounded-Sweet Leaf acts on the solar plexus slightly, like Wood Betony. This experience suggests that Sweet Leaf acts deeply on the senses.

At any rate, more than anything, Sweet Leaf is a great medicine for Meniere's and tinnitis. Between my students, friends and myself, we have improved or cured well over a dozen cases. There have been only three or four failures. Some people have needed to take it for a long time.

One of my herbal friends in New England started to use Sweet Leaf for Meniere's and tinnitis and had much success with many people. In only one case did it not work. She believed this was because the person had been dosed with radiation in the past. She did, however, help him with another problem. Just as he was leaving, he mentioned that he was having a difficult time with a tenant upstairs. (He lived in the downstairs of a duplex he owned.) He was afraid to kick her out because she was a spiteful, vengeful person who knew all the legal loop-holes and would make trouble for him.

My friend gave the fellow Sweet Leaf for the Meniere's and a spray bottle with some Agrimony in it. (Remember how we use that for "interference.") He sprayed it all around his apartment and the one occupied by the tenant. In two days she complained how she hated the house. She gave her notice and moved out that very day. The whole thing was not only a great relief to the landlord but a remarkable testimony to the influence of a plant. My herbalist friend said, "Don't tell anybody about this or they'll run me out of town on a rail." So her name remains unknown, though I would like readers to know that these strange, miraculous healings and magical shifts happen to other people as well.

Back to Sweet Leaf and a more scientific approach. During a lecture attended by one of my friends, ethnobotanist Dr. Jim Duke noted that, based on its chemistry, *Monarda fistulosa* should be one of the best candidates as a remedy for Alzheimer's Disease. Personally, I don't know much about plant chemistry, but this made sense to both myself and my friend. Sweet Leaf has such a deep, searching, cleansing, building, and restoring influence on the nervous system. It helps subtle nerve processes which are associated with the ability to perceive, appreciate, and express beauty and harmony in life.

The Passion Medicine

It took me a long time to understand the personality of Sweet Leaf, though now it seems transparent and clear to me. This is the medicine that helps us appreciate beauty and deal with passion. Such a problem is so deeply human, and must be widespread, but I had never thought about it as something an herb could heal or influence.

One time I was leading an herb walk in Wisconsin. I gave a sprig of Sweet Leaf to the woman nearest me and went on talking. In a few minutes she said in a concerned and confused tone, "What was that supposed to do?"

"Uh, well," I stammered, "what did it do to you?" I was expecting her to say that her throat was swelling up or see was having a tachycardia attack and we needed to bring her to the Emergency Room. Fortunately, I was pleasantly disappointed.

"When you gave it to me I suddenly heard this whole symphony orchestra playing this beautiful piece of music. It went on for a minute or two before dying away." She said all of this as if something wrong had happened. She was a passionate person who, however, sometimes mistrusted having strong feelings.

I forgot this experience for a few years, but it came back to me when I began to appreciate the personality of this wonderful plant. I also remembered the sixteen-year-old aspiring dancer. Sweet Leaf is a medicine plant which helps us to sense beauty around us and also helps us deal with the passion that is stirred as a part of our human nature.

Nature's Medicine

Sweet Leaf is one of the primal healing plants of North America. It illustrates one of the seven great truths which we confort on the medicine path. I mentioned these seven lessons in my book, *Seven Herbs, Plants as Teachers.*

The first lesson on the path is that Nature is alive. She offers her goods to us. These include the beauty and richness of the land and of all natural beings. Each is supplied with some part of this richness. We are stimulated by this beauty. We are endowed with passions and loves which attract us to different people, callings, places, and things. We need to work with the resources of Mother Nature to live and follow our calling. We need to do this in a way which is respectful. If we do not respect our Mother, we are worthless. Sweet Leaf teaches us to perceive beauty, to trust and go with our passion to create something else that is beautiful, and to respect the sources of our inspiration.

There is, within each of us, a little piece of Mother Nature. Our personal life is a fragment of the All Life. It is a precious gift which we should not take for granted. This too we should treat with respect. It would be better if we did not burn up this gift of life in wasteful pursuits, though it seems to be our nature to do so.

This little sliver of life is like a drop of mortal oil which burns from birth to death. When the oil burns out, the flame goes out and the life is over. The old alchemists had an idea that the volatile oils in flowers were a food for this "mortal oil" which kept alive this "wick of life."

Alchemical doctors like Paracelsus liked to give Lemon Balm *(Melissa officinalis)* as a general tonic; it is one of the European herbs which contains the most essential oils. Melissa was believed by the common people to be an elixir of longevity.

Sweet Leaf is probably the best American analog of Lemon Balm. I like to think the volatile oils contained within it feed and cleanse the "oil of life" burning within. The volatile oils of Sweet Leaf are sometimes valuable as a food which need to be consumed from time to time. I have known a few people who have to consume Sweet Leaf or similar culinary herbs with lots of volatile oils on a regular basis in order to remain healthy.

Remember that the remedies that are sweet, full of juiciness, beau-

377

ty, and aroma are the deer medicines. The mints and other plants, with their fine, sharp-edged stems, are also lumped together in this group. Indeed, any plant which helps us to understand and cope with beauty is a deer medicine, or (if it is used as a love charm) an elk medicine. Sweet Leaf is used as a perfume so it is also a love charm. It grows in the kinds of places which the deer frequent, in old fields near the edges of woods, where feeding and hiding are hardly a breath away from each other.

Preparation and Dosage

Sweet Leaf should be picked when the flowers are at their peak. Fortunately, this plant is in bloom for about a month in July and August. The flowers, stalks, and leaves are all used. The herb is just as good fresh or dried. Leave the roots in the ground to grow another year. Since I am accustomed to using tinctures, I make mine by macerating the fresh or dried herb in vodka. For some reason, it does not turn out well if brandy of equal proof is used. The dose is small: one to three drops, one to three times a day, as needed. In acute fever, one may need give it continuously. (If you use this plant for burns you have to add your own supply of saliva.)

Wild Bergamot is used in the culinary arts and it has no known toxicity. It is classified with the many safe mints used in cooking.

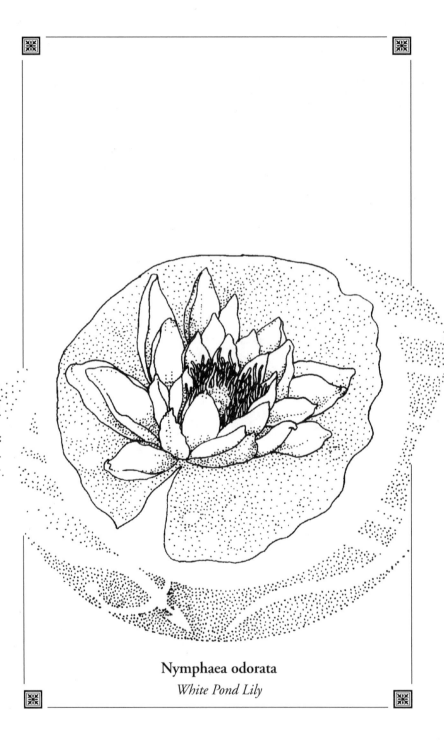

Nymphaea odorata
White Pond Lily

Nymphaea odorata

White Pond Lily

The beautiful water lily is native to Europe, Asia and North America. There are several different species which have been used in herbal medicine. The appearance and properties of these half dozen species are very similar. Water lilies have been used since antiquity in European herbalism, and likewise by the American Indians. Separate traditions in different parts of the world have generated similar ideas about the uses of this plant. Furthermore, the traditional Western concepts fit perfectly with the profile of "kidney *yin* deficiency," which is so important in Traditional Chinese Medicine. The dovetailing of different traditions shows how the basic strength, perspective, and validity of ancient, traditional, and folk medicine throughout the world. Although cultures may be totally unrelated, they still look to natural patterns in the organism, and what do they find? The same patterns.

The common water lilies of Europe are the White (*Nymphaea alba*) and the Yellow (*Nuphar lutea*). They have been shown to contain considerable starch, tannins and several alkaloids. Water lilies have long been used as food and medicine in Europe. Dioscorides and Plinius speak of them. Even at this early date they were already known for their ability to diminish sexual desire and stop the flux of various fluids from the body, thus restoring stamina. (This is what the Chinese would call "deficient kidney *yin*.") Water lilies were used by Indian and pioneer doctors, and a few homeopathic provings were made, but the plant was largely forgotten by professional doctors by the late nineteenth-century. Today, *Nymphaea* is largely used by herbalists for vaginal itching and discharge.

381

These rather limited indications were received from Samuel Thomson; otherwise, the use of Water Lily might have died out altogether.

"Kidney *Yin* Deficiency"

The correlation between traditional Western indications for Water Lily and the traditional Chinese concept of "deficient kidney *yin*" is so remarkable that we can discuss them together. The "kidneys" are more or less equivalent to the sexual-urinary tract. The fluids or *yin* of the body are low or deficient, so that they cannot sedate the heat, resulting in generalized irritation and overexcitement. There may be a further loss of fluids due to heat: night sweats, diarrhea, and loss of sexual fluids are common. There may be loss of sperm, urine, prostatic fluids, vaginal discharges or excessive menstrual bleeding. Generalized weakness and debility are common, with weakness of the lower back and knees in particular. There may be a flush of heat in the afternoon. Often the cheeks are red: the so-called "hectic flush" or "malar flush." The pulse is usually rapid and nonresistant, as the heat is "having its way with the system." These "*yin* deficiency" fevers were known in the older Western textbooks as "hectic fevers." Now compare these indications with the use of Water Lily.

Gerard (1597) gives an eloquent introduction to this plant. "The Physitions of our age do commend the floures of white Nymphaea against the infirmities of the head which come of a hot cause: and do certainly affirme, that the root of the yellow water lily cureth hot diseases of the kidnies and bladder, and is singular good against the running of the reines," that is, uncontrolled discharge of urine or sperm. "The root and seed of the great water lilie is very good against venery of fleshly desire, if one do drinke the decoction therof, or use the seed or root in powder in his meates, for it dryeth up the seed of generation, and so causeth a man to be chaste, especially used in broth with flesh. The conserve of the floures is good for the diseases aforesaid, and is good also against hot burning fevers." The leaves of either water lily "laid upon the region of the backe in the small, mightily cease the involuntary flowing away of the seed called Gonorhea, or running of the reines."

Gerard felt that the white kind was the stronger of the two. "Water Lillie with yellow floures stoppeth laskes, the overflowing of seed which commeth away by dreames or otherwise, and is good for them that have the bloudie flix," or dysentery. However, "water Lillie which the white floures is of greater force." It also stays the whites and external bleeding.

Culpeper says that this plant is "under the dominion of the Moon, and therefore cools and moistens." He does not specifically mention the applications to the sexual sphere, but recommends them to stay "all fluxes in man or woman," and also "for those whose urine is hot and sharp," and to "procure rest and to settle the brain of frantic persons." Preparations of the flower and leaves are used externally on inflammations and hot swellings. The moon represents the habitat of water lilies, since the moon rules all terrestrial waters in astrology. In addition, Culpeper is thinking of how the water lilies nourish, cool, and build up the waters of the body, thus stopping fluxes.

Nuphar lutea was given a homeopathic proving by a Dr. Petit of France, in the middle of the nineteenth-century. After further experience he was able to support these scanty provings with a handful of case histories. His account can be read in Hale's *New Remedies*. *Nuphar* produces such symptoms as "weakness; restlessness; diminution of the strength; and flush." (This sounds very much like a description of the hectic flush associated with "*yin* deficiency.") The mental symptoms are quite interesting. "Excessive moral sensibility, giving one great pain on witnessing the suffering of animals," yet "great impatience at the slightest contradiction." Headaches were prominent, a painful sensation of weariness in the stomach with slow digestion and wind colic. Early morning diarrhea was prominent, resulting in further exhaustion. Impotence or excess desire, sexual exhaustion, and aggravation from sex, especially in men. Nocturnal emissions. After ten or twelve days, small itching blotches like psoriasis appeared on the skin. There was also "sensation like flea-bites in different parts for several days."

Dr. Petit provides a number of case histories, of which one will suffice. A man had been suffering for nine years from involuntary seminal secretion during sleep, while defecating and when urinating, without erection. He was pale and languid. He took *Nuphar* for a month. "His paleness diminished, his general weakness disappeared by degrees, and his digestive functions took a new start. At the same time the pollutions ceased, erections came on, accompanied by a decided propensity for the generative act, and before the thirtieth day of the treatment he was able to satisfy it with success, and without fatigue." So that was a happy ending.

The Underwater Panther

The American water lilies were widely used by the Indians for food and medicine. The Menomini Indians informed anthropologist Huron Smith that this plant belongs to the spirits of the Underneath. This is perhaps not surprising, for a huge chunk of the root, dragged up from the nether reaches of a muskeg swamp by a moose or beaver, looks like some monstrous sea serpent hurled from the weird mansions of the Underworld. The plant is especially linked with the Underwater Horned Serpent, the great totem of the Grand Medicine Society. This fantastic animal, which lurks in our northern waters, is also called the Underwater Panther. It is an archetypal cousin to Behemoth, the Sea Monster of Old World origin.

The Underwater Panther is one of the largest and most powerful residents of the Underworld. Like Behemoth, it is a being or symbol representing and personifying the waters of the world. It is the primal waters of the world.

The Menomini remark that water lilies generate the fogs that hover over lakes. This is not a matter of inconsequence, since the Great Spirit is said to be most readily observed in these intangible mists which arise from time to time. This demonstrates how the forces that arise from below meet the forces which descend from above, like yin and yang, in order to make visions of important things available. In fact, this mist represents the faculty of seership or imaginative vision, in which images reflect spiritual truths. In the Water Lily we see an overactive imagination and susceptibility to lascivious images.

What Water Lily does for the cosmos it does for the individual. It was used by the Indian for many of the same problems as the Europeans. It fortifies the misty and refined fluids, so that a balance of opposite forces may be achieved, particularly in the nether reaches or sexual area of the organism. The root is large and starchy, containing much carbohydrates, mucilage, and tannins so that it makes an ideal topical dressing for external sores and inflammation, also acting through the system to soothe and tone the mucosa and the attendant internal surfaces and organs.

The American water lilies were quickly taken up by the white settlers, who fortified their own valuable traditions with native lore.

Unfortunately, they were too conceited and fearful about religion to learn about the Underwater Panther.

Water lily was well known to the early colonial doctors, the "fathers of allopathy," as we may call them. Cutler (1785) says that the roots of the native lilies were used, "in the form of poultices, for producing suppuration in boils and painful tumors, and are very efficacious." Dr. Jacob Bigelow (1817), who went to the trouble of writing a three volume materia medica, mostly to indulge his skepticism about various native medicinals, gives a glowing report on Water Lily. "The roots of this plant are among the strongest astringents, and we have scarcely any native vegetable which affords more decided evidence of this property. When fresh, if chewed in the mouth, they are extremely styptic and bitter." This statement which reveals a poorly trained sense of taste, plus a lack of knowledge about the truly powerful astringents and styptics in the vegetable kingdom, such as Wild Geranium and Oak. Compare Bigelow's superficial analysis with Dr. Cook's assessment below. "The roots are kept by most of our apothecaries, and are much used by the common people in the composition of poultices."

The officinal species in herbal medicine is generally considered to be the White or Sweet-scented White Water Lily, named *Nymphaea odorata*. This has a wide range, growing from Newfoundland to Manitoba, south to Florida and Louisiana. The Yellow Pond Lily (*Nymphaea advena*) is also used. It is even more widely distributed, from Labrador to the Rocky Mountains, south to Florida and Texas, west to Utah.

Dr. William Cook (1869) gives a lengthy account of *Nymphaea odorata*. "These roots are mildly and very pleasantly astringent, slightly stimulating, leaving behind a tonic impression, and with just enough mucilage to make their action rather soothing. The yellow is rather more stimulating than the white." Here is someone who had a trained sense of taste.

"Their influence is expended upon mucus membranes, excessive discharges from which are lessened by them; while tenacious discharges are loosened, ulcerative conditions healed, and the tone of the structures improved. Their action is quite gentle, but persistent; and they never leave behind that dry condition incident to the use of geranium and astringents of that class." Such articles more accurately deserve the term "styptic."

"Sub-acute dysentery and diarrhea are the maladies for which they have been most used, and they are truly excellent in such cases; but they may be employed with equal, if not greater, advantage in all mild forms of leucorrhea and prolapsus, with a tendency to ulceration of the cervix." They are beneficial either orally or by vaginal injection. "Also in catarrh of the bladder, lingering congestion and aching of that organ, and chronic irritation of the prostate gland with gummy discharges." Local applications are beneficial for subacute and chronic inflammation of the eyes and mouth, ulcers associated with lymphatic weaknesses, irritation, and foul discharge, of a mild nature, including venereal ulcers.

Water lily roots were long used as a food in both northern Europe and northern America and this nourishing property shines through in the medicinal sphere. "They influence the assimilative organs," continues Cook, "and may be employed to great advantage in those forms of scrofula which present weakness of the bowels and a tendency to curdy diarrhea."

The term scrofula in this instance would refer to a general stagnation and swelling in the lymphatic structures. "Scrofula" has been too narrowly defined by modern interpreters to mean suppurating and tuberculous glands, especially in the neck. It is clear from the descriptions of the old authors, and the actions of the plants they used to treat "scrofula," that they were often just referring to a generalized lymphatic stagnation and hypertrophy.

Nymphaea odorata was given a homeopathic proving by a Dr. Cowles, who was the only subject. The symptoms produced were not exactly those noticed in the proving of *Nuphar lutea,* yet they still fit under the same general heading of kidney *yin* deficiency—or Sea Monster deficiency, if you like. More of a head cold and sore throat kind of a situation was setup. There was again the morning diarrhea. There was a slight increase in sexual desire, weakness of the back, and involuntary passage of urine, with feeling as if it was not all expelled. "Lascivious dreams."

In my experience, the single most important symptom is the rapid, nonresistant pulse.

Preparation and Dosage

Rafinesque (1830), who immigrated from Europe as a young man, says that the properties of the American lilies are similar to the European, "but much more efficient and decided." Cook believed the white flowered variety was better for internal use, the yellow flowered for external. Millspaugh says that the "European species differs but slightly from our *N. odorata.*" It is doubtful that he was able to compare them in person, as was Rafinesque.

The fresh root, gathered in the fall, is sliced thin and dried. "The form of infusion is the best for internal administration, in most cases; made by pouring a pint of boiling water on two drachms of the root, of which one or two fluid ounces may be given every two hours," says Cook. "No iron implement should be used while preparing it."

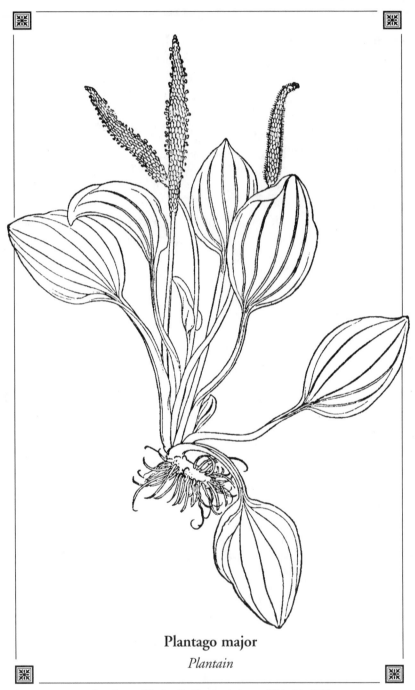

Plantago major

Plantain

from Leonard Fuchs, *De historia stirpium,* published in 1542

Plantago major
Plantain

This common weed, growing between cracks in the sidewalk and on paths well beaten by traffic, is an Old World native, but has spread to all continents in the last few centuries. In locations as diverse as North America and the South Pacific it has been called "Whiteman's Footprint."

There are several members of the genus *Plantago* used in herbal medicine. *Plantago major* is the most common. It is used interchangeably with *P. lanceolata*. The first has a broad leaf, somewhat like a wide tongue, the second has a lance-like leaf; both are also called Ribwort. These plants were prominent in the medicine of the early Anglo-Saxons. *P. psyllium* is the source of Psyllium seed, used as a mucilage and mild laxative in herbal and allopathic medicine.

Plantain is the type of common weed which is a perennial favorite in folk medicine. It is widely available, safe to use, and easily applied to a variety of common complaints. Plinius mentions it, for example, as an important remedy for boils. "Plantain, applied with salt, five-leaf (*Potentilla*), and the root of the great clot-bur," is the remedy of choice, he relates. This is still sound advice. He also used Plantain for the most severe kinds of shingles, when the horrible blisters arch around the middle of the torso and threaten death. "To prevent this extremity [of death], plantain is thought to be a sovereign remedy, if it be incorporat with fuller's earth."

Dioscorides gives additional indications. *Plantago* is drying and binding he says, stops the flux of blood, carbuncles, herpes, and other skin eruptions, including "all malignant and leprous, running and filthy vlcers." It is also benefical for swollen glands, including the parotids, pains in the ears, griefs of the eyes, bleeding gums, and "doth cleanse the vlcers of the mouth." He remarks that it acts on asthma, consumption, the stomach, dysentery, epilepsy, and "stranglings of the womb." Galen classified Plantain leaves as cold and dry in the second degree, meaning that it is cooling to hot, inflamed tissues and drying when there is a flux or discharge. It is still classified in this manner today in Arabic medicine. Plantain was thought to have particular affinities to the head and genital regions.

Plantain continued to appear in nearly every herb book, down to the present. Gerard attempted to strain out the superstitious uses when he wrote his account. "I finde in ancient Writers many good-morrowes, which I thinke not meet to bring into your memorie againe; as that three roots will cure one griefe, foure another disease, six hanged about the necke are good for another maladie, &c. all which are but ridiculous toyes."

Plantago major was introduced to the homeopathic audience by Dr. Edwin Hale about 1870. It received a homeopathic proving shortly after, which demonstrated the validity of the traditional applications. It was widely used in botanical, eclectic, and homeopathic medicine at the turn of the century. Dr. J. H. Clarke speaks quite glowingly of this little plant, often ignored in homeopathic texts. Plantago "is one of the most useful of *local* remedies in homoeopathy." Here it is most commonly used as a salve, in the manner employed by herbalists. With this local application he has seen it cure erysipelas, poison ivy, erythema, burns, scalds, swollen glands (especially of the breasts), bruises, incisions, bites, and frostbite.

The "Herbal Drawing Agent"

Plantain is, first and foremost, the primary "herbal drawing agent." Although conventional medicine does not imagine such a faculty, there are several plants which are known to herbalists for their ability to pull splinters, dirt, pus, and infection out of wounds. Plantain is probably the chief representative of this group. Exactly what chemical constituents allow for this faculty is not clear, but we see it in the signature or natural history of the plant itself. Plantain grows on hard, compacted ground, showing that it has an ability to pull nutrients from the hard-packed soil. What it can do for itself, it can do for us.

Father Sebastian Kneipp describes how Plantain has long been used as a folk medicine on wounds. "When the country people have wounded themselves at their work they seek quickly for ribwort leaves, and do not cease squeezing until they have forced a few drops out of the rather stubborn leaf. This sap they either put directly on the fresh wound, or else they moisten a little rag with it, and place it on the wounded part. If the leaf refuses its medicinal sap, and only becomes soft and rather moist with rubbing, they place the soft leaf itself on the wound."

"Is there any danger of blood-poisoning in this proceeding?" the good Father asks. This is his expression for tetanus. He says it will prevent this disastrous complication. "The plant sews the gaping wound together as with a golden thread, and like rust never gathers on gold, so all putridness and proud flesh flies from the ribwort."

One of my students studied under an old herbalist in Minneapolis, now deceased. A fellow came to him after he had fallen off a motorcylce and skidded along the road. His ankle looked like chopped meat, the wounds were full of dirt, and the doctors had no idea how to clean them out. The herbalist juiced up some Plantain leaves and poulticed the wound throughout the day. The next morning the inflammation was down and the wound was clean.

Plantain leaves are placed on bee stings, insect bites, and snakebites to draw out the venon. "A woman with only one arm came to me in great distress," wrote Dr. Shook. "She had been stung by a bee on the only hand she had left. Several years previously, she had been similarly stung by a bee. That time she had gone to a doctor because the whole arm was swollen and she was in grave danger." The doctor lanced the swelling and drained the pus, but the arm had to be amputated. "This lady was in abject despair, believing she would lose her other arm." We can well imagine. There was some Plantain outside Dr. Shook's door. "I picked some of the leaves and gave them to the woman, telling her to wash and crush them, make a poultice and apply to the part where she had been stung. Next day, this lady returned to thank me and pay for my advice. The hand was entirely well."

The Anishinabe herbalist Keewaydinoquay of Garden Island in Lake Michigan told a rather remarkable story about Plantain. A woman tagged along on an herb walk she was giving one summer. Keeway-dinoquay pointed out Plantain as a drawing agent, especially beneficial for removing venom. The woman returned to Florida. Several months later she was out with two friends in a garden when they ran into some black widow spiders—a nest of them, probably. They were all bitten and decided to go to the doctor the next day. The one woman remembered about Plantain, chewed up a leaf, and put some on the bites. The next day the other two women were dead.

Tongue, Gums and Teeth

William Coles (1657) classified Plantain under the mouth, because of the great affinities this plant has to that cavity and because the leaf looks like a tongue. This sounds a bit fanciful, but it hits the mark because Plantain is a medicine of great importance for the mouth, gums, and teeth. It is an excellent general tonic for the gums, pulling out infection and toning the tissues. There are many people who are afflicted with infection about the roots of the teeth, which may or may not respond to dental surgery. Plantago has a remarkable ability to draw out the infected material. This use goes back in eclectic, homeopathic, and botanical literature.

I have seen Plantain draw pus and infection from the roots of teeth and the empty sockets several times in the most remarkable manner. Following the extraction of a molar, a friend of mine got a rapidly spreading infection extending from the socket up into the maxillary sinus, the nose, and perhaps towards the brain. Only a few hours had passed and she was in excruciating pain. She called me and asked what she should do. "Why don't you go to the emergency room," I replied. She thought I was joking. She pulled my arm until I suggested she get some dried Plantain leaves (it was winter), roll them up, and place the wad under the socket. This promptly reduced the pain and several hours later brought away "six huge gobs of pus like caterpillars."

My friend Susan had a tooth disintegrate one Saturday morning during a Memorial Day weekend. It was impossible to get a dental surgeon except at the emergency room—even that promised to be tough. By the time I arrived her face was red, hot, and sweaty, there was a shooting pain from the root of the teeth up into the brain and she was in excruiating pain. St. John's Wort and Plantain tinctures placed on a cotton ball or swished in the mouth relieved the pain, removed much infected material, and kept the whole thing manageable until Tuesday morning.

Respiratory Tract

Plantain is a moist, cool herb. Distinctive, long fibers run through the leaves. They contain mucilage and fiber. The former soothes and cools irritated tissue, mucus membranes, and the skin. The latter stimulates the peristaltic action in the bowels and the activity of the mucosa of the alimentary tract generally. There is also a subtle effect on the nerves. Plantain not only soothes inflamed nerves, but can help bring back damaged nerve function. This property is reflected in the doctrine of signatures: long, nerve-like veins run through the leaves—as any young child can testify.

Plantain has an affinity to all mucus membranes, which it cleanses and disinfects, just as it does the skin. For this reason it has been used for respiratory inflammation. It lessens irritation, cools, lubricates, and removes phlegm.

I have used it where the cough gave the impression that there was something like a fine splinter stuck in the side of the bronchial tube or trachea, provoking the cough. A twelve-year-old girl had a dry cough from age three months, the cause of which could not be found. I thought it sounded like a particle was stuck in there and gave Plantain. She was cured in a week. Another man had a chronic irritated cough which had been bothering him for three years. "When did it start?" I asked. Since I wasn't a doctor he decided to be honest. "Well, I was stopped at a traffic light on my bike. When the light turned this big truck spewed all this exhaust at me and I breathed some of it in. Ever since then, I've had this cough." Plantain tincture cured completely. "Prozac," says the doctor.

Plantain is also beneficial where there is a well seated infection producing mucus. "The dried leaves of ribwort yield likewise a splendid tea against interior phlegm-obstructions," noted Father Kneipp. He liked to combine it with *Pulmonaria officinalis,* a plant most useful in very deteriorated and infected conditions in the lungs. This is a good match for Plantain.

In the winter of 1995-96 there was a very bad flu that often lapsed into pneumonia. One woman I was trying to help had an especially severe case. I had to recommend that she go to a doctor and get antibiotics. Even then, she still teetered on the brink of respiratory failure for months. I tried various things with little success. One of my students even sat in to observe and got sick herself! By spring, six months after the initial attack, she was still experiencing respiratory distress whenever she went off the antibiotics, so I sat down with the intention of remaining until we had the right remedy. About an hour and a half later I decided to try Plantain. This turned the corner. It brought up an enormous amount of dark green, smelly phlegm and she started to get better. "It drew out all that infected material," was what she said six months later. That was when I was trying to help her again with respiratory oppression and infection. The Plantain drew out the mucus and was very important to her healing, but it still did not cure.

Culpeper says that Plantain is "held an especial remedy for those that are troubled with the phthisic, or consumption of the lungs, or ulcers of the lungs, or coughs that come of heat."

Large Intestine

Plants which have a red-purple color are often suited to conditions where there is toxic heat or low-grade septic conditions. They often act upon the large intestine and portal circulation draining off that area. Some of our most important detoxifiers figure here: Dandelion, Burdock, Echinacea, and Plantain. The latter has long been used for removing pus and infection. In addition, the fiber content of Plantain makes it a gentle stimulant to the bowels, so that it exercises the intestines and furthers elimination. Plantain is a cousin of Psyllium seed, used as a bulk agent for the bowels. Thus, it is considered a laxative; yet the old authors also spoke of it as a drying agent for diarrhea and dysentery, so it acts both ways as a regulator. At the same time, the mucilaginous qualities soothe and coat the membranes. Finally, as a drawing agent, Plantain seems to pull stagnant materials out of the colon. In short, we have a remedy which stimulates the activities of the intestines, coats and soothes the walls, detoxifies the blood supply, and assists elimination.

The old authors often mentioned the action of Plantain on the intestine. Culpeper says it "prevails wonderfully against all torments or excoriations in the guts or bowels," and Gerard notes that it "stoppeth the boudy flix and all other fluxes of the belly." It also acts strongly on the uterus and genitalia, removing heat and stopping excessive bleeding. Culpeper says it is specific for hot conditions in the uterus.

Preparation and Dosage

It is best to pick Plantain fresh and juice the leaves, for internal or external use. An infusion can also be made from the fresh or dried herb by pouring a pint of boiling water over an ounce of leaves. The tincture can be used in a dosage of one to thirty drops. For teeth and gum problems, gargle. The salve is beneficial for external use.

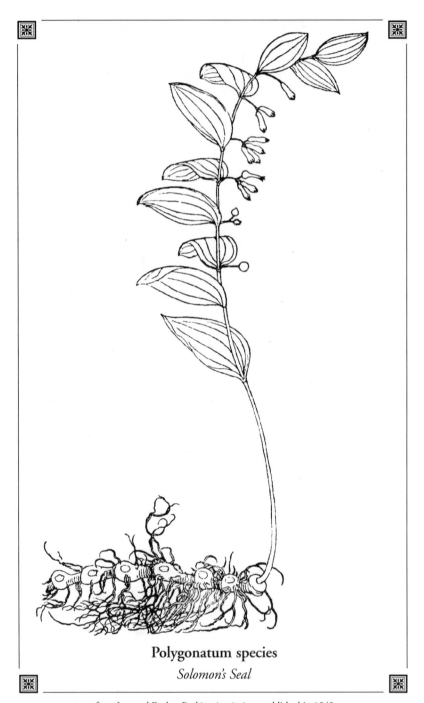

Polygonatum species

Solomon's Seal

from Leonard Fuchs, *De historia stirpium,* published in 1542

Polygonatum multiflorum
Solomon's Seal

Solomon's Seal is a member of the Lily family native to lightly wooded areas in North America, Asia, and Europe. It is sometimes found in open glades, sometimes in shadier woods. There are a number of different kinds, all of which appear to have similar properties.

The name *Polygonatum* means "many-jointed," referring to the nodes on the stems and the jointed roots (or actually, rhizomes), which look like a knarled mass of knuckles in some instances, and like a series of vertebra in others. When the stem dies back at the end of the season it detaches from the root leaving behind a round mark that looks like a little "seal." Each year, a new unit of root is generated and a new stem rises up. Thus, there is a mark for every year the plant has been growing. These little "seals" reminded people of the sigils or enscribed circles used by magicians to invoke spirits. King Solomon was associated with wisdom in the Bible, and later with magic. Hence, this plant was called *Sigilum Salomonis* or Solomon's Seal.

In the North American woods True Solomon's Seal (*Polygonatum* sp.) has to be differentiated from False Solomon's Seal (*Smilacina racemosa*), a plant which grows in the same places and has a similar appearance. The flowers of True Solomon's Seal appear at the joints while the False has them in a terminal cluster at the end of the stalk. The first has blue berries, the second red. Also, the leaves of True Solomon's Seal fold around the stem like muscles attaching to a bone while the leaves of the other arise from a little node on the stem. The roots of the False are smaller than the True, but also look like knuckles and vertebra with little seals on them. Both of these plants have valuable medicinal properties. However, we will be concentrating on the True Solomon's Seal in this chapter.

The ancient writers did not value Solomon's Seal highly. Dioscorides recommended it as a poultice to seal green [fresh] wounds, but Galen considered the whole plant to be poisonous. He was wrong: only the berries are toxic. Gerard noted these statements. "Galen saith, that neither herbe nor root hereof is to be giuen inwardly," he writes. "But note what experience hath found out…of late dayes, especially among the vulgar sort of people in Hampshire, which Galen, Dioscorides, or any other that haue written of plants haue not so much as dreamed of." He goes on to describe how it is a remarkable remedy for a wide variety of muscular and skeletal problems. Gerard deserves the credit for bringing Solomon's Seal into modern literature. He concludes his account, "Common experience teacheth, that in the world there is not to be found another herbe comparable to it." I absolutely agree.

The North American Indians also used Solomon's Seal for muscular and skeletal problems. They also utilized it as an important food and as a soothing agent for the mucus membranes. These uses were picked up by a few black and white practitioners in the South, but the plant is generally unknown in popular American herbalism at the present time. Solomon's Seal achieved its greatest fame, however, as a magical charm.

Muscular and Skeletal System

Solomon's Seal has an extraordinary influence on the muscular and skeletal system, affecting a wide variety of problems relating to tendons, ligaments, bones, joints, bruises, breaks, calcifications, decalcifications, and so on. I learned about its properties in a most remarkable fashion.

One evening I was teaching a class on flower essences. There were several chiropractors in attendance. One of them asked if there was an herb for "ligamentous looseness." I didn't know what that meant, so he explained. When an adjustment is made it may pop out because the ligaments are loose. That makes it difficult to keep adjustments in place. I told him I'd look into the question. The next day I was reading Gerard's *Herball* (1597). Under Solomon's Seal I found the following statement:

The root stamped and applied in manner of a pultesse, and layd upon members that have been out of joynt, and newly restored to their places, driveth away the paine, and knitteth the joynt very firmely, and taketh away the inflammation, if there chance to be any.

Later I confirmed that it worked incredibly well to tighten or loosen tendons, ligaments, attachments, and joints. Eventually I started to use it in all manner of muscular and skeletal problems and I have finally come to view it as the single most reliable, useful, and foolproof remedy that I have ever come across. Many of my students and friends feel the same way about it. Solomon's Seal is suited to conditions where the ligaments and tendons are loose or tight; it adjusts the tension on the connective tissue to the right level. This prevents injuries and corrects old traumas. It also feeds and lubricates the ligaments, tendons, muscles, and attachments, making the muscular and skeletal system stronger and more harmonious in its actions. It has many related and additional uses which we will discuss.

A most dramatic case illustrating the use of Solomon's Seal in tightening tendons came my way shortly after I started to use it. A woman in one of my classes had an adult son who was suffering from a stretched ligament in the ankle. The doctors estimated that it was over an inch too long and recommended surgery to cut out the elongated part and sew the ends back together. The man decided against that option, though the condition was painful and debilitating. I recommended Solomon's Seal and Horsetail, but she recommended Solomon's Seal and *Rhus tox.* Somehow he ended up taking Solomon's Seal and homeopathic Calcium carbonate, which was also a good idea. The stretched ligament was back to its normal size in one week. No surgery was needed.

I have seen so many cases of stretched, loose, or tight tendons cured by Solomon's Seal that I can hardly count them—probably over a hundred. I remember one man in his forties who had been a cornerback on a famous college football team. He had all sorts of problems from old injuries—sprains, strains, broken bones, a separated shoulder, etc. Solomon's Seal made him feel almost completely free of pain and flexible in a short time. One of my friends was recently trying to help an elderly man with limited motion in the wrist due to an old injury. He also had a floating and detached patella in one knee. After one day, both conditions were considerably less troublesome; in a short time he was returned to complete function.

Solomon's Seal also joins and seals broken bones. Gerard continues, "Among the vulgar sort of people in Hampshire, if any of what sex or age soever chance to have any bones broken, in what part of their bodies soever; their refuge is to stampe the root hereof, and give it unto the patient in ale to drink; which sodoreth and glues together the bones in very short space." They also give it to their livestock for the same purpose. Gerard adds that it "sodoreth and glues together the bones in very short space, and very strangely, yea although the bones be but slenderly and vnhandsomely placed and wrapped vp."

Solomon's Seal is one of the few remedies that has the "intelligence to set bones," as I call it—the ability to get the bone in the right place. Mullein also has this property. I generally use Solomon's Seal in combination with Comfrey and Boneset to heal broken bones. Recently my eighty-seven-year-old grandfather broke a collar bone. It was not healing up—often a problem with older people—until we gave him this formula. The doctor was very pleased with the result.

Solomon's Seal not only helps calcify and strengthen bones, but it also will decalcify unhealthy deposits. Gerard says that it is useful "against inflammation, tumors or swellings that happen vnto members whose bones are broken, or members out of ioynt, after restauration." I have used it dozens of times to correct bone spurs. These are usually the result of tensions on the muscles and tendons, causing unnatural pressures and hence, overgrowth of the bony tissues. Solomon's Seal corrects the tensions and then the spurs disappear. It has cured bunions as well. Solomon's Seal also has some effect upon the cartilage as well. I use it in combination with Horsetail, which rebuilds cartilage. It may be that Solomon's Seal indirectly helps the cartilage to regenerate better by adjusting the tensions on the joint. These two remedies together will often cure joints damaged by torn ligaments and deteriorated cartilage. They can be given externally, as well as internally.

Gerard also notes that Solomon's Seal is an excellent remedy for bruises from blows or falls or "gotten by stripes," that is, whippings, or "womens wilfulnesse, in stubling vpon their hasty husbands fists." We are reminded that Gerard's information about Solomon's Seal comes from poor people in the south of England, where feudalism was still entrenched and servants and women were often treated as chattel. Solomon's Seal not only helps remove congealed blood, but also draws out infected material and dirt.

As a direct result of Gerard's testimony, Solomon's Seal found a niche in English herbalism. John Hill wrote in 1751 that it is a "vulnerary of the very first rank." Even William Cullen (1781), the advocate of exotic and toxic drugs, recommended it for hemorrhoids. Unfortunately, it is almost forgotten in English and American herbalism today.

The American authors were not generally aware of the use of Solomon's Seal as a remedy for the muscular and skeletal system. Dr. William Cook (1869), who renders an otherwise brilliant account of its affinities in regard to internal organs and tissues, was barely acquainted with this side of the plant. "The fresh roots, bruised and boiled in milk, make a fair external application to bruises, light burns, lingering sores of an erysipelatous character, and other affections of the skin where there is a stinging sensation." (This would include poison ivy.) Cook and other American herbalists recommended it particularly for female problems, leucorrhea, vaginitis, pelvic weakness, and painful menstruation.

The Indian people, on the other hand, were well acquainted with Solomon's Seal. It was an important food staple and is still used as a trail food. In addition, it is considered to be a fine remedy for muscular and skeletal problems.

The doctrine of signatures completely confirms all of these uses. The roots or rhizomes look like knuckles, vertebra, and joints. The seal looks like the place where the femur rests in the hip joint socket. The white color of the rhizomes resemble bones. In fact, the dried root separates into an inner and outer layer like the periosteum covering the bone—a signature for dried out, brittle bones and bone healing. The healing power is thought to penetrate all the way down to the marrow of the bone in Chinese herbalism. The white rhizomes yield a gluey mucilage which relates to tendons that, as age advances, become gluey and get stuck together in adhesions which prevent full range of motion. The leaves join around the stems, like muscles attaching to the bone and the flowers—later the berries—also arise from these joints. The stalk rises up at a ninety-degree angle, the signature of Wolf Medicines (Agrimony, Werewolf Root, St. John's Wort)—thus, an example of a "spirit signature." The stalk leans over, which is a signature indicating that this is a plant for debility and nutrition. The rhizomes are rich in nutritious sugars and carbohydrates, as well a soothing mucilage. These signatures point us towards the next sphere where we can use Solomon's Seal.

The resemblance to the socket of the hip joint is a very significant matter. Ancient people—we see this in the Hebrew Bible—placed their hand under the thigh or hip joint when they made oaths or swore to tell the truth. They considered the joint of the hip to be the place where covenants, magical agreements, or "spiritual documents" are "stored." Jacob was hit on the joint of the hip and lamed when he fought with "beings divine and human," receiving a new name and covenant.

Wolf Medicine

One day Susan called me. Her big husky dog had diarrhea and was rapidly developing weakness in the rear hip joints, so that he couldn't stand comfortably. I brought some Solomon's Seal over in my pocket. The moment I came inside the gate, the dog looked at me, struggled up to his feet, walked across the yard, and sniffed my pocket. I gave him the Solomon's Seal then and there. He was well in two days and never had those problems again.

Not only dogs, but wolves like Solomon's Seal. (It is sometimes called "Wolf's Milk" in German.) Ancient people probably observed that this medicine toned up the joints and the digestion, both of which areas are strained by the lifestyle of the wolf. The horizontal rhizome under the ground, with the vertical stalk rising up from it indicates a wolf medicine.

Solomon's Seal also has a profound effect upon the mucus membranes and digestive tract. The root is sweet, the temperature is cool and moist, the overall impression is chewy, fibrous, and slightly mucilaginous. The sweet taste indicating a nutritive aspect and the cool, moist elements demonstrate lubricating and cooling properties. The Chinese herbalists use Solomon's Seal as a remedy for convalescence from fever, when the heat had consumed the fluids and emaciated the flesh. The Ayurvedic physicians use it to tonify the primal fluids of the body.

William Cook was one of the few American physicians who gave a knowledgeable account of the action of Solomon's Seal. "Its mild taste has created an opinon that it is nearly inert as a remedy; but in its own place it will be found among the most desirable articles of the Materia Medica," he writes. He used it principally as a moistening mucilaginous agent to coat and sooth the mucosa.

Its influence is expended slowly, and is chiefly directed to the mucus membranes; and it is soothing to these structures, diminishing excessive mucus discharges, and exerting upon them a gentle tonic impression. These qualities fit it for use in all sub-acute and chronic irritation and weakness of those tissues, where the system is not profoundly depressed, but the local difficulty is with general feebleness and irritability. The local and general nervous tissues seem also to feel this soothing and strengthening action. The mucus structures of the vagina and uterus are particularly influenced by it; and it is one of the most desirable agents in all ordinary forms of leucorrhea, simple prolapsus, and female weakness in general. Its combination with suitable tonics will secure from the latter a more distinct influence upon the uterine organs, and I prize it very highly in all such conditions. Though not of itself sufficiently stimulating to meet very depressed cases, its association with such more postive agents as hydrastis and viburnum will obtain happy effects. It exerts a good impression on the kidneys, bladder and prostate gland; relieving them of lingering congestions and catarrhal discharges. Though little used with reference to its action upon the lungs, it will be found a superior article in coughs during convalescence, and in chronic coughs with local feebleness, especially when the expectoration is rather free and the respiratory passages sensitive. In those cases it may be combined with such agents as prunus, lirodendron, and lycopus. It is a good soothing agent in irritable piles, where a decoction may be used freely; and may be used to much advantage in chronic inflammation and pain in the bowels, and in chronic dysentery. Very large doses will gently move the bowels.

Cook gives the following recipe for vaginitis.

Bruised roots of Solomon's seal, three ounces; boiling water, twenty ounces. Macerate in a covered vessel, with a gentle heat, for an hour; then add caulophyllum [Blue Cohosh] and grated orange-peel, of each a drachm; in ten minutes strain and express, and add two ounces of

Sherry wine. This is an elegant tonic preparation for monthly leucor-rhea, especially when menstruation is somewhat painful. The wine may be omitted. Dose, two fluid ounces three or four times a day.

In addition to acting as a nutritive agent on the muscles in general, Solomon's Seal has a gentle regulating effect on the heart muscle. It contains convallarin, a cardiac glycoside also found in its cousin Lily of the Valley (*Convallaria majalis*). Both of these plants have a nice rhythmic arrangement of flowers on the stalk, but Lily of the Valley contains a large amount of convallarin, while Solomon's Seal has just a trace. This is a compound closely related to the *Digitalis* glycosides used in cardiac treatment, so Lily of the Valley has now been banned for internal use. Solomon's Seal has just a small amount of this substance, and can be safely used as a mild cardiac tonic.

The Wolf Medicines usually have a ninety-degree angle in their construction, indicating an affinity to making profound changes or turns in life. They help bring a person to a transformative place, or help them go through the change, or help them adapt to a change that has already occured. The ninety-degree angle represents joints in the organism, and key-joints in the path of life.

High John

There is a mysterious plant called "John the Conqueror Root" or "High John the Conqueror" in the deep South, particularly among Black folks. People use it as a charm, sometimes worn in a bag around the neck or on the person, to ward off psychic manipulation or bad luck and attract good things. It is actively used for "conquerin"—that is, psychic manipulation—by people who dabble in that sort of thing. The rest of the population wears it in self defense.

The name "High John the Conqueror" reflects Afro-American folk-lore. High John was a slave who escaped from the planatation system, ran away into the woods and swamps and through conjuring could never be found. They sent dogs after him, but he was invisible. When trouble came up on the plantation he would always know about it and help through his magical powers. The roots he doctored with were named after him: "High John" and "Little John." Just to keep would-be magicians on their toes, a number of different roots are called by these names.

Destiny is a possibility, a fork in the road, where we have the opportunity to associate ourselves with something new. It knocks on our door and waits for an answer. If we are alert, we will see the omens, the magical signs, which point out the way to a new, better life, more in line with our sense of destiny. Then we can take the plunge and get on the new road. The new path leads to who we really are. High John helps people see the omen, take the risk, rise to the occassion, get a new start.

I believe in magic. It was Solomon's Seal that brought me to my home on Sunnyfield Road. One day I was teaching a little herb class in a public park, just outside the gates of a wildflower garden in Minneapolis. It's against the law to pick plants in public parks, so I fudged a little and picked a plant outside the gate, but still on public land. I wanted to show my students how the roots looked like bones and knuckles.

I was holding up a nice little chunk of fresh root when an "unmarked park ranger" bore down on me and started yelling. "There's a fifty dollar fine... How could a person like you, in a position of authority teaching people, pick a plant in the park..." etc., etc. It happens that I entertain a different ethic with regard to plants. I believe we not only have to perserve them, but taste, touch, smell, see, and interact with every part of them. Nevertheless, it was humiliating. (Shame is one of the best ways to "conquer.") And it is the job of Park Rangers to protect plants.

At that moment I knew that if I was ever going to be able to teach about herbs in the right fashion, I was going to have to have my own little patch of ground. I needed to dig the little guys up and pass them around. At that very moment the impulse was born in me to start looking for a home with enough land for a garden. That led me to Sunnyfield Herb Farm.

I looked for a house in the city, in the country, in the east, south, north, and the west. My students out in Minnetrista, west of Minneapolis, said, "You've got to get an herb farm out here." I thought, "Sure, how could I afford a farm out in horse country, where everybody holds down a six figure income." But things have a way of working out.

One of my students, Suzanne, was a real estate agent. We drove around, but I didn't see anything I liked. Then I went to housesit at another student's place, out on Game Farm Road. To pass the time, I drove back and forth on various country roads. One day I went down

Sunnyfield. I had been avoiding it because there was one little farm that I always loved and never thought I'd be able to buy. I had been to a party there fourteen years before. "Who'd want to sell it?" I thought. "And how could I afford it?"

This time when I drove by it was for sale. "Maybe there's just two or three acres around the house," I thought. "I could afford that." When Suzanne looked it up, it turned out it was drastically reduced in price. There was a guest house on the property, in the life estate of Aunt Esther, the aunt of the heirs. She got to live there until she died. The whole seventeen acres of rolling fields, bird-infested marsh, and spotty woods were for sale.

The heirs had been trying to sell the farm for three years without success. None of the rich people shopping for horse farms in the area wanted to be entangled with a life estate. But I liked Aunt Esther. When I noticed the astrological ephemerides and Rosicrucian books in the bookcase, I knew we were cut from the same stock.

Sometimes, as the years passed, I would worry about whether I could keep up on the payments and the ever-bourgeoning property taxes, but a little voice would pop up and say, "It is your destiny to live here."

Preparation, Toxicity, and Dosage

The rhizomes should be picked during the fall, after the berries drop. True Solomon's Seal is available in herbal commerce but is seldom found in commercial preparations. I have made my own tincture by cutting up the rhizome and macerating it in vodka. It is so sweet it will make brandy into a syrup. Cook says the roots "yield their qualities to water and diluted alcohol; are much impaired by heat; and undergo deterioration by long keeping." The dose of the tincture need not be great, one to five drops is usually sufficient. The berries are toxic.

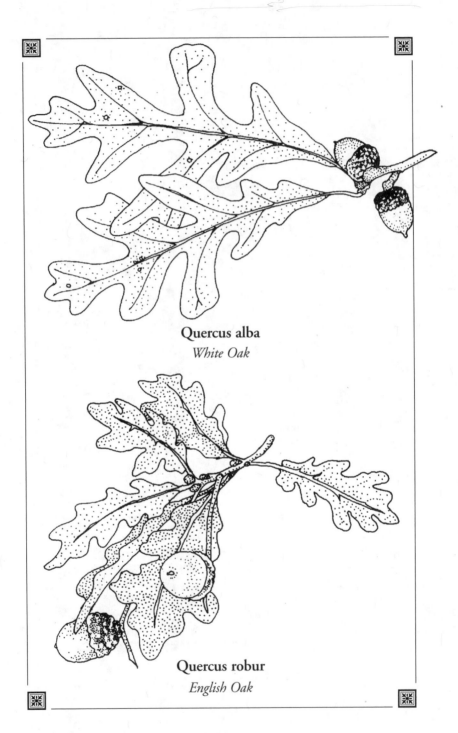

Quercus alba
White Oak

Quercus robur
English Oak

Quercus alba
White Oak

Throughout the world, and since the most remote periods, various kinds of Oak have been used in herbal medicine. Most parts of the tree contain high quantities of tannins, used for their astringency. In American herbalism the White Oak (*Quercus alba*) is the officinal plant. In European medicine the English Oak (*Quercus robur*) is used.

The English or European Oak has been utilized in medicine since antiquity. Hippocrates, Dioscorides, and Galen testify to its virtues. The principal uses recorded by Dioscorides are still prominent today: stomach problems, dysentery, spitting blood, and bleeding from the womb. The Renaissance authors continued to value it highly. Mattioli (1563) recommends Oak for fluxes of blood and semen, spitting of blood, stone in the kidney and bladder, blood in the urine, suppression of urine, flooding menstruation, and vaginal discharge. Culpeper (1653) says it "is one of the best remedies that I know of for the whites in women." And it continues to be valued today in European medicine. Dr. Rudolf Weiss (1985) recommends Oak bark as a compress in weeping eczema, ulcers on the legs, contact dermatitis in the early, weeping stage, inflammatory eye conditions, and inflamed hemorrhoids.

These uses depend upon the tannins contained in the tree. A more subtle concept of Oak was developed by Dr. Johann Gottfried Rademacher in the early nineteenth-century. He removed the astringent tannins by distillation to produce a "spirit" or essence, which he called *Quercus glandium spiritus* (spirit of acorn). He gives an extensive account of its use. His work was picked up by the innovative English homeopath, Dr. J. Compton Burnett, who developed the use of the medicine further. A later English homeopath, Dr. Dorothy Shepherd, published an account of her experience with Burnett's indications in *A Physician's Posy*. Finally, *Quercus robur* is the Oak which Dr. Bach collected and used as his flower essence. The mental state associated with the tree by Dr. Bach fits well with the ideas of Rademacher and Burnett. (It is quite possible that Dr. Bach was influenced by Burnett's work.)

"The Mighty Oak is Broken Down"

The story of the development of the more subtle understanding of *Quercus robur* by Rademacher and Burnett is entertaining and educational. It illustrates how it is possible to develop knowledge about a remedy through purely empirical means, such as careful observation, deduction, and experience rather than from pharmacology, homeopathic provings, or theory. Rademacher found out about the remedy by accident, "in a wonderful way," as he says. Burnett provides a translation in his *Diseases of the Spleen* (1896):

> *Many years ago (I do not remember the exact time) a working carpenter, who had previously lived in Credfeld, came to seek my advice for his bellyache, which was of long standing. According to his own statement, he had long been under Sanitary Councilor Schneider in Credfeld, who was not able to help him, and so sent him to Professor Gunther in Duisbery. Ten journeys thither were likewise in vain.*
>
> *I tried my usual remedies for seemingly such cases, but to no good; and as I noticed he was a good cabinetmaker, and dabbled a bit in upholstery, I told him it would be a good plan if he were to hire himself out to a country squire as joiner, thinking that the food of the servants' hall would suit his sick stomach better than the beans, black bread, and potatoes of the master carpenter. The good fellow followed my advice, and lived with a squire for many years; and I heard nothing more about him. Finally, he married the parlor maid, and settled here in this town as a joiner. One day when visiting his sick wife I remembered the old story of his bellyache, and wanted to know how it then was. "All right," said he, "I have not had it for years." It seems that a local surgeon, being one day at the squire's, told him to get some acorns, and*

scrape them with a knife, and then put the scrapings into brandy, and leave them to draw for a day, and then to drink a small glass of this spirit several times a day. He did as he was advised, and was forthwith relieved, and very soon entirely freed from his old trouble.

Rademacher knew enough about the barber-surgeon to know that he would not be able to describe anything much about the remedy, so his investigation of the medicine took a different course.

As I had in the meantime become much more cunning, I questioned the joiner himself afresh as to the kind of his old pain, particularly as to the part of the belly where the pain was last felt when he had had a bad attack. He was in no doubt about it, but at once pointed to the part of the belly nearest the left hypochondrium. So I very shrewdly suspected that the abdominal pains were really owing to a primary affection of the spleen, in which notion I was strengthened by remembering that the best pain-killing hepatic and enteric remedies had done him no good.

To get as soon as possible to the bottom of the thing, I set about preparing a tincture of acorns, and gave a teaspoonful five times a day in water to an old brandy drunkard, who was sick unto death, and of whom I knew that he had suffered from the spleen for a very long time, the spleen being from time to time painful. He had likewise ascitis, and his legs were dropsical as far as the knees. It occurred to me that if the acorn tincture were to act curatively on the spleen the consensual kidney affection and its dependent dropsy would mend. I soon saw that I had reckoned rightly. The urinary secretion was at once augmented . . . the tension in the praecordia became less and less, and this hopelessly incurable drunkard got quite well, much to the surprise of all who knew him, and, honestly speaking, much to my own surprise also.

Having thus put the spirit of acorns to such a severe test . . . I went further, and used it by degrees in all sorts of spleen affections, and that not only in painful ones, but in painless ones, in the evident ones, and in those of a more problematical kind. Gradually I became convinced that it is a remedy, the place of which no other can take. More particularly is it of great, nay, of inestimable value in spleen-dropsy.

Rademacher assigned about one third of all dropsies to the spleen, the remainder to the kidneys and heart. In relating the spleen to edema he agrees with Traditional Chinese Medicine. The spleen is a part of the

411

lymphatic system, and is therefore to be associated with stagnation of lymphatics and lymph fluid. This in turn is associated with sagging of venous structures.

Rademacher found that the tincture worked best if it was distilled, so that the astringent principle had been removed. It is clear, therefore, that it is a deeper, more essential property of Oak he was using. He also made some interesting observations about its effects on patients:

> *Certain few people feel, as soon as they have taken it, a peculiar sensation in the head, lasting hardly a minute or two, which they say is like being drunk.*
>
> *With a few people, particularly with those who have suffered from old spleen engorgements, diarrhea sets in after using it for two or three weeks that makes them feel better. It seldom lasts more than a day, and it is not weakening, but moderate. Hence it is not needful either to stop the acorn-water, or to lessen the dose.*

Burnett realized that *Quercus* had the potential to be a homeopathic remedy for drunkenness. "When we regard it from the pathogenetic side as producing…a cephalic state resembling alcoholic intoxication, and then from the clinical side as having cured an abandoned drunkard, it looks very much as if we had a remedy homoeopathic to alcoholism." And he went on to prove that this was the case, giving several of his case histories, in his inimitable style.

"Colonel X., aged 64, came under my observation on January 15, 1889, broken down with gout and chronic alcoholism, and pretty severe bronchitis. Heart's action irregular; liver and spleen both enlarged; and he complained bitterly of a gnawing in the pit of the stomach. His gait was unsteady and tottering, his hand quivered, and altogether; he was in a sorry plight. The poor fellow had lost his wife, and had for a good while tried to rub along with the aid of a little Dutch courage, in the shape of nips of spirits, for which he was always craving. Severe windy spasm; no sugar, no albumen." Burnett put him on ten drops of the spirits of acorn, three times a day. A month later, "he is chirpy again, and has no craving for whiskey." Months afterwards, he heard that the colonel was in fair health and still free from the craving.

Burnett was treating another patient for necrosis of the nails and a weak heart, when the patient confessed that "he thought he took too much sherry *in nips*." Burnett was reminded of the colonel: "He was

never intoxicated...but still never free from the effects of his nips."
Again, ten drops of the spirit of acorn was given in water, morning and
evening. "This brought out a good deal of gouty eczema of scalp, poll
and backs of hands," but the drinking was controlled.

The wife of another officer wrote Burnett for help with her husband. He denied drinking, but the wife said, "I can always tell by the
look of his eyes; they are so yellow, and puffy underneath." Cured with
a month of *Quercus*.

It would not be necessary to quote any further cases from Burnett,
but his diction is so entertaining that I find it hard to stop. In addition
to being a fine homeopath, he was the father of the eminent novelist,
Dame Ivy Compton-Burnett.

"A noble Nimrod, about 40 years of age, a very free liver, and
plagued with attacks of gout, came under my observation in the spring
of 1891 for varicose veins of the lower extremities, starting originally, it
seemed to me, from an enlarged spleen, which was seemingly left after
typhoid fever. Knowing his mode of life, and on account of the spleen,
I gave him Quercus for a month, 10 drops at bed time, and then noted
'He likes his medicine, as it keeps his bowels very regular.'" It improved
the veins, disposed of some rings under the eyes, and hot feet.

"A country squire, from the shire of Moonrakers, bachelor, 60
years of age, was accompanied to me on October 3, 1893, by his brother, resident in London. This gentleman was so very ill that his case was
regarded as quite hopeless. He was not capable of stating his own case,
and hence his brother did it for him. Patient was flushed, and in much
pain over the eyes and in both rib regions. Stooping caused very great
pain, worse in the left hypochondrium. Both liver and spleen notably
enlarged. He is exceedingly nervous, very depressed, glum, taciturn, and
moved to tears by almost anything. He could not walk without support,
on account of his great giddiness. His breath was in the highest degree
disgustingly stercoraceous (*merdeux*), so much so that I very nearly vomited when examining him. He was personally unknown to me, and I had
no history of him, but that smell of breath is an unmistakable sign of the
chronic tippler." He was quite sober, "but took frequent nips, particularly when confined to the house by wet weather." (Worse from damp
tends to indicate the spleen.) After one week on *Quercus* his symptoms
were dramatically better, the breath normal, and in six weeks he went
home "perfectly well." And Burnett gives one more case, but I might as

413

well let readers obtain his little books, *Diseases of the Spleen* and *Gout and Its Cure*, where all this is written.

As a colorful medical writer, ready to poke fun at all schools of medicine including his own, Burnett's work was enjoyed by home-opaths, allopaths, and eclectics. One physician who picked up on *Quercus* was Dr. Dorothy Shepherd, another English homeopath. In *A Physician's Posy* she gives a selection of her own cases, justifying Burnett's indications. She confirms that *Quercus* is singularly suited to sherry-tip-plers who are never really drunk, but never free from the influence. Shepherd had a sympathy for female patients and observed that it was especially suited to middle aged women who were lonely and took to the bottle in place of companionship. (Indeed, Burnett's cases seem to indi-cate an element of loneliness.) The cases she gives are, however, those of men—and ones very much like Burnett's. There was the "traveler in spirits, broken down in health," the "black sheep of a well-to-do fami-ly...down on his luck and disappointed with life," and "that dear old sinner, the once brilliant actor," etc., now "a repulsive specimen." The last patient stopped using the spirit of acorn because it ruined his taste for brandy and sherry! Shepherd also gives a case which was merely splenic, not alcoholic—"a retired army man who suffered from bouts of a special tropical intermittent fever, which had produced an enlargement of the spleen." Nat. mur. 6c cured the intermittent and *Quercus* cured the swollen spleen.

Next in line to teach us about Oak was Dr. Edward Bach. He may have heard of Oak through homeopathic channels, but his knowledge of the plant ultimately came from his attunement to its psychological qual-ities. According to Bach, Oak is suited to persons who fight against their disease and problems, for years even, never giving up, yet never succeed-ing. (The "fight" element reminds us of these retired military officers, so commonly described by Burnett and Shepherd.) "Much balance is lost, mental and physical," he continues. The mental symptoms may include "severe nervous breakdowns, or such types of insanity which can be described as completely unbalanced (where there is great loss of control); and the same in the bodily state, where the patient loses control over parts of the body or its functions." And this sounds like some of the cases cited by Burnett and Shepherd.

Dr. Bach points out that physical symptoms are analogous to the mental. Oak is suited to strong, disciplined persons who are broken down by long-suffering and serious ailments. Although they have a strong personality, they fall. "The mighty oak is broken down," I like to say. The pathology centers around the "spleen," or lymphatic system. In Traditional Chinese Medicine the spleen is said to be responsible for "holding up" the tissues and organs. In the Oak person, not just the organs but the personality fall. The strong integrity we associate with the Oak tree is lost. And yet, usually we see it in some area of their life—as Dr. Bach says, they keep fighting on.

The following case history, from my own records, demonstrates the unity of the physical and mental symptoms. A forty-six-year-old man came to me because of some pretty severe edema which was starting to develop from the waist down. He was also suffering from pain in the right side, above the pelvic bones, but well below the area we would associate with the liver and gallbladder. The pain seemed to be in the viscera or intestines. It was not appendicitis. He had swollen glands in the inguinal crease and edema extending down most of the right leg and around both ankles. There was much pain and swelling about the right knee, where there was an eruption with dry skin and itching, covering an area about the size of the palm of his hand. There were several smaller patches on this and the other knee. The eruption felt hot and dry. Some swelling and eruptions on the knuckles of the left hand. When he was ten, the patient fell from a horse and ruptured his spleen. The organ was removed to prevent him bleeding to death. The present symptoms had been developing over the last half year since his best friend died, his business expanded, he was working twelve-hour shifts on his feet, and he moved his family and household to a different city. He had a strong personality, little given to worrying about his health. At the beginning of the whole trouble he had experienced an uncharacteristic urge to drink which he acted on for about a month, but which went away. The tongue was swollen about the sides, pale towards the front, purple towards the back, and covered by a fine yellow sticky coating. Lips were a little blue-purple.

This was clearly a case where the spleen organ system was not functioning. It was not "holding up the organs," and the blood and lymph were stagnating due to poor circulation. There was probably some intestinal prolapse and the cardiovascular system may also have been weakened. The descriptions of both the European and American White Oak seemed to fit. I recommended Oak flower essence internally, White

Oak bark externally in a bath, Cleavers tincture internally, and Cleavers herb externally per bath. The Cleavers was for local lymphatic reabsorption, the Oak for the source of the problem. Our friend reacted quickly. He felt much better after a few hours and most of the symptoms, serious as they were, disappeared inside three weeks.

Some homeopaths will probably ask, "How do you know whether it was the Oak or Cleavers that did the job?" I know which did what, because I know the plants. My information is not based on theory, but on observation of plants, people, and cures. Oak does one thing, Cleavers another. It is true that we would not really know which Oak did the trick—I was counting on both.

One thing I have learned about Oak is that it is virtually a specific for edema resulting from the removal of lymphatic glands or the spleen (as in this case). White Oak bark tincture, internally or externally, is an excellent medicine for women who have had lymphatic glands removed near the breasts, resulting in edema down the arm or nearby. I have seen this work repeatedly.

The following symptoms are the specific indications derived from Rademacher, Burnett, Shepherd, and Bach. Intoxicated feeling, giddiness, trembling hands, fluttery nervousness. Nervous breakdown; mentally and physically broken; alcoholism. Face flushed; rings under the eyes, puffy and yellow. Tongue thickly coated and foul, breath putrid. Tongue and lips purple or blue. Swollen spleen and liver; pain in the left side; dyspepsia, stomach ache; constipation, diarrhea, intestinal prolapse, anal fistula, hemorrhoids; varicose veins. Edema of the lower extremities. Gout; eczema.

American White Oak

The White Oak is a beautiful tree native to the Eastern Woodlands of North America. There is a quiet integrity about it and the leaves are colorful in the fall. It has a light bark and wood—woodworkers named it "White Oak." It is perhaps the most astringed looking member of the clan, for the bark looks as if stretched around the trunk. The barks of various Oaks, but especially this one, were—and are—used by the American Indians in herbal medicine. The inner bark was at one time officinal in American medicine. It is still an important medicine in herbal medicine, and many of us practicing herbalists would consider it an indispensable agent in the clinic.

Quercus alba was classified as a "simple astringent," by Dr. William Cook (1869). "But while this quality is predominant, it contains a distinct tonic principal of the slowly stimulating character." For this reason, it not only disciplines loose tissues, but gives them a better permanent tone. It is tempting to think that the very hard Oak has a mineralizing aspect; many writers consider it nutritive. It is also antiseptic. Ellingwood (1919) notes, "white oak bark is used locally, in decoction, for the general purpose of an astringent, but it is also tonic and antiseptic, and possesses specific powers." The specificity of Oak comes out, as we have seen, in relationship to broken-down and ruined systems. As an antiseptic, it not only disciplines lax, atonic tissue, but cleanses out putrid conditions and waste materials. (Burnett noted several symptoms of deterioration in the nails and the terrible breath.)

Ellingwood gives a general overview of the most common uses of Oak. "The agent is of value in epidemic dysentery, acute and chronic diarrhea, obstinate intermittents, pulmonary and laryngeal phthisis [tuberculosis], tabes mesenterica, great exhaustion of the vital powers from disease, profuse, exhausting night sweats, colliquative sweats in the advanced stages of adynamic fevers, and debility, and severe diarrhea in sickly children, scrofula, gangrene, ulcerated sore throat, fetid, ill-conditioned and gangrenous ulcers, relaxed mucus membranes with profuse discharges, bronchorrhea, passive hemorrhages, relaxed uvula and sore throat, spongy granulations, diabetes, prolapsus ani, bleeding hemorrhoids, leucorrhea, menorrhagia, hemoptysis."

Starting with the mouth and working down, primarily through the alimentary tract, we may follow Ellingwood on the principal uses of White Oak, filing in here and there from other sources. "I have depended upon a decoction of white oak bark one ounce to the pint of boiling water, to which I have added after straining, a dram of boric acid, for all ulcerations of the mouth or throat, both in the early stages and in many chronic cases. It is surprising how many simple early throat troubles this will abort, and how frequently it will prevent suppuration in tonsillitis. Combined with Yellow Dock, it has cured for me the severest cases of nursing sore mouth that I have had, after other lauded remedies had signally failed." Other practitioners have used Oak by itself as a gargle in aphthous sore mouth, putrid sore throat, and diphtheria. Herbalist Alma Hutchins (1992) notes that it removes "excess of stomach mucus, which causes the common complaint of sinus congestion, postnasal drip, etc." However, the principal use of White Oak bark is to tone the intestines. Ellingwood continues, "In severe epidemic dysentery, a strong decoction of white oak bark, given internally, in doses of a wine glassful every hour or two, the bowels being first evacuated by a cathartic of castor oil and turpentine, has effected cures where other treatment had proved of little or no avail." When given internally in diarrhea and dysentery, "it should be combined with cinnamon or another astringent aromatic." It is useful in cases where nutrition is compromised due to the poor condition of the intestines and the severe loss of fluids. Tabes mesenterica, marasmus, scrofula, "and diseases attended with exhaustion, baths medicated with white oak bark, accompanied by brisk friction, have restored the waning powers of life." Ulcerations of the bowels, prolapse, hemorrhoids, anal fissure, and fistula can also be treated. Alma Hutchins uses the less astringent "distilled water of the buds" for leucorrhea, womb problems, hemorrhoids, and prolapsed rectum (sitz bath). The bark tea she recommends for "often dangerous fistulas on the rectum."

White Oak bark also acts on the mucus membranes of the respiratory tract. It is useful in both acute and chronic conditions. Hutchins recommends it for sinus congestion and discharge, inflammation, burning fever, and infection. It is also beneficial in serious, chronic illness. "In pulmonary and laryngeal phthisis a very fine powder of the bark may be inhaled," says Ellingwood. It pulls the tissues together and establishes healthy recuperation, stopping uncontrollable bleeding and discharges.

An anonymous publication, *Herb Success Stories* (1980) mentions a number of impressive case histories demonstrating the dramatic action of White Oak bark. One woman wrote, "My teeth had all come loose, and my mouth was becoming misshapen. The dentist told me that he was going to have to pull all my teeth and probably do some surgery on my jaw. I got started on white oak bark, packing it around my teeth at night and rinsing my mouth out with a tea solution made out of the white oak bark in the daytime. Within three or four months my teeth were all solid. As I was doing this I reshaped my mouth with my hand, pushing the teeth back until they were all perfectly spaced and solid in my mouth. I didn't have to have any surgery."

Another woman related, "I'm a firm believer in white oak bark. I have had problems with varicose veins since I had my first baby. I'm on my feet an awful lot, and these veins used to erupt and become like little red prickly dots that itched like fire. I took vitamin C and vitamin E for years, but sometimes I had absolutely no relief. So I went to white oak bark. I had hemorrhoids too. I used the white oak bark and didn't ever have to take sitz baths. I took four white oak bark doses in the morning and four in the evening, and I don't have hemorrhoids or varicose veins anymore." She helped another woman with similar problems. "A woman, about seven months pregnant, heard about how herbs had helped me. She thought she wasn't going to carry this child, which was her sixth. She had enormous varicose veins dangling like grapes. She was a thin woman. I suggested to her to take sitz baths with the white oak bark and to take heavy internal doses. So she did. She wrapped her legs, and in a week she was no longer with the wraps and was carrying the baby beautifully. She had no more pain and no more problems. She delivered the baby. Then a year later she had another baby—you know, people never learn. She used the white oak bark, and it carried her right on through." She also treated "a large woman who's in the restaurant business and is on her feet a lot. She's never without white oak bark."

Large, nodulated, ugly varicosities, of a blue-yellow color, that "look like grapes," are an excellent keynote symptom, pointing to White Oak (or European Oak). I remember one case where a fifty-six year old man came in with the complaint of impotence. He seemed reasonably healthy and happily married. I could discover no particularly strong indications until I noticed that the veins in the wrists were somewhat nodulated. I asked if he had varicose veins and he showed me some nice examples on his legs. He took Oak flower essence (the European kind) and was completely cured of both conditions within six months.

From the experience of myself and others, I believe that Oak has a remineralizing influence. I have used it for bone deterioration, and I know of a chiropractor in my neighborhood who has used it (with good diet) to stop dental caries!

Preparation and Dosage

The usual preparation is made from the inner bark of the White Oak. It has been prepared as a tea, tincture, or in capsules. The inner bark yields its properties to water, and to a lesser extent in alcohol. The decoction is made by boiling one ounce in a pint of water for fifteen minutes. The usual dose of the tincture is ten to fifteen drops. There is no particular toxicity, but a large dose would be very astringent and puckering. In contrast, Rademacher pioneered in the manufacture of the spirit of acorn and Dr. Bach made the Oak flower essence, both of which work on the more energetic level, often accomplishing the same thing as the astringent.

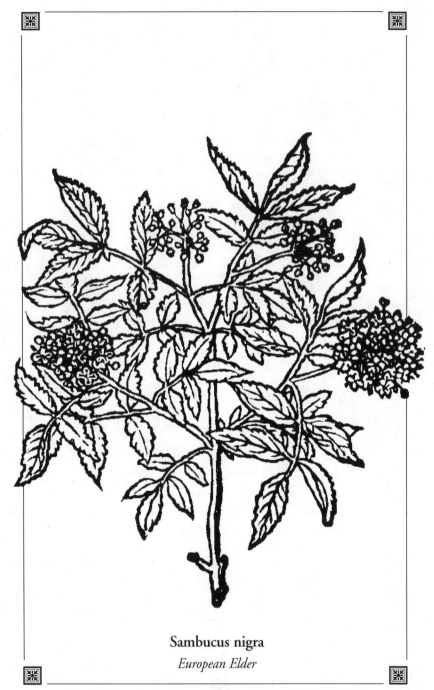

Sambucus nigra

European Elder

from *Herbarium Imagines Vivae,* published by Christianus Egenolphus, 1535

Sambucus canadensis
Elderberry

Elderberry is a small tree or bush common to pastures, meadows, and light forests. The most prominent species in Europe is the Black Elder, *Sambucus nigra.* This is one of the premier plants utilized in the herbal medicine and folklore of Europe. There is also a smaller kind, *Sambucus ebulis,* or Dwarf Elder, which is less commonly used. In North America we also have two kinds of Elder, one of which is the superior. *Sambucus racemosa* grows on upland soils, flowers in the spring, and has red berries. It is the most toxic Elder; children have died as a result of making toys from the wood, so it is not used in herbal medicine. The other one is *S. canadensis,* the medicine of choice for North American herbalists. It grows on low soils, flowers in mid-summer, and has dark purple berries.

There seem to be no particular properties which distinguish the medicinal use of American Elder from the Black. "Our species is not sufficiently distinct from the European," writes Charles Millspaugh (1893). They have been used interchangeably. Both of these sister-plants received incomplete homeopathic provings and are used in a moderate sort of way in homeopathy. There are slight differences in the physical properties, however. The Black is somewhat larger than the American, so that it approaches the height of a small tree. This explains the European tradition of its use as the wood from which the Holy Cross was made or the tree on which Judas hanged himself. This sort of idea would make little sense in America, where the humble Elder is a modest bush easily broken under light pressure.

The lore surrounding the Black Elder is immense and mysterious. Legends lie thick about its humble branches. All parts of the plant have been used in folk medicine, sometimes in slightly different ways. The traditional medicinal uses were recorded in a wealth of detail by Martin Blochwich in 1633. Modern authors continue to contribute significant insights, and the homeopathic literature is not too small. It is difficult to know where to begin with this medicine plant, but it would not be a bad idea to start with—

The Little Elder Mother

Elder is endowed with a heavy, somewhat narcotic and rank smell: Shakespeare called it "the stinking Elder." This exhalation has a mild influence on the mind and senses. The plant is considered slightly psychoactive and this undoubtedly contributed to the many mysterious traditions associated with it.

The generic name *Sambucus* comes from the Latin term for a musical instrument—the Pan pipes—which were originally made from the hollow stems. Anything which was held in the hand of the Lord of the Hunt—the Guardian of the Animals and the spouse of the Lady of the Underworld—ought to be powerful indeed. Plinius says that the country people thought the most shrill and haunting music was made by the *sambuca*.

In northern Europe the Elder was associated with a powerful female being called the Elder Mother, the Hylde-Moer, or the Lady Ellhorn. It was considered a potentially fatal mistake to pick the plant without making an offering. The most common practice was to ask for some of the plant in exchange for notifying the Elder Mother that one's body would eventually be returned to the earth. In England, Elder wood crosses were placed on the new grave in hopes that it would bring the departed person peace. They are also affixed to doors and windows to disappoint "the Charms of Witches," as Blochwich says.

Elder is one of the significant trees in the Underworld lore of Western Europe. The gist of the legends say that the Elder serves as a doorway to the Underworld, or magical fairy realm. The tree is sometimes identified directly with the Queen of the Netherworld, or occasionally the King. These persons are sometimes said to dwell in the Elder tree, or again, a historical person may be identified with a particular

Elder tree, where he or she was taken into the Underworld. It is considered perilous to fall asleep under an Elder: one may be stolen to another world—and not necessarily returned.

Hans Christian Andersen incorporated the lore of the Elder into his fairy tales. In *The Daughter of the Marsh King* he describes an extensive, impenetrable fen, in the midst of which there is a lake. An Elder tree bends down over the lake. We learn variously that here the Marsh King has his throne, or that the Elder is the Marsh King himself, or that the tree is the door to the Underworld, where the Marsh King rules. Through this door a desperate mortal woman is driven. She becomes the captive of the Marsh King. The story revolves around the daughter of the woman and the King. She must assimilate her human and supernatural origins, her pagan and Christian roots, and redeem her mother from captivity. In *The Little Elder Mother,* the tree serves Andersen as a metaphor for the poetic genius, the origin of fairy tales. A little boy who has been sloshing around in puddles all day is given a cup of Elder tea by his mother and sent to bed. The old man boarding upstairs drops by and is implored to tell a fairy tale. It is not entirely clear whether he tells a story or the boy falls into a light dream. The Little Elder Mother takes him on a journey to faraway lands in the south. When the story is over, or the boy awakens, he comments that it is hot in the southern regions. His mother, noting the perspiration on his skin, agrees that he has been to hot countries and is satisfied that her herbal tea has done its work.

The name Elder has been traced to an Old English word *aeld,* meaning "fire." This is thought to relate to the use of the hollow stem as a smoking tube, or perhaps a tube to blow on newly kindled fires. Elder pipes were probably used for leech craft and priest craft. However, a more mundane idea may have been behind this fiery name: after all, Elder is as an herbal remedy for fever.

When Christianity appeared, Elder came to be associated with both Jesus and Judas. After his crucifixion, Jesus went down into the Underworld to free the souls of the dead who had been stored there during ages past. This is a recurrent motif in folklore, called "the Harrowing of the Underworld." The Elder, as tree-doorway to that realm was a natural addition when the story of Jesus reached Europe. The Underworld in its negative phase, as the abode of the unfortunates who stray from their paths and get caught by powers greater than themselves, fits the story of Judas.

According to tradition, the person who journeys into the Underworld is faced with three choices (see *The UnderWorld Initiation*, by R. J. Stewart). It is possible to remain in that enchanted world. Another choice is to take the difficult road of return to Middle Earth ("ordinary reality"). On this road one becomes a mediator of gifts from that magical realm to everyday society. The last choice is to take the easy road that "some say leads to heaven, but others say leads to hell," as expressed in the ballad of Thomas the Rhymer. The spiritual gifts gained on this journey can entice an individual so that they are put to personal use and one falls into a state of spiritual corruption.

The imagination is often ignored by people concerned with making a living amid the dust and thorns of the material world, but it is the channel of communication from another dimension. Tubular plants such as Elder and Angelica have long been associated with the shamanic journey to the Underworld in Eurasian folklore.

The taboos surrounding the Elder probably originate in a remote period when it was still understood that it was not safe to accidentally journey into the Netherworld in imagination or dream. Despite these cautions, Elder wood was used for a variety of purposes. Small crosses are made from branches cut between the joints and bound together by red string, or sometimes red bark. The wood is gathered on the last day of April. This is also an excellent day to gather the leaves for medicine. As Blochwich says, "The common people keep as a great secret in curing wounds, the leaves of the Elder, which they have gathered the last day of April."

Planting an Elder in the corner of an herb garden is considered to be beneficial to the medicinal plants growing there because the Elder serves as a sort of tutelary spirit for herbs. The stinking leaves are also thought to repel insects. It is, however, much more difficult to transplant an Elder into the garden than one would suppose. One of my friends found out by experience. She went out in her woods, identified a small Elder, and enlisted a friend to help dig it up. She is an experienced woodswoman and herbalist, so the adventure which followed was rather strange. "I don't know how the Elder did it, but after digging for forty-five minutes, when we almost had it out of the ground, we found that it was another kind of bush!"

Hippocrates, Plinius, Dioscorides, and Galen gave accounts of the medicinal properties of Elder. The Hippocratic writers relied upon it in a wide variety of uterine problems. Dioscorides used the Black and Dwarf Elders interchangeably. "There is ye same virtue & use in them both, drying, expelling water, yet bad for ye stomach." The leaves and stalks taken as potherbs "purge phlegm, and choler." The root is good for edema and viper bites. It also "softens ye Matrix and opens ye passages & sets to rights ye disaffections about it." Externally, it is used on hot swellings, dog bites, and hollow ulcers. Galen classified Elder as drying, gluing, and moderately digesting of corrupt material.

It is rather surprising that the old authors do not make more of the strong emetic and purgative properties of the plant. The use of these qualities comes over to us from the folk medical side of the tradition.

The Renaissance authors, drawing on popular sources, added many additional uses. Gerard comments, "It hath not only these faculties [mentioned by Galen], but others also; for the barke, leaues, first buds, floures, and fruit of Elder, do not only dry, but also heate, and haue withall a purging qualitie, but not without trouble and hurt to the stomacke." Dr. Blochwich (or Blochwitz) published a curious little volume in Latin in 1633, translated in English as *The Anatomie of Elder*. He drew on sources in folk medicine and professional literature to flush out an account of Elder spanning 230 pages.

Elder was so widely used in folk medicine that it was said to comprise an entire pharmacopoeia of the common folk. Shakespeare ranks it with the worthies of medicine. "What says my Aesculapius? My Galen? My heart of elder?" Blochwich compares it to the premier medicines of the era. "What the more sober and learned Chymists have attributed to their manifold Medicinal Mercury, Antimony, Vitriol, we may admit, admire, and acknowledge in our Elder."

The account by Blochwich is comprehensive. He tells us that every part of the plant contains medicinal properties, and that many complaints, from toothache to the plague, can be cured with Elder. The dried or fresh flowers, green or ripe berries, seeds, buds, leaves, fresh shoots, inner bark, outer bark, wood, pith, root, and a fungus growing on the tree called "Jew's Ears," were prepared in all sorts of different ways—by syrup, tincture, distillation, extract, wine, oil, water, vinegar, conserve, decoction, infusion, hot and cold tea, bath, powder, salt, oil, salve, smoke, amulet, etc. Authorities from Hippocrates down to this period are cited by Blochwich. He also credits "common women" who keep their knowledge as a "great secret."

Elder continued to occupy a place of importance in the herbal materia medica and has, even in the last decade, reasserted its old position of importance as a popular remedy for the flu. Among the modern authors, Dr. Edward Shook gives a detailed account.

As in European tradition, the American plant came to be used, part by part, in different ways. "In domestic medicine this plant forms almost a pharmacy in itself," comments Millspaugh. Some of the curious traditions surrounding the tree were carried over to the New World. J. I. Lighthall, "the great Indian medicine man," denounces the idea that the bark peeled upwards causes vomiting while it purges when peeled downwards. He says the difference is due to the size of the dose. "In large doses it will vomit, and in smaller ones act as a gentle purgative." He still records the different uses of the flowers, hot or cold. "Take the flowers and make a hot tea, and give it freely, and it will produce sweating," writes Lighthall. "Take the same amount and give it cold, and it will run off on the kidneys." In American herbalism the berries came to be used as a blood tonic in anemia. This is perhaps one of the few differentiating points in the Old and New World traditions. The inner bark made into a salve is used to break up congealed blood and swellings. Peter Smith, the "Indian physician" from "the Miami Country" says a cold decoction of the stalks is a good remedy for boils, because they "cool the blood." The pith is used as a moxa by Indians, and the hollow stalk has been used as a medicinal smoking tube in America, as well as Europe.

The Tubular Remedy

Chris Hafner, an acupunturist and herbalist in Minneapolis, first taught me about this medicine. He pointed out the affinities it has to stagnation of blood and fluids, also to infants and young children. These insights give order and sense to the accounts found in folk tradition, modern herbalism, and homeopathic literature. They also fit nicely with the doctrine of signatures.

The hollow tubes of the young branches not only point to the use of this plant in journeying, but show affinities with the tubes of the body, especially the blood vessels and pores of the skin and membranes. Elder has a powerful influence on the blood, to remove the stagnation found in bruises and boils. It also decongests heat and stirs up the blood in the interior, bringing it to the surface to remove heat and toxins. The stuffy, narcotic smell of the Elder reminds us of something closed in, needing aeration, and this is what *Sambucus* accomplishes for the body in open-ing the circulation. It completes the job by opening the pores of the skin to bring the heat and fluids out, also stimulating the kidneys. It has long been used for stagnant fluids and edema dependent on renal insufficien-cy. This makes it a remedy for cold conditions, as well as hot. Elder is the characteristic remedy when we see bruises that are blue and swollen from blood and fluid retention, especially of the wrists and ankles. It has long been used for old people with swollen ankles, and works especially if the skin is tinted blue.

Elder has a deep action on the other tubular structures of the body, including the respiratory tract, digestive organs, and pores of the skin. It is an ancient remedy for opening the lungs and bringing up mucus. Homeopathy notes that it is beneficial for children who wake in the night, gasp for breath, can't breath, turn blue, retain a blue look in the face. It is sometimes used for childhood croup.

The respiratory effect, combined with the diaphoretic capacity to open the pores of the skin and bring on perspiration, points to its use in preventing or curing recent flus, coughs, and colds. It acts both ways, to bring on perspiration when the pores are closed and the skin is red and hot, or check immoderate sweating with a cold surface. (Compare with *Arctium* and *Monarda*.) It also has a positive effect on many kinds of skin problems, including erysipelas, roseacea, eczema, and boils.

Elder was long used as an emetic and purgative to stimulate the stomach and bowels. Here the tubes also come to mind. In smaller doses it acts as a tonic restorative and antispasmodic, soothing and toning the tissues of the digestive tract. It possesses a mild nervine relaxant proper-ty which makes it appropriate in stomach problems, indigestion, bloat-ing and gas, colic and even convulsions. Elder increases activity and secretion, so that materials are moved along at a better rate, digestion is enhanced, congestion and stagnation are removed, and the portal circu-lation is opened up. This gets heat and congestion out of the deep inte-rior from around the intestines, decongests the liver, and moves the stool. It is not necessary to induce vomiting or purging to get *Sambucus* to act gently and slowly to improve these kind of conditions.

Elder has a mild sedative effect on the nerves (which are also tubes), augmented by its ability to sedate heat and irritation. It has been used for "wild ravings" and wakefulness, as Blochwich tells us. This also

429

reflects the relationship to journeying and imagination. Very often it will settle the heart, spirits, and blood, reducing the pulse somewhat in frequency and force. Finally, *Sambucus* acts upon that great concentration of tubes, the kidneys, to stimulate activity. It is used to remove edema, especially in the legs and ankles.

If there were only one indication I could give for Elder it would be the puffy, mottled aspect of the skin, so that there is a look of fullness with reddish-blue marbling over a pale surface. In Black people there is a darker marbling over lighter skin. This congestion appears most striking in the meatier parts of the legs, thighs, and forearms. If this symptom is present *Sambucus* is the remedy, no matter what the disease.

Chris taught that *Sambucus* is the remedy for infants, just as *Chamomilla* is the remedy for babies. In utero, the circulation of the blood and removal of waste products is conducted by the mother, but all of a sudden the newborn has to do all the work on his or her own. The peristaltic action is not always up to full operational capacity in the infant and there may be chaos in the movements of fluids, blood, and waste materials. Chris pointed out that Elder is particularly indicated when the infant is blue and swollen over the bridge of the nose and the skin of the checks is dry and red. The tubes aren't working so well, from the kidneys to the intestines to the skin. This kind of complexion is an indication of a tubercular taint, according to homeopathic experience. *Sambucus* is most active in the beginning and end of life—infancy and old age. The passageways to the Underworld are more open then.

Young Elder wood forms a light, hollow tube filled with pith, but in the older branches the wood thickens and the pith almost disappears. This reminds us of how the bones thicken as a child matures, especially how the fontanels close over, bringing an end to infancy. Elder is the remedy for the period of life up to the closure of the fontanels. It strengthens the baby in infancy, so that there is better transportation of fluids and blood through the tubes, while the bones grow in a healthy manner. It is, likewise, a remedy for old age.

Because Elder improves oxygenation of the blood, breathing capacity, respiratory problems, and kidney function, Chris suggested that Elder might be a preventative for sudden infant death syndrome (SIDS). Studies show that poor kidney function and not getting enough air during sleep (due to position, among other things) contribute to this problem. I thought this was a very good suggestion, and keep an eye out for indications for this remedy in the very young. This is not, of course, the only factor. Statistics show that ninety-seven percent of all infants who die from SIDS had a vaccination within twenty-four hours.

Boericke gives a good account of the respiratory symptoms associated with *Sambucus nigra* in homeopathy. The child is easily frightened, wakens with fear, suffocating, starts with fear, is not easily placated, is sensitive to impressions and images, which frighten. "See images when shutting the eyes." The child wakes with a sense of suffocation around midnight, is frightened, cannot breath. Face blue and clammy, or dry with heat and redness. Suited to the sniffles of infants; nose dry and stuffy. The child cannot breath when at the nipple, due to stuffed nose. Sweating during the day, dry heat of the skin at night. Extremities cold, blue, swollen.

Dr. Erastus Case, a turn-of-the-century homeopathic physician in Connecticut, recorded a nice little case of the sort that fits in here. A girl child, twelve-hours-old, was seen on December 5, 1896. "Respiration was established with difficulty at its birth, but the cause was not recognized. There have been several periods in which the breathing was suspended so long that the face became blue, and life seemed extinct. By closely observing the babe the nature of the trouble was found to be spasm of the glottis." One dose of *Sambucus nigra* in a high potency was given. "A few attacks followed much shorter and less severe, none after twelve hours. Since then she has been well."

Here is a good case history from my own notes, showing the properties of *Sambucus canadensis* as an herb tea. Elder was not widely used as a pregnancy remedy in the Old World, as far as I can tell, but it was utilized in this capacity by the Eastern Woodland Indians. According to Charlotte Erichsen-Brown, the Iroquois used Elder for particularly difficult cases, where other remedies had failed and the life of the mother and infant were at stake. This usage did not come over into professional or lay practice in nineteenth-century America.

Acting on this tip, I used *Sambucus* with success in a difficult pregnancy. The sister of my friend Susan was just starting into the eighth month. The baby had stopped moving, and in alarm, she went to the hospital. The fetus was still alive, but the mother was frightened, having lost her first child to SIDS. There was another scare—she went to the hospital again—but the baby was still fine. Another week passed. I didn't meet with the mother, but worked through Susan. She said that her sister was blue around the eyes. "In fact, she was born a blue baby." She was craving oxygen and wanted to go into labor, but felt too weak. I thought about the mix of symptoms. Perhaps the baby was inactive because it was not receiving enough oxygen. I had Susan pick up some dried Elder flower tea (*Sambucus canadensis.*) They sat down together and had a cup. Though barely dilated, contractions started right then and six hours later a healthy baby boy was delivered.

The Anatomy of Elder

In order to chronicle the innumerable uses of *Sambucus,* let us take a look at the various uses of the different parts of the plant, then the conditions which Blochwich and tradition, down to the present, associate with the plant.

Flowers. The properties of the flowers change according to whether they are fresh or dried, or served hot or cold. The fresh flowers are more purgative. "They likewise trouble the belly and moue to the stoole," Gerard explains. If dried, however, they loose these purgative properties. "The vinegar in which the dried floures are steeped are wholsome for the stomacke: being vsed with meate it stirreth vp an appetite, it cutteth and attenuateth or maketh thin grosse and raw humors," meaning catarrh or phlegm. They are also prepared as a wine. The vinegar and the wine, with the simple infusion, are the preparations most commonly used by Blochwich.

The hot infusion of the dried flowers is the preferred preparation to induce sweating and drive out fever. Henry Box, a famous English Quaker herbalist in the early part of the twentieth century, states: "For colds, influenza, fevers, inflammation of the brain, pneumonia (inflammation of the lungs), stomach, bowels or any part, *this is a certain cure. I have never known it to fail,* even when given up and at the point of death." He had lived through the perilous influenza epidemic of 1918. "It will not only save at the eleventh hour, but at the last minute of that hour. It is so harmless that you cannot use it amiss, and so effectual that you cannot give it in vain" (quoted by Shook).

"The cold infusion of elder flowers is a very fine remedy for sore and inflamed eyes," says Dr. Edward Shook. "It is also given as a general treatment for acidity, scrofula, and glandular enlargements taken internally... and applied outwardly for sprains, bruises, swollen glands, mus-

432

cular soreness, stiffness, rheumatic pains, and so forth."

Leaves. These are more stinking and insipid than the flowers. Blochwich reports, "There are some that say the leaves only of the Elder doth mollifie and discuss Schirrus [cancerous] tumors by Signature; because it groweth in dark and shadowy places."

"The leaves of the elder plant, although very effectual in dropsy, are not recommended because of their nauseous taste and somewhat drastic purgative properties," writes Shook. "We find that we get ideal results with the bark and berries and that, therefore, the leaves are not necessary for internal use."

"The leaves are, however, extremely valuable made into salves or oils for outward applications to wounds, burns, sunburn, bruises, contusions, sprains, and for many skin affections, acne, itch, etc.," Shook continues. He mentions the use of leaves gathered on the last day of April, as a folk remedy for hemorrhage. "The leaves [are] boiled soft in linseed [i.e., flaxseed] oil, for the relief of piles." A similar ointment was concocted by the London College of Surgeons at one time. Shook used his ointment for "purulent sores, ulcers, infected wounds, and so forth." The oil he used on hemorrhoids, burns, wounds, and as a cosmetic for enhancing the skin. He compounded fresh leaves of Elder, Plantain, and Wormwood to make a salve agreeable for "tumors and swellings, muscular rheumatism, stiff and aching back and so forth." All of these preparations, formulas, and uses were originally mentioned by Martin Blochwich in 1633.

Inner Bark. "The yellow middle [inner] bark is commended by his signature for the yellow Jaundice," continues the exuberant Blochwich. It was widely used as a purgative for the gallbladder, stomach, and intestines in folk and premodern medicine. He reports an old folk belief: "The commons are fully perswaded, and call experience to witness, that if those middle barks be pulled downward from the Tree, it emptieth the body of evil humors by purge; if they be pulled upward, it worketh by vomit." This tradition was still widely kept up in nineteenth-century America.

"The bark should be dried and kept for several months before use," says Shook. "The fresh bark, like cascara sagrada is violently irritating and poisonous to children." It causes spasms and cramps more readily than the other parts of the plant, and therefore cures them. Hence, it is used in biliary congestion, constipation, spasmodic asthma with copious phlegm and stringy mucus, epilepsy. It also acts on cardiac and renal dropsies.

As a purgative, Elder acts on the intestines, but it should be used in smaller doses for a cumulative effect, rather than the sudden gush. Gerard has much to say about the use of Elder as an intestinal remedy. The tender leaves, "taken in some broth or pottage open the belly, purging both slimie flegme and cholericke humors: the middle barke is of the same nature, but stronger, and purgeth the said humors more violently." It is used to remove "choler ànd waterie humors," and is specially good for the dropsy.

The leaves and bark are also used locally for swellings or injuries. They remove heat and inflammation from infections and boils, closed cuts, and infected ulcers. Elder cools and decongests the blood. By decongesting local accumulations of blood and fluids, it opens the channels of the nerves, hence has been used for neuralgic pain. Finally, it is good for arthritic pain in older subjects with stagnant blood and fluids.

Berries. These have a property not found in the other parts of the plant; they are used as a tonic to build up the blood and combat anemia. For this purpose they may be combined with blackberries. However, both the berries and the oil expressed from the seeds were used for many of the same purposes as the other parts of the plant.

Dr. Shook says the berries cleanse and gently purge the stomach and bowels, promote perspiration, remove cold, sore throat, nasal congestion, bronchial catarrh, and asthma. A syrup taken at night "promotes pleasant perspiration and is demulcent to the chest."

Seed. "The facultie of the seed is somewhat gentler than that of the other parts," says Gerard. "It also moueth the belly, and draweth forth waterie humors, being beaten to pouder, and giuen to a dram weight: being new gathered, steeped in vineger, and afterwards dried, it is taken, and that effectually, in the like weight of the dried lees of wine [tartar], and with a few Anise seeds." This preparation "helpeth those that haue the dropsie. But it must be giuen for certaine daies together in a little wine, to those that haue need thereof." The dried berries are "good for such as haue dropsie, and such as are too fat, and would faine be leaner, if they be taken in a morning to the quantity of a dram with wine for a certaine space." Blochwich also relied on the "oyl expresst of the kernals" for such purposes.

Pith. "Note," says Blochwich, "that the pith of the Elder being pressed with the finger, doth pit, as Hydropick feet do." Thus it is, by signature, a remedy for hydropsy, edema, or water retention. "The pith being cut and swallowed, is commonly much praised for moving urine, and purging those dregs," which cause the stone. "I know a man who being troubled with the Ascitis and Stone, by the perswasion of a Country-woman, used only this pith" to cure himself of kidney pains and edema. Blochwich then gives a formula called "stone-break spirit of the Elder," which he traces back to Matthiolus. Thin shaves of pith are infused in the spirit of the berries, pressed, and strained. To this, Juniper berries are added. "In the difficulty of making water, and in the not making water at all, these Medicines are excellent."

The pith dried and pressed or squashed, says Gerard, "is good to lay vpon the narrow orifices or holes of fistulas and issues, if it be put therein."

Fungus. Not having seen one of these, I must rely upon the account by Gerard. "There groweth oftentimes vpon the bodies of those old trees or shrubs a certaine excrescence called *Auricula Iude*," he says. He incorrectly translates this as "Jew's Ear;" the correct translation refers to Judas. "It is soft, blackish, couered with a skin, somewhat like now and then to a mans eare." This curious article attracted much attention and was used in medicine. It "hath a binding and drying qualitie," notes Gerard. "The infusion thereof, in which it hath bin steeped a few houres, taketh away the inflammations of the mouth, and almonds of the throat in the beginning, if the mouth and throat be washed therewith, and doth in the like manner helpe the uvula."

Blochwich gave an account of every possible use of Elder known up to the time of his writing in 1633. He drew from all the old sources, such as Hippocrates and Dioscorides, from the more modern and "Chymical" authors, and also from the "Country People," "Matrons" and "she-Montebanks," whoever they were. From this we get an overview of the uses of Elder in traditional herbal literature which is quite unique. Let us follow Blochwich, organ by organ.

Head. "In mitigating the pain of the head, and removing distempers thereof in women, we use happily the Cake of the flowers of the Elder, left in the Vesica [vessel] after the distillation of the water; it must not be burned." This preparation also "rarifieth the skin." If there is heat

435

associated with the head pain, "some use rose cakes bedewed with the vinegar of the Elder," or simply the vinegar on the head externally.

A decoction of the flowers induces sleep, if rubbed on the legs and arms before bed. Blochwich recommended Elder flowers and Poppy seeds for "raving and wakings." *Sambucus* evidently works by sedating heat which is agitating the mind. The vinegar of Elder flowers, "recovers those as it were, from death, that are subject to swounings and faintings upon every the lightest cause or occasion." Here it may be operating as a blood tonic, or as an anti-hysteric.

Epilepsy in infants, children, and adults "expects its most specifick cure, almost from the Elder." A compound of Elder flowers, Linden flowers, and Peony root is used during the convulsion. (Peony is an old specific for epilepsy.) Blochwich treats us to a case history from his own experience. "An infant, which being Taken sometimes with Epileptick fits, each day, with a great deal of crying and pain of belly," with yellow-ish-greenish stool, was brought to him for help. He observed that the mother's milk was "serous and thin," and thought this to be the source of the problem. He recommended Elderberry wine and burnt Hartshorn for the mother, "which cured all."

Blochwich also mentions the use of an amulet in the treatment of epilepsy. "In the month of October, a little before the full moon," pluck a twig of the Elder and cut the part out between two joints. Cut into nine pieces, tie up in a linen cloth, and bind above the heart with thread. Tighten until the thread breaks, remove the amulet with an instrument, and bury in the ground so nobody can touch it." Considering the strong smell of freshly cut Elder, this amulet may have medicinal properties.

Apoplexy and palsy, or stroke and paralysis, as we would now say, also come under the positive influence of Elder. Blochwich outlines a formula made from Sage, Marjoram, "Ivy arthritica," Cowslip flowers, Lily of the Valley, and spirit of Elder. This is for the apoplexy of old men, he notes, not that from head injuries or brain fever. If the stroke has caused a paralysis or "palsie of the sides," he recommends Elder, Sage, and Greater Burdock. Rub the affected limbs with Elder.

Eyes, ears, nose, and throat. Dried Elder flowers in Rose water are applied to the eyes, "to mitigateth opthalmicke pains, and strengtheneth the sight." It did much help "in a more vehement tumor of the eyelids, whereby the whole eye was hid."

Elder and Chamomile flowers are combined and used as a fomentation for ear pain. Elder flowers and Oregano are used for difficult hearing. "The same vapor takes away the tingling, whistling, and other sounds of the ear," says Blochwich. (*Origanum* is one of the closest analogues to *Monarda fistulosa,* which often palliates or cures tinnitus.)

The juice of the recently pressed Elder leaves in a little wine, dropped into the ears, "doth cleanse the filth of the exulcerate ears." Likewise, Elder leaves are used for ulcers in the nose, even in "a greater exulceration" with proud flesh. (Here we see the use of the leaves for external surfaces.)

"The best Water of the Flowers of the Elder, often drawn up in the nose, doth help the smelling, that is diminished by some great sickness."

As we approach the mouth, throat, and conditions of the upper respiratory tract, Blochwich shows more dependence on folk tradition. "The Common Women, so soon as they suspect any Disease in the Throate of their young ones," wash the tissues with a preparation made from the fungus. It helps likewise the ulcers of gums and throat, the ulcers of small pox, and swollen tonsils. A decoction of Elder flowers is used for heat and inflammation in the tonsils. And, "women with great success, give [Elder wine] to their coughing unquiet Children." This is also beneficial for older people. Elder is accounted "a great secret amongst women" to treat such hoarseness as proceeds from a catarrh, and so to "make a clear voice." It is also used for "the Cough and hoarseness proceeding from heat in feavers."

Elder was a highly regarded medicine for the treatment of toothache. "No one Medicine sooner easeth this great pain," he quotes Raymond Minder. The wine and vinegar of the dried flowers are again used. The common people made toothpicks and spoons from the Elder to prevent toothache. This may have some practical effect, but it is heightened by the use of magic. "The common people take of these elder tooth-pickers...and glew them to the Trunk of an Elder," while it is being irradiated by the morning sun, then "pull away the bark, and cover the place with rosin of the Pine." In this manner, they "cure all toothaches." Blochwich notes, "'Tis not apparent by what vertue this is done." He speculates that the toothpicks stimulate the gums and let a certain amount of blood. (*Sambucus* also acts as a blood purifier, removing heat and toxin from boils and abscesses.) "But we leave every man to his judgment." Thank you.

Respiratory Tract. Elder is an important remedy in pulmonary problems, from the simple sore throat and hoarseness, to asthma and tuberculosis. The infusion of the dried flowers or the syrup of the flowers or berries are especially recommended. Blochwich describes a simple preparation of Elder flowers, berries, or buds with honey and vinegar to help expectoration when there is shortness of breath and asthma. "In a great dyspnoea" or a "suffocating catar," he recommends a formula of Elder, Elecampane, Orris Root, and Fennel Seed. Elder is also beneficial for what Blochwich describes as "that wild Cough, where corrupt matter is [expelled], and more corruption feared." This is probably a description of tuberculosis. Elder proves sedative to these conditions by removing fever and quieting the nervous system.

Digestive Tract. A plant which acts both as an emetic and as a purgative must have a powerful action on the digestive sphere. On a more subtle level, it works by decongesting stagnant blood in the portal circulation, as well as removing heat and toxicity. As a sedative, it also relaxes the nerves envolved in peristalsis. As a tonic it can build up weak, cold conditions.

Blochwich says that heartburn is treated with a mild emetic made from Elder, while the colic is cured by spirit of Elder and Chamomile. He knew of "a Churchman, who by this spirit in a short time dissapateth the Collick, which had been long with him."

Colicky symptoms in the abdomen are highly characteristic of *Sambucus.* I have a number of case histories to demonstrate this. A woman down the road from me was suffering from severe lower back pain, heartburn, and colic for over a year. She had puffy, mottled skin on the forearms and thighs. Mother tincture of *Sambucus canadensis* in doses of three drops removed the symptoms from the start. The back, which had been injured, improved in part. Several weeks later I saw another woman who was suffering from some kind of subclinical intestinal problem. She had been to the doctors until they ran out of tests. One told her to take Prozac, the other said she would have to wait until the problem manifested as "something," before they could treat it. The patient's subjective impression was that the condition centered about where the small and large intestines meet, and was "festering." The symptoms started about a year ago, at which time she also gained alot of weight. There was intermittent colic and lower back pain. *Sambucus canadensis* immediately improved the intestinal situation and over a few months she lost weight as well.

438

Blochwich gives a very nice formula for those of a "weak, cold Stomach, and of hard digestion:" Calamus root, Ginger, Mint, Fennel seed, Anise seed, and Elder berries. This combination ought to be very soothing, due to the presence of all those carmatives with volatile oils.

The crystalline salt of Elder, a preparation made by burning the marque left after distillation of the spirit, is used to cure worms, says Blochwich. Elder was used both for diarrhea and constipation. It was specific for a kind of flux where semi- or undigested food passed in the stool, also for bloody dysentery. Here it may be used in combination with Tormentil root and Plantain leaf, another very good formula, though the leaf of Cinquefoil or Agrimony could be used instead of the root of Tormentil. It is also beneficial for tympanitic or flatulent distention, here taken with Fennel and Anise seed. The leaves are used for constipation. "There is nothing more excellent to ease the pain of the Hemmorhoides than a fomentation made of the flowers of Elder and Verbasie [Mullein] or Hony-suckle in water or milk." Blochwich supports this by reference to two cases healed in this manner. The outer bark is used for anal prolapse.

Elder, as we have seen, also has an action on the gall ducts, which it purges. Here Blochwich recommends a combination of Elder and Wormwood, with exercise.

Kidneys. Elder was widely known for its ability to remove edema and correct problems in the kidneys. It is used for both a cold, pale edema, and a hot, inflamed kind with scanty urine.

Blochwich gives several dramatic case histories of different kinds of edema cured with various preparations of Elder. A citizen of Haina, after two years of fever, became "leucophlegmatic" (pale, swollen, and weak). He was cured by the use of Elder and Wormwood to purge, then Elder and hartshorn to sweat. "His whole body did detumifie; a more lively colour, and laudable appetite did return."

In reference to ascitis, or edema in the abdomen, Blochwich says, "There is no man that doth not perceive that the Elder is of great virtue in this disease." And "where the bowels are more hot, and the urine more red, which is oft-times a deadly token in Hydropick [dropical, edemic] persons," Elder is also beneficial. Here the green leaves, or dried if necessary, are used externally, especially on inflammatory edema in the feet or ankles. "But seeing these fomentations are tedious, it is enough to carry the green and dry leaves of the Elder in the stockings." He knew of a "great lawyer" who was cured in this manner. This type of approach is essentially homeopathic and shows the power of the herb to remove serious disease in minute doses.

Blochwich goes on to relate a case which was particularly famous in his region. "A grave Matron," aged about sixty, suffered several weeks from "a white flux of the belly," followed by edema and weakness. She was given up for dead, but took Elder flowers in conserve and was cured. She lived to be eighty years of age, "to the great wonder of all those that saw and heard."

Female System. Hippocrates used Elder for many kinds of female problems. Blochwich listed these traditional uses, plus others based on his own experience. He describes the use of Elder in many kinds of uterine problems, including swollen womb, inflammed uterus following child birth, ulcers of the womb (here use Flaxseed and Elder), excess flow of thin blood, clotting and coagulated flow, and cramps.

Blochwich gives a case of cancer of the womb cured with Elder, although it is difficult to be sure that the diagnosis was correct, since the details are not given. However, this shows that the same theory of coagulated blood was recognized in Europe, as it was in India, China, and the Americas, as a cause of cancer. He describes "the Scyrrous disposition of the matrix, where the cram'd humor is hardened into a Scyrrous" tumor.

The use of Elder as a general tonic for the newborn is also mentioned by Blochwich. "A handful of Elder flowers well dried" and macerated in wine is used as a general sort of cleanser by people of "the best sort," who "wash their new-born babes" with it to remove congested humors in the stomach and joints.

Joints. The old Western doctors, like their Eastern counterparts, believed that arthritis was largely caused by "humors" getting stuck in the joints, condensing and causing inflammation and swelling. This is a condition in which Elder is again appropriate. "A linen cloth dipt in the distilled water of the leaves and flowers of the Elder, and applied warm wonderfully asswages the pain, unlocks the pores, digests the matter and strengthens the nervous parts." He recommends putting the dried Elder flowers in vinegar, "where the colour and heat is greater," so that the medicine can penetrate better. Where the joints are cold, spirit of Elder flowers (alcoholic distillation) is preferred.

Elder is also beneficial for gout. "I know a man, that whensoever he is troubled with the Gout useth only this unction," made from cream, fine meal, and Elder leaves worked into the consistency of a poultice and applied hot.

Skin. Elder is used in febrile diseases where the pores need to be opened or there is a rash. It is also beneficial for chronic conditions such as erysipelas, rosacea, eczema, scabies, psora, itch, boils, carbuncles, and herpes. In all of these cases, the idea is that Elder opens the pores and removes filthy humors from the interior.

Blochwich mentions several kinds of serious skin disease cured with Elder. A baker's wife "could not go out of dores by reason of the abundance" of hot pustules on her feet, black towards the middle and red to the outside. She was cured with Elder flowers macerated in milk. Elder is also used by "she-Montebanks" who cure "eating herpes" and "have gained largely" thereform. Blochwich knew of a woman who, taken with "the Rose" or rosacea, applied an extract of the berries to her chest. This "provoked sweat moderately," and using no other remedy, "but a knot of red fine linnen, wherin Elder-flowers are sewed," she cured herself of the disease.

A specific remedy for erysipelas, according to Blochwich, is the new Elder flowers, or the old if necessary, in the milk of a red cow, or at least a cow with red spots, drunk several times in the wane of the moon. As a general remedy to cleanse the putridities in the interior that create the scab and psora Blochwich recommends a salad of the buds in the spring (this is probably a scurvy remedy), or Elder flowers, Borage, and Chicory.

A most interesting approach is to use "an amulet made of Elder, on which the Sun never shined, if the piece betwixt the two Knots [joints on the twig] be hung about the patients neck." Blochwich adds, "I learned the certainty of this experiment first from a friend in Lipsick; who no sooner err'd in diet, but he was seized on by this disease [erysipelas]; yet after he used this Amulet, he protested he was free; yea, that a woman to whom he lent it, was likewise delivered from this disease." Blochwich suggests that the reader decide for himself whether or not such devices work, or by what means.

I have myself used Elder tincture internally in infants and children with rough, red, dry skin (sometimes diagnosed as eczema), especially where the "meaty tissues" of the cheeks or on the forearms are involved.

Fever. Elder is used for just about every form of fever, from the touch of flu to the plague. "The common people, as soon as they find the first touch of a Fever, they take the Rob [berries] of the Elder in Vinegar, Spirit, or water of the flowers thereof," in order to sweat and remove the initial contagion. It is also beneficial for intermittent fever or flu with relapsing chills. Elder flowers in honey and vinegar may be given before the fit. "The Polychrest powder of Elder buds" in whey, purges the yellow and black bile, as well as phlegm and serous humors, and thus treats the tertian and quartan ague, that is, intermittent fever. In addition to this, Elder treats "continual and burning" fever, "where the heat is more intense, and great drought tormenteth the Patient." Here it is given often, to extinguish the fire, cut the gross and tough matters, purge the humors, and sharpen the recuperating appetite. It also is used to control the "spotted fever," including "the Pox" and measles, the rash of which indicates the presence in the interior of filthy humors that need to be removed. Finally, Elder was used in the most dreaded fever of all, the plague. "A little sponge being wet in the vinegar of Elder, and carried in a hollow globe made of Juniper-wood," probably around the neck, and so smelled, "mightily strengtheneth the spirits against the impression of the infections contagion." Indeed, even just a few drops of the Spirit of the flowers taken daily or at the beginning of the plague, pestilence, or spotted fever, can prevent or curtail it. Elder washes were also used on the plague buboe or swollen glands and on ulcers of the glands.

Blochwich goes on to give a case history of some kind of "plague" cured in his homeland. "When in Anno 1626, the Plague was raging in Haina, and many of the infected were troubled with head aches, ravings, and wakings; a worthy man told me, he found no readier help to dissipate those venomous vapours, and bring sleep in his own and other bodies; then after giving of several medicines, to bind their heads about with the flowers of the Elder."

Wounds, Hemorrhage, Contusions, and Ulcers. Elder is used to stop hemorrhage, prevent pain, hurry recovery of punctured nerves, "discuss the black bloud" in contusions, take the heat out of burns, and sooth and cleanse "deep, perverse, and fistulous ulcers." The latter usage is credited to Dioscorides; here the powder of the leaves is sprinkled into the fretting ulcer. Elder is also used for the stings of wasps and bees, anointing the part with the oil of infused flowers or kernals. Viper bites are treated with Elder roots or berries in wine.

Acting on Chris Hafner's tip that Elder is beneficial when the tissues are swollen and blue, I always think of this medicine especially for bruises and injuries to the wrists and ankles, where the contusions tend to retain fluids.

The use of Elder in domestic medicine was so common and extensive that Hahnemann, the founder of homeopathy, worried that people were getting poisoned by the constant use of the tea. He proved the medicine (giving small doses repeatedly until it produced symptoms), showing that the Elder (*Sambucus nigra*) can produce many symptoms. He then wrote vigorously against the folk healers and housewives who used Elder as a cure-all. He fails to note that the provings verify many of the traditional uses.

Preparation, Toxicity, and Dosage

Maude Grieve and Dr. Edward Shook give directions for collection and preparation of the various parts of the Elder. Taking into account folk traditions and pharmacological differences, it appears that the various parts of Elderberry act in somewhat different ways. I have a preference for the flowers, which have a nice smell and are not as active as the bark and leaves. The tea made from the dried flowers is nice, or a tincture from the fresh flowers. This would be the American species. I have also used the low homeopathic potencies of both kinds.

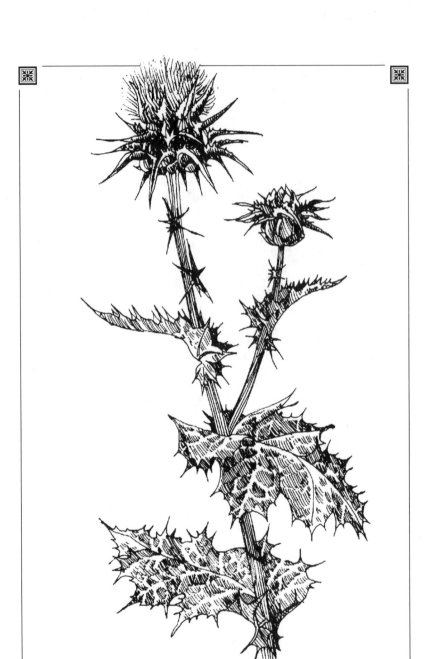

Silybum marianum

Milk Thistle

Silybum marianum
Milk Thistle

This is "a stately and very beautiful plant," writes Culpeper. "If brought from a remote part of the world, it would be much esteemed in our gardens." The common names are Milk Thistle, Our Lady's Thistle, and St. Mary's Thistle, the latter a translation from the German *Mariendistil.* The ribbons of white running through the leaves were said to spring from a drop of Mother Mary's Milk. The plant was used as a galactagogue, though today its cousin Blessed Thistle (*Cnicus benedictus*) is more often employed in this capacity.

Milk Thistle is a member of the Aster family native to southern and western Europe but cultivated and naturalized in the Americas. It is particularly at home along the Pacific coast from northern California to British Columbia. In many places it will self-seed in a garden, but not grow wild. Originally classified as *Carduus marianum* in the older literature, in modern times it was subjected to a nomenclatural change in order to bring it in line with more recent findings in botany, so it is presently known as *Silybum marianum.* The older name is still used in homeopathy.

All parts of the plant are nontoxic and the leaves have been eaten as a food. They make a delicious salad, tasting like the highest quality lettuce greens, with a firm, crunchy, desirable texture. Unlike lettuce, they remain edible throughout the summer, if one likes a faintly more bitter taste. The thorns have to be cut off each leaf, so it is worthwhile as a table green, but not as a marketable crop. The stalks, flower receptacles (resembling artichoke), and seeds have also been eaten.

Milk Thistle was known to the ancient authors as a food and medicine. Plinius stated that the juice of the herb mixed with honey was a remedy for "carrying off the bile." It is still used to decongest the liver. Milk Thistle found its place in medieval Catholic folk religion and medicine. The herbalists of the Renaissance gave it a thorough treatment. By this time its use in clearing "obstructions from the spleen and liver" was well established, but the popularity of foreign and toxic drugs pushed Milk Thistle aside after the beginning of the eighteenth century. Interest was rekindled by the Paracelsian revivalist, Johann Gottfried Rademacher (1772-1850). He is generally credited with inspiring the modern phase of interest in German medicine. Rademacher correctly stated that the most active ingredients were in the seed coat.

Rademacher first learned about this plant in 1809. He had been called to attend a woman suffering from abdominal pains centered in the cecel region. He could not determine whether it was gallstones or induration of the liver. Although he had seen a good many cases like this before, his efforts were ineffectual. Hectic fever with coughing supervened, the face took on a muddy, yellow disposition, insomnia joined on, and emaciation set in. These symptoms suggested tuberculosis complicated with hepatic symptoms. No one expected the patient to live. At this point Rademacher remembered that Stahl, an eighteenth century doctor, had praised the seed of *Carduus marianum* in respiratory complaints associated with hepatic fevers. Rademacher gave the woman a tea and she recovered completely. Subsequently, he found Milk Thistle useful in cases where there was congestion, induration, and inflammation of the liver or spleen, accompanied by hemorrhagic tendencies. *Carduus* would usually effect a cure when there was blood in the sputum, stool, urine or excessive menstruation, when these conditions were accompanied by swelling and congestion of the liver and spleen, with pains in the sides. He also used it to cure gallstone colic. Milk Thistle became one of Rademacher's organ-specific remedies, exhibiting an affinity for the liver and spleen.

Rademacher's work was popularized for English readers towards the end of the nineteenth century by the colorful London homeopath, James Compton Burnett. *Carduus marianum* was one of the remedies he learned about from Rademacher. In 1887 a "young lady of sixteen summers," was brought to Burnett by her mother, suffering from severe bouts of vomiting which had been going on for three months. She was sometimes roused from her sleep by an attack. "Her constitution had been damaged by diphtheria, and eighteen months previously she had had varicella." Burnett was able to relieve the vomiting, but the abdominal pains got worse. "There the thing still was: I had relieved the symptoms but I had not cured the real primary seat of the same. I then did what might with advantage have been done before the treatment was begun, viz.: I made a careful physical examination of the bare epigastrium and of the two hypochondria." This revealed a greatly swollen spleen and liver. The vomiting was merely a reflex symptom caused by crowding on the stomach. "Here I fell back upon my Rademacherian experience with Carduus." He gave five drops of the mother tincture of the seed in a tablespoonful of water, morning and night. "The generally improved appearance of the young lady after she had been a month under the Carduus was very striking, and repeatedly remarked upon by friends." What sixteen year old girl would not like that! The condition was completely cured.

Burnett's experience, combined with homeopathic provings that had already been undertaken, went far to popularize this remedy in homeopathic circles. His works were also read by allopaths and eclectics, and the remedy was taken up by members of all these schools. Meanwhile, there was continuing interest in Germany.

The eclectics continued to develop a picture of the *Carduus* pathology. The last edition of King's *Dispensary* (1898) give the following as characteristic symptoms:

> *Dull aching pain over the spleen, which passes up to the left scapula, associated with pronounced debility and despondency, splenic pain, with no enlargement or with enlargement, when there are no evidences of malaria. Congestion of the liver, spleen and kidneys. General bilious conditions accompanied with stitches in the right side, with hard and tender spots, in this locality, gall stone, jaundice, hepatic pain and swelling.*

I was called into consultation by telephone to help one elderly woman who had been hospitalized for over a month, teetering on the brink of death. Her original complaint was a serious edema, followed by extreme weakness, then a rash of classic liver symptoms: bitter taste in the mouth, indigestion, pain in the hepatic region, and mild jaundice. At this juncture we gave *Carduus marianus* 3x and the hepatic symptoms quickly disappeared.

The eclectics continued to build up their knowledge of the properties of *Carduus*. Ellingwood noted in the *American Eclectic Materia Medica* (1919):

> *Harvey, in the California Medical Journal, says the indications are so plain that a tyro can prescribe it with certainty. It is indicated where there is venous stasis, the true veins enlarged and clogged with blood. This is true of either the large or small veins. He says he cured once case, where the veins from the hips to the toes were as large and as hard and twisted as Manila Rope. They could be felt through the clothing. He cured completely a varicose tumor in the popliteal space [behind the knee]. It was about four inches long, and three inches wide. The skin of the neck and hands was discolored. There was a troublesome chronic cough with the expectoration of large quantities of offensive matter. He believed these symptoms to be associated with disease of the spleen. He had observed these colored spots in other cases, and sometimes found long continued soreness and tenderness of the joints of the feet. Carduus, in five-drop doses three or four times a day, cured all the symptoms in this case, restoring the patient to perfect health. The remedy acts slowly and must be persisted in.*

Rademacher noted a hemorrhagic tendency, but Burnett and the eclectics found a congested, swollen, varicose condition. As with Yarrow, we see in Milk Thistle a mastery of the opposite conditions of hemorrhage and congestion of blood. This again illustrates how herbs encompass antipodal actions within their operation.

Pharmacological research on the active components in Milk Thistle began in Germany about 1960. This led to the isolation of a substance called silymarin, the "active ingredient." Subsequent research showed that it was a mixture of substances called flavanolignans. Laboratory and clinical research demonstrated that silymarin prevented the destruction of liver cells, increased the production of new liver cells, and increased the level of glutathione, an amino acid which helps to detoxify poisons and process hormones. Milk Thistle has, therefore, been viewed primarily as a liver medicine. It is principally used to protect the liver cells against damage from chronic drinking, drug taking, poisoning, hepatitis, and mushroom poisoning.

However, viewed against the background of tradition and historical use, Milk Thistle appears to be primarily a spleen/lymphatic remedy, acting secondarily on the portal and hepatic systems. To trace the disease process from the traditional standpoint, we see that weakness of the lymphatic system results in poor assimilation and nutrition which gives rise to weakness, congestion, stagnation, and prolapse of abdominal viscera. Veins are turgid and congested. Varicose veins, hemorrhoids, pelvic congestion, menstrual problems, blood stagnation, and hemorrhage may be a consequence. Stagnation in the portal circulation results in congestion and induration in the liver and other organs in the abdomen, such as the pancreas and the spleen. There may be die-off of hepatic cells, thickening of bile, and the appearance of gallstones. Poor liver function and pelvic congestion can lead to pre-menstrual stress and difficulties during pregnancy. The spleen, as part of the lymphatic system, is involved as well. Mental symptoms calling for Milk Thistle indicate an association with the spleen. Gerard mentions "melancholy" and King's *Dispensary* says "despondency." These emotions are typical of the spleen, not the liver, which is commonly associated with anger and frustration. These sorts of conditions occur in association with serious, chronic diseases, as the case histories cited by Rademacher, Burnett, and Ellingwood indicate.

At the present time, Milk Thistle is widely marketed as a "liver remedy." My own experience suggests that Milk Thistle is an excellent liver and abdominal medicine in serious cases. I have used it only three times: in every case the person was seriously ill or even facing death. I mentioned this to my friend Margie Flint, an herbalist in Marblehead, Massachusetts. She has used Milk Thistle extensively in people with cirrhosis of the liver from alcoholism. She agreed entirely: Milk Thistle is usually only indicated in serious cases.

Milk Thistle and Death Cap Mushroom

One of the most interesting facts about Milk Thistle is that it is a specific antidote to the Death Cap or *Amanita phalloides* mushroom. This usage was known in folk medicine for centuries. The mechanism by which it works has now been demonstrated by modern research and clinical use has shown its extreme importance.

Death Cap contains powerful hepatotoxins that decimate liver cells in a short time. The usual symptoms are intense abdominal pains, nausea, vomiting, and fetid diarrhea. Death occurs in thirty percent of the cases. A few people have been brought back from the edge of death by transplanting the liver. Clinical studies undertaken in hospitals in Germany, France, Austria, and Switzerland have shown that Silymarin cut this mortality rate almost in half. Today Milk Thistle is used in German medicine as the specific antidote for *Amanita phalloides* poisoning. It is not used in the United States because the introduction of a new drug would require millions of dollars in tests to satisfy FDA standards, and no American company would undertake the cost on a drug which could not be patented.

Although I do not have a great deal of experience using Milk Thistle in lymphatic and hepatic complaints, I have relied upon it to save the life of a friend suffering from acute *Amanita* poisoning. And who else could that be but Susan?

In the summer of 1991 it rained all season long, providing a perfect environment for many mushrooms to flourish. The television news shows were warning people not eat *Amanita phalloides*. It was springing up all over the place, often in people's yards. As luck would have it, Susan bought a mushroom identification book, went out in her back yard, and nibbled on a fungi. She took two small bites, about the size of a little finger nail each, of an immature specimen of *Amanita phalloides*. Considering her small body weight (eighty-four pounds), the fact that she was a Crohn's disease patient with yards of abdominal scar tissue and adhesions that could easily rupture from vomiting, and that the immature fungi is more poisonous than the mature, this was quite enough.

After three hours Susan started to feel like she had the flu: chills alternated with fever and she experienced achiness in the joints. Half an hour later she started to suffer severe abdominal pains, with vomiting and black, fetid diarrhea. She called the county poison control center. They recommended the emergency room. She also called me, and even waited an hour and a half for me to return the call. By this point in her life Susan trusted the herbalists more than the doctors. As usual, she was justified: herbalists have an antidote for mushroom poisoning in Milk

Thistle which doctors in the U.S. do not. I said, "This sounds like fun" and rushed over.

By the time I got there Susan was lying on the bathroom floor, prostrated with dry heaves, fading in and out of consciousness. Another friend had arrived. I took one look at the mushroom and didn't need to wonder about its identity. I gave the antidote and we headed to the hospital. All I had was a quarter ounce of Milk Thistle seeds. She tried her best to chew it.

As we drove off Susan mumbled, "I can see the Other Side." A few blocks later she added, "They're coming to take me." Just before we got to the hospital she said, "It's the right herb."

We got Susan to the emergency room and sat in the waiting area. They immediately gave her an anti-emetic intravenously and put her on a heart monitor. She was having convulsions, the monitor was going wild, the doctor, nurse, and orderly were all standing by expecting to do cardio-pulmonary resuscitation. All of a sudden the convulsions stopped and the monitor settled down to show an ordinary heart beat. The three attendants looked at each other, at her, and at the equipment. They fumbled with the dials. The nurse had some intuition. She grabbed a Milk Thistle seed off Susan's clothing, stuck it in her face and asked, "So what's this?" That was the first reason Susan didn't want to go to the hospital. "I don't know," she said quickly, but they were all over her clothes and in the froth around her mouth, so she thought better. "Uh...its the antidote." The staff didn't say anything.

Paul and I were still sitting in the waiting room. Finally, a pleasant and dedicated nurse, the kind of person that emanates the sort of feeling you would like in all hospital personnel, came out and said to us, "Your friend is going to be all right. We're going to keep her in Intensive Care tonight, but you can go up for a visit."

We met Susan in her new room. "I don't wanna be here," she complained. "They won't let me smoke and they tried to put me in the same room I was in last time." (That was when she was in a coma for three months, following an ileostomy and overmedication on morphine.) We urged her to stay. All of a sudden a doctor burst into the room. It was apparent he had just been called in from home and was learning about the case from the notes on the clipboard he grabbed off the door. Leafing through, he asked, "What's the problem?"

"I ate a poison mushroom."

"Where'd ya get it, Lunds?" he asked sarcastically. (Lunds is a famous grocery store chain in Minnesota. The hospital is in the inner city and he evidently thought she was a drug overdose.)

"No, I found it in my back yard."

The doctor didn't say a thing, but for some reason I could read his mind. It was like there were letters spelling out thoughts over his head. "Oh oh, this woman's crazy," was what he was thinking to himself. He continued to leaf through the notes. "This says you have Crohn's disease," he almost shouted. "How do you know this isn't a flare-up of Crohn's?" Susan said she knew the difference. "Who's your regular doctor?" he asked. This was the second reason Susan didn't want to be checked into a hospital. "Well, uh...I saw Dr. Smith at Park Nicolett a year ago."

"What!" our medical friend exploded. "You haven't been to a doctor in over a year? And you have Crohn's disease! You're supposed to check in once a month!" Again, I could read the words over his head. I expected them to say something like, "My God, what's wrong with you," but to my surprise they said: "Oh my God, I'm the primary health care provider!"

The interview wasn't going well. Susan kept arguing that she wanted to go home. The doctor was very up front about the situation. "I could let you out, but it would be against your medical recommendation. That would be fine with me, but I'd have to write it down in your file that way." I told her she would be better staying there. Finally, our advisor put his medical foot down. He addressed Susan sternly: "You and I are prisoners here tonight. I don't want to be here and you don't want to be here, but we're both stuck here until morning." I thought, "Wow, an honest doctor," but our other friend thought he was callous. In a moment we were ordered out of the room.

The next morning the doctor was more friendly. He had seen the computer print out of Susan's medical records, complete with the gunshot wound that barely missed the heart, the Crohn's disease, the peritonitis which had gone untreated for two weeks when the small intestine burst (due to medical incompetence), the ileostomy, the over-medication on morphine which caused a three-month coma in the room next to the one she was currently camped out in, and the absurdly low potassium levels the night before which should have killed anyone. The whole case was just an oddity and he was relieved to be going home with nothing worse than a weird story.

I do not believe that toxicological tests were run on the mushroom we brought in, but the staff was extremely impressed with our "herbal antidote." Susan's potassium level had gone as low as 2.3, well below the 3.0 level where death is expected. A few years later a doctor was looking at her charts. "My God, I've never seen anybody who had this many green sheets in her records and was still alive." (Green sheets indicate days spent in the Intensive Care Unit.) "We'd have to shoot her to kill her," he joked. Then he read the part about scar tissue from a gunshot wound complicating the ileostomy. "Oh, I see that's already been tried."

A few days after Susan got out of the hospital, I told my friend Gina at the little Indian craft store about the incident. She happened to ask, "I was exposed to hepatitis at a powwow this weekend, is there a remedy for that?" Well, as a matter of fact, I replied, Milk Thistle is the remedy for that. And of course, I had some in my pocket. I had gone on a Milk Thistle shopping spree just to be sure, since I only had a few seeds when Susan got sick.

One would think the story ended there, but of course it didn't. Later that day Gina was telling a friend about the mushroom poisoning over the front counter of her store when a woman walked up from the back of the room. "Excuse me," she said, "but I work in—Hospital emergency room and the nurse who handled that case is my best friend." They had read over the pamphlet I left on Milk Thistle when we brought her in. She said they were keeping a supply of Milk Thistle in their locker. "But that could cost you your license!" said Gail. "We'd rather lose our license than a patient," the nurse replied. "Each year a few people die from eating that mushroom."

A Further Adventure With Milk Thistle

The next spring I planted Milk Thistle in Susan's garden. It took us a while to realize that the little green leaves were coming up right where she had picked the mushroom the year before.

A few weeks later I went out to housesit for some friends in Minnetrista. I transplanted some Milk Thistle out there as well. This was at the time when I first saw the little farm for sale on Sunnyfield Road. I went over to the home of my real estate agent, Suzanne, and we prepared an offer. Meanwhile, one of her sons was having terrible medical problems.

Kurt had been an alcoholic since his teens. This eventually resulted in pancreatitis. He happened to fall into the hands of a particularly wretched doctor. The man removed half the pancreas. For a year Kurt stopped drinking and the pain was relieved. Thinking it wouldn't matter anymore, he started up again. The pain came back. When he stopped drinking, there was no improvement. "Well," said the doctor. "We could inject poison into the celiac nerve and kill it so that you won't feel the pain." They went ahead with that idea, but injected too much poison and killed nerves all over the place. Because of the nerve damage Kurt now had severe diarrhea. Over three months he lost twenty-five pounds. Besides, the pain in the pancreas got worse. The doctor now suggested that they remove the rest of the pancreas.

Kurt decided to get a second opinion. He finally let his mother help him. They drove down to the Mayo Clinic in Rochester, Minnesota. "What!" said the doctors down there. "Take out the pancreas? You'd die of hemorrhaging on the operating table." They didn't know what to do. One doctor suggested a bland diet, another laughed at that idea scornfully. While they were having a conference up in a big tower, Kurt got up and wandered over to the window. As he was staring out, a hawk flew up and smashed into the plate glass window right in front of his face.

Kurt and his mother returned home. She called me, explained the situation and asked for my advice. While Suzanne was pouring out the whole, complicated story, I kept hearing the words "Milk Thistle, Milk Thistle," in my ear. It was so strong and unusual, I didn't know exactly what to say. "Are you thinking of any particular herb?" I asked Suzanne. She replied, "Milk Thistle."

There are few things as soothing to the stomach and hypochondriac region as the fresh leaves of Milk Thistle, so I sent Suzanne out to get some at the place where I had been housesitting. It was about two miles down the road. Kurt started taking them on Friday. By Wednesday the diarrhea had stopped and he had gained five pounds. The pancreas was no longer painful. I came out to make an offer on the farm and look over his condition.

In the end, we got the farm.

A few weeks after moving in, I was back in Minneapolis attending a class taught by one of my friends. His classes about herbs were interspersed with odd comments about the behavior of witches, difficulties in the personal lives of shape-shifters (especially when they become senile), or the loss of a certain shade of yellow in medieval Venetian trade beads. "John," as I will call him, mentioned that he was looking for an apartment to rent. A woman in the audience raised her hand. "We have a house for sale if you want to move west." Just to humor her, John asked where it was. "Minnetrista," she replied. He and I almost fell out of our chairs. It was only two miles south of my new farm. Well, my friend didn't buy the house, but he stayed out there for a few months with the owners, Mark and Michelle, trading his vast array of knowledge for room and board.

Next spring I got a call from Suzanne. She had a feeling she should call me. "Kurt's interested in this house over near Halstead Bay." She described it. "I know that house," I exclaimed. "That's where John used to live!" She had taken classes from him as well.

Kurt and his wife got the house. At the closing, Mark was telling Kurt about all the little quirks in the home. "There's these pennies in the windows," he explained. "They're for, uh, they're for…" He didn't know what to say, but Suzanne finished the sentence for him: "They're to keep the witches out." She guessed who put them there and knew why.

Well, you could have heard a pin drop, Suzanne later confided. The two real estate closers and the other agent sat bolt upright in their chairs. Meanwhile, Mark and Suzanne had a fine conversation.

After the signing, on the way out the door, Suzanne's husband turned to her and said, "Where do you come up with these people?" The truth is, as Suzanne and I have found out, they're all over the place.

Preparation and Dosage

Silymarin is found in the leaves and seeds, but is highest in the seed coats, which is the officinal part to be used. From this, an infusion, extract, powder, or tincture is made. Dose is about five to sixty drops of the tincture. As an antidote in mushroom poisoning, it would be best to use a concentrated extract of the seed in powder or tincture so that the patient can get the silymarin into the blood quickly. In Europe it is given by hypodermic.

I only had a small amount of the unprocessed seed when I helped

Susan, but it still worked. This, of course, is what traditional herbalists would have had to work with. My friend Halsey Brandt pointed out, "You know, considering the amount of seed coat Susan was actually able to get into her system, that was almost an infinitesimal dose. It is really kind of homeopathic."

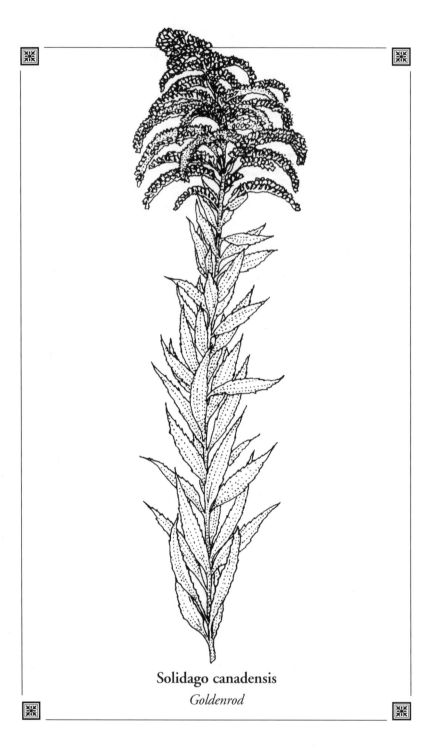

Solidago canadensis

Goldenrod

Solidago canadensis
Goldenrod

S *olidago* is a genus in the Aster family, native to the temperate regions of the world. In Europe there is only one indigenous species, *S. virga-aurea*. There are about forty-five species in North America, depending on which botanist one is talking to. They blend into each other and are notoriously difficult to classify. One of the most distinctive is *Solidago odorata*, a beautifully scented Goldenrod native to the Midwest. There is also a salty Goldenrod native to the coast of New England and some down in the Southwest that are resinous. The Indians used the sweet kind as an incense and it was, for a time, official in the U.S. Pharmacopoeia.

One of the most common kinds of Goldenrod is *Solidago canadensis,* which is more or less officinal in North American herbalism. It can easily be identified because it is the one Goldenrod with galls on the stems. Studies of this species have been undertaken and show that it possesses somewhat more of the active ingredients than the European variety, so it is certainly useful.

The spire of golden-yellow flowers that top the rod-like stalk towards the end of summer give rise to the common name Goldenrod. This is also the meaning of the Latin *virga aurea.* The name *Solidago* comes from the Latin *solidus + agere,* meaning that it "causes to solidify, or bring together" the lips of a wound. *Solidago* was one of the main wound-remedies prominent during the Middle Ages. Since then it has been largely forgotten like so many other fine woundworts of the period: *Sanicula, Alchemilla, Ajuga, Prunella,* etc. It was at one time known as *Consolidae saraceniae* because its wound-healing properties were learned from the Saracens.

Gerard (1597) comments, "It is extolled above all other herbes for the stopping of bloud in sanguinolent ulcers and bleeding wounds; and hath in times past beene had in greater estimation and regard than in these dayes." Why did it fade in popularity? "I have known the dry herbe which came from beyond the sea sold . . . for halfe a crown an ounce. But once it was found in Hampstead wood . . . no man will give half a crown for a hundred weight of it."

The strong affinity of *Solidago* for the kidneys became apparent at a later date. "This herb is a very old and good kidney medicine," wrote Rademacher. He says it would be just as silly to call it a "diuretic" as to call *Nux vomica* or *Chelidonium* a "cholagogue." It does not just cause diuresis, but brings the kidneys back into a healthy condition. The kidney-affinity is also well represented by Maria Treben.

European homeopathic physicians were interested in *Solidago* and it was given a modest proving. They continued to use it as a kidney remedy. Clarke writes, "the grand keynote of this remedy lies in the condition and the action of the kidneys and the quality of their secretions. Diseases arising from or complicated with defective action of the kidneys are very likely to be benefited." *Solidago* is employed on pretty much the same indications in both homeopathy and herbalism. However, it is little known to the modern homeopath.

Goldenrod flowers and leaves were used in European folk medicine, according to Ludwig Kroeber, as remedies for diarrhea, scrofula, asthma, cough, chronic catarrh, spitting of blood from the lungs, bedwetting, jaundice, throat problems, ulceration of the gums, teeth problems, ulcers, and swellings. Similar uses are recorded from the American Indians, according to Frances Densmore and Victor Vogel: fever, colds, flu, respiratory problems, hemorrhage from the lungs, tendency to tuberculosis, pain in the chest and back, sprains or strains, especially with edema, stoppage of urine, cramps and convulsions, wounds, especially with blood coming from the mouth, ulcers and jaundice. One of my Anishinabe friends says that her old grandmother called it "Female Medicine" and used it for menstrual problems, cramping, excessive bleeding, and as a specific for diarrhea. "It worked every time, like magic." (The variety she showed me was not the *canadensis*.)

Most of these uses trace back to poor kidney action, as Clarke said, either directly or indirectly. Even the poorly healing wounds and ulcers reflect an unclean condition of the body probably dependent on the kidneys. The bleeding probably stems from heat agitating the blood, which the kidneys are not cleaning. The menstrual problems show the close relationship of the kidneys to the sexual organs.

The kidney medicines are generally either masculine in character (Rattlesnake Master, Indian Hemp, Gravel Root) or feminine (Goldenrod, Lady's Mantle, Queen Anne's Lace). Goldenrod pulls the blood into the kidney from the vessels; Gravel Root balances the solids and minerals; Lady's Mantle allows the more refined fluids back into the bloodstream, condensing the urine; while Queen Anne's Lace pulls the coarse substances out into the ureters and on down to the bladder. Rattlesnake Master and Indian Hemp support the "fire" of the kidneys, the adrenals, so that the fluids will be pumped along and the fire kept hot. Goldenrod and Lady's Mantle support the *yin* or water, sedating the heat and maintaining the fluids. Water Lily and Lady's Slipper, also very feminine plants, build up and tonify the *yin* or fluids. Well that, at any rate, is my personal mythology of kidney remedies.

A Golden Staff to Lean On

The flavor of the leaves are fairly bitter and slightly pungent, the temperature slightly warm, the impression felt upon the stomach. The leaves are used as a bitter to stimulate the stomach and alimentary tract. The flowers contain a higher proportion of volatile oils, which make them more pleasantly pungent and less bitter. They act more on the respiratory tract. The flavor of the roots is sharply pungent or peppery, moderately bitter, warm in temperature, and stimulating in impression. They act as a strong stimulant to the kidneys.

All summer long, while other plants are flowering, Goldenrod is steadily raising its single stalk towards the sky. Finally, around the middle of August the golden-yellow spires appear. Both a staff and a spire are included in the picture. It is like the tarot card showing a man walking along a road with a heavy burden upon his back, a walking staff in his hand. His head is bent down, so that he does not see a church spire rising in the distance which shows that his destination is within reach. The message of Goldenrod is to endure to reach the goal.

The root tells a similar story. Ojibwe herbalist Kathleen Westcott said to me, "The Ojibwe doctor does not just look at the above-ground part of the plant, but also at the roots. If you dig up Goldenrod during the growing season you will notice that the rootlets go downwards into the soil all summer long. When the weather starts to get cold it sends the roots out sideways, forming a compact mass just under the surface. It is as if the plant was storing for winter." There is a message here of free growth, then of change in order to prepare for a difficult time. The root holds onto the earth, just as the foot of the traveler cleaves to the path with determination to reach the goal.

A similar story is told by Maria Treben about the typical Goldenrod patient and the effect of the medicine upon the kidneys. A fifty-two-year-old man huffs and puffs his way up her stairs to the first floor and throws himself into a chair, fighting for breath. The kidneys are exhausted. He says he has cirrhosis of the kidneys. She gives him an herb tea containing Goldenrod and Yellow Dead Nettle and the condition is eventually cured. Treben goes on to explain that the kidneys work off all our emotions. When we are going through a trying period the kidneys process our emotions in the same manner that they process the blood.

It has long been recognized that *Solidago* is a kidney medicine. The Goldenrod problem begins with a lack of endurance, a lack of strength to persevere through difficulty, an inability to process what is necessary to get to the end. The kidneys get weak and they are unable to suck in the blood in order to process it. The sodium-pump that establishes a suction drawing blood into the kidneys is evidently weakened. The kidneys fail to remove uric acid from the blood, it builds up in the system causing irritation of the tissues and a general preponderance of irritating materials to soothing fluids. This results in scanty, dark, turbid urine. As this urine runs through the urinary tract it causes irritation of the passages resulting in cloudy and burning urine as mucus builds up to protect the inflamed passages. Often, the kidneys are sore, tenderness is felt over them, they ache and feel distended, and the lower back is tired. These symptoms may be associated with chronic nephritis, cystitis, or prostatitis. Since the uric acid cannot leave through the kidneys, it is thrown off through the bowels, skin, and lungs, resulting in irritation of the intestines and diarrhea; irritation of the skin, ulcers, sores, acne, and scrofulous conditions; irritation of the respiratory tract, red, inflamed eyes, mucus in the lungs, and finally bloody sputum. The liver, which depends on the kidneys to remove irritant matter, becomes inflamed and symptoms of "liver fire" appear. Goldenrod is well suited to patients with exhausted kidneys which can no longer pull in the blood. They have tired lower backs and tired feet. The motto of the Goldenrod patient is "I can't make it, where's the nearest chair."

Solidago is often called for after disease has exhausted the body and the kidneys can't process the buildup of waste material. Rademacher writes, "Goldenrod has proved excellent in acute gastric fevers when the urine became dark and turbid, although the patient had been getting better. The improvement had reached a standstill, or was not moving fast enough. A decoction of the Goldenrod brings the sick kidneys to a normal condition and makes the urine clear and normal again."

In terms of traditional Chinese medicine, the *Solidago* pathology begins as kidney *chi* deficiency (lack of energy in the renal process) and turns into kidney *yin* deficiency (lack of fluids to lubricate and soothe the tissues) and goes on to produce liver *yin* and lung *yin* deficiency. The typical symptoms of liver and kidney *yin* deficiency are usually present: rapid, slightly wiry and weak pulse, reddish tongue, malar flush across the checks, irritated eyes, and hectic fever. There are also symptoms of heat in the blood, as the blood becomes infected. Hence, *Solidago* was used for septic infection in wounds, such as gangrene. I have seen it help patients with Kaposi's Sarcoma.

The following case histories particularly bring out the psychological profile of *Solidago*. A four-year-old girl was brought in by her mother. She had red eyelids and mild conjunctivitis, some scruffy sores on the scalp, and was both listless and uncooperative. It seemed as if something had disturbed her. It turned out that several days previously she had learned about the existence of sex from a little boy. Her mom confirmed for her that yes, men and women had to join together for babies to be born. Her problem seemed to date from this realization. I looked at the girl in this light. The look in her eyes gave the impression that she had had a vision of the ramifications of this knowledge and seen the pain that would arise from the difficulties of interaction between the sexes. *Solidago virga-aurea* 12x completely cured the physical symptoms and cheered up the mind. I don't know if there is any cure for the complications between the sexes.

Shortly after this, a three-month-old baby was brought to Crescenterra, where I then worked. She had an unusually developed sense of personality. The problem was that she couldn't look at anyone other than her mother or father without cringing in fear and pain. With her parents she was completely happy. The eyelids were a little red and I remembered treating her father with *Solidago virga-aurea* 12x for hay fever the fall before. As I watched her, my impression was that she was too sensitive to face people. *Solidago virga-aurea* 12x cured the mental and physical symptoms. The mother latter reported, "she needs the remedy when she's in a 'covenants broken' frame of mind." It almost seemed as if the little girl had an awareness of the difficulties that would accrue on the path of life.

In my practice, *Solidago virga-aurea* comes in most handy for hay fever. Along with *Apis mellifica*, Propolis, *Arundo mauritania*, Silicea, and *Ambrosia artemisiafolia,* the majority of cases will clear up. I know of no better remedy for cat allergy, although it will not cure every single case—just almost every case. Boericke describes the eyes just right: "red, inject-ed, watery, stinging, burning." The eyes of the *Solidago* patient look like a person who has just gotten out of a swimming pool. There is a gener-alized redness of the conjunctiva. There are not the bright red blotches of *Euphrasia,* the glazed, painful red of *Pulsatilla* (or sometimes *Euphrasia*), or the blood-shot blood vessels of *Ambrosia.* With this there is congestion, sneezing and running of the nose, redness and irritation of the skin. *Solidago* often has welts from allergy, a fact not mentioned in the literature I have seen. This makes it comparable to *Apis* in many cases where there are welts.

Preparation and Dosage

The leaves are picked during early summer, flower tops during the latter part of the summer and early fall. The root is taken during the fall. The leaves are used to make the tea. The flower tops make a nice tincture in brandy.

The bulk herb, the tincture, and the lower potencies can all be used, and possess about the same traits. Material doses are probably bet-ter when there is real kidney disease, but in milder cases they tend to cause aggravations, such as conjunctivitis. The potencies work better for the allergies.

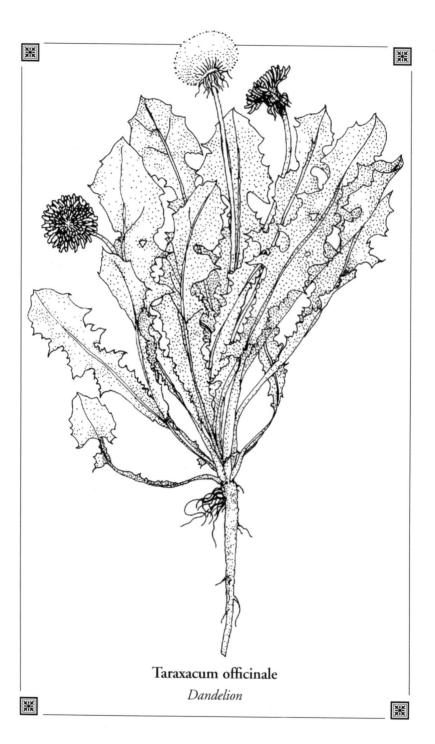

Taraxacum officinale
Dandelion

Taraxacum officinale
Dandelion

This extremely common flower is a favorite in Western folk medicine. It is used in a general sort of a way as a "liver cleaner," "blood purifier," and diuretic. The indications given in the literature are of a vague and general nature, although it seems to work as a general cleanser in an admirable fashion. Often, a few months on Dandelion can really tone up the hepatic structures, remove stagnation, jaundice or gallstones, improve digestion, decongest the portal system, and remove difficulties caused by heat rising to the skin. It also seems to act on the waters of the body, gently promoting lymphatic activity and definitely correcting problems in the urinary tract originating with stagnant, damp heat. There are many additional uses. An excellent account of Dandelion in given by Susun Weed.

Dandelion occupies a more specific, narrow position in the Chinese pharmacopoeia. It is used as a remedy for clearing heat, especially "liver fire" and "fire poison" (abscesses, boils, sores, etc.) However, this does not seem to account for all of its actions in traditional Western usage.

Hahnemann took an interest in *Taraxacum* and gave it a homeopathy proving. He did not seem to have used it much and it was omitted from the kit he was working with at the time of his death. Subsequent homeopaths seem not to have used it a greal deal either, but by the end of the nineteenth century a few useful guiding symptoms had been developed.

As far as can be determined at the present time, Dandelion seems to have a small scope when used in a specific or homeopathic manner. Perhaps this can be enlarged upon in the future. When used as a general "liver cleanser," as it is in Western herbalism, Dandelion may accomplish much, but it is difficult to determine exactly what it does in any given case. It is a medicine illustrating the differences between the specific and a general approach.

Boericke gives one of the best accounts found in homeopathic literature. He mentions the affinities to the liver and kidneys long associated with the remedy, and also gives several important characteristic symptoms. The most important is the "mapped tongue." There are not too many remedies which have this. His description of the mapping is very exact, and I have verified it in my own experience almost every time I have used *Taraxacum.* "Tongue covered with a white film; feels raw; comes off in patches, leaving red, sensitive spots."

As time passes, I become more liberal in my definition of a mapped tongue, and find that *Taraxacum* works when the tongue coating is yellow or white, when there is little coating, when there is prominent excoriation of the tongue body, showing the characteristic "mapping," or when there is barely any sign of this.

Another characteristic symptom Boericke mentions is pain in the sterno-cloidal-mastoid muscle. Unfortunately, a portrait of the conditions and patients in which these symptoms would appear is not included by Boericke. Let me try to provide one from my own experience.

The mapped tongue of *Taraxacum* gives one the impression that there are turbid fluids and mucus in the system being baked down by heat into a film. In traditional Chinese medicine, the mapped tongue indicates that there are turbid fluids precipitating into mucus. These block the circulation of fluids and heat builds up. This produces a simmering, low-grade heat, like fire smoldering in wet leaves, not the robust sort of heat (like *Achillea.*) *Taraxacum* is, therefore, a remedy for low, simmering heat and dampness in the system. I have seen *Taraxacum* clear out this sort of condition in well over a dozen cases.

All of these people suffered from similar conditions. Their entry complaint was usually "sinus infection" or "allergies." It appeared that they had a chronic infection in the bones around the sinuses, eyes, and ears. The mastoid process is often tender, the sterno-cloidal-mastoid muscle also sore. In three people there was also lumbar pain. One actually came on the entry complaint "backache caused by allergy medication." (I don't think she had the etiology down correctly—I think the allergies were themselves the causative agent.) All of the people had a history of antibiotics (for sinus infection), desensitization shots (for allergies), or tetracycline (for acne.) I would have to presume that the infections they were suffering from were driven from the sinus cavities into the soft parts of the bones in adjoining areas (such as the mastoid.) *Taraxacum* may be considered as a specific remedy for patients suffering from low-grade, internalized heat lingering in the bones of the face and head around the sinuses, ears, eyes, and neck. It also has an effect on the kidneys and bladder. One person experienced pain in the bladder and achiness generally, much relieved by urination, which was frequent and copious. (This symptom more or less appears in the homeopathic provings.) In my first half dozen cases I gave Dandelion tincture (whole plant or root), in doses of five drops. This is one of the slowest-acting remedies I have ever seen. Although most of these people felt immediate improvement, the condition only slowly improved over several weeks or months. One person felt she had made no improvement at all—yet, she never had her allergic symptoms again. Later, I started to use the homeopathic potencies and they worked as well.

The mental state in these people differed widely. Two complained of being "bitchy," one felt (and looked) dull-minded, and one was nervous. All of these symptoms show a connection to the liver (anger, nervous tension and auto-intoxication.)

Taraxacum seems also to have a relationship to a certain type of high fever. I am not sure of the exact indications, but here are two short case histories. My friend, Kathryn Thorngren of Lake City, Minnesota, saw a five-year-old boy who had been suffering from a serious high fever for two weeks. Nothing the doctors gave him made any impression on the case. She gave *Taraxacum* tincture, and within twenty-four hours the condition was entirely dissipated. About the only clear symptom she could give me was: hot head, cold hands and feet, which is found in the homeopathic materia medica.

My friend Dennis Anderson, a homeopath in Mondovi, Wisconsin, is well versed in the relationship between minerals, the soil, and weeds. He says that Dandelion prefers a decalcified soil. The thick taproot pulls up calcium from down below and brings it to the surface. This fits in with our observation that Dandelion helps infections seated in the bones. It also led me to use Dandelion in cases where decalcification was the chief entry complaint. In one case, a woman had infected root canals extending up into the jaw, which was infected and decalcified, according to X-rays. I gave Dandelion and White Oak bark (for gum disease) and the results in one month were remarkable. The dentist literally ran out of the room when he saw the X-rays and exclaimed to his assistant, "Look at the difference between these X-rays. The bone is recalcifying." At the time I thought it was only the Dandelion that did the job, but now I believe that Oak bark also helps recalcify the bones.

Preparation and Dosage

Dandelion is unusual because its medicinal contents and properties change more radically than most other medicinal plants, depending on the season, crop, and other environmental factors. It is likely that no two preparations of the plant are identical. There is also much variation from one part of the plant to another. The leaves are more diuretic than the roots, which perhaps have a greater affinity to the liver.

Hahnemann used *Taraxacum* in single drop doses of the tincture. I have used the tincture and 6x. A tincture made by soaking the chopped roots in brandy produces what I think of as a very good tasting product. The bitterness of the roots is sweetened up by the brandy.

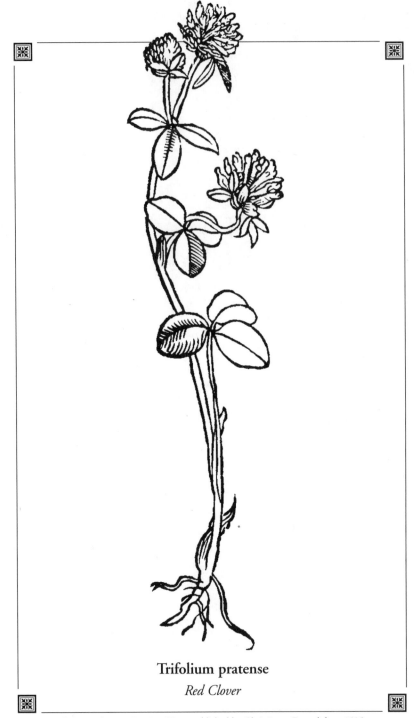

Trifolium pratense

Red Clover

from *Herbarium Imagines Vivae,* published by Christianus Egenolphus, 1535

Trifolium pratense

Red Clover

This common roadside flower is a member of the Legume family widely grown as an animal feed. It originated in central Asia and was spread through cultivation to all parts of the world. It is widely naturalized throughout the world, although it tends to die out unless the area where it is growing receives a mowing once a summer. The flowers are the part used. They flower in early summer, when the weather is still cool, straggle on till fall, and bloom again.

Red Clover flowers are sweet and tasty. They may be plucked as a snack as one walks in the fields. Because they have a medicinal action on the salivary glands causing a slight stimulation, they quench the thirst. Thus, they are an excellent remedy for the herbal forager in the fields. Picked and dried in the semi-shade they make an excellent, sweet tea. It is also possible to preserve them in alcohol, but most people prefer the dried flowers used as a tea.

Defining the Properties of an Alterative

Red Clover has a long history of use in herbal medicine. It is used as a "blood cleaner" and "blood thinner" on rather general grounds, often in combination with other detoxifiers like Burdock and Yellow Dock. All of these plants are classified as "alteratives," a name which means that they "alter the body in some way." Generally, such remedies act on the lymphatics and the liver to remove metabolic waste products. Each alterative has a different affinity to structures and processes in the body and today, from a position of greater knowledge, we can be more specific about their actions. The word "alterative" is not very satisfying.

Australian herbalist and naturopath Dorothy Hall, in *Creating Your Herbal Profile* (1988), gives an excellent account of the affinities and uses of Red Clover, showing most exactly what kind of an alterative it is. She demonstrates that it has a special affinity to encysted glands. She discovered this through personal experience.

When she had her youngest child Hall was afflicted with severe mastitis. The doctors in the hospital gave her antibiotics. After the infection subsided there was a hard lump, which was explained to her as "scar tissue." Sixteen years later, now an experienced herbalist, she was fasting and taking Red Clover tea. The lump swelled up, became quite red and painful, and she realized that it was not scar tissue per se, but an encysted gland. She added some detoxifying herbs like Burdock to help her system and the lump faded away.

Hall went on to gain a deeper understanding of the properties of Red Clover. She explained that it is the remedy for encysted glands, where the body encysts or calcifies around a swelling in order to isolate toxic materials. A single swollen gland may remain for a long time or it may suddenly break open, releasing a trail of noxious materials which cause an ongoing pernicious fever that is difficult to track down to a source. I soon had the opportunity to put this new information to use.

My brother in Anchorage, Alaska, was stricken by a very serious fever that burned away perniciously for about five months. He had to stop working and was actually incapacitated. The doctors checked him for everything, including AIDS and immunological problems. He consulted with me by telephone but my guesses were inadequate. He went to a local naturopath who also failed to get results, and back to the doctors, of course. Finally, he called me again.

I went over the symptoms carefully but could still not understand them. Finally I simply asked, "What do you think the problem is?"

He answered without hesitation. "Well you remember how I had impacted wisdom teeth as a kid? They were removed surgically, but the next year I had a cyst in the neck. That was also removed, but I just feel like there is something left in there." Right away, I knew exactly what remedy would cure. Red Clover tincture cleared up the fever in five or six weeks and he returned to his usual, sterling health.

Although the encysted gland had long ago been removed, I gave

Red Clover to my brother because it was the remedy which should have been given then. This is an old technique used in homeopathy, based on the idea that the vital force has a memory of the initial problem and carries the trauma on long after one would expect the problem to have disappeared.

Red Clover has an affinity to the glands about the neck, under the ears towards the back of the neck. Here it should be compared with Cleavers. However, it tends towards single swollen glands, not numerous swellings, like Cleavers. It has an affinity to the parotids and the salivary glands in the back of the mouth. Red and White Clover have long been used, especially in homeopathy, as specifics for parotiditis, or mumps. The homeopathic provings and initial clinical experiences also showed that Red Clover acts strongly on the salivary glands, removing congestion, unplugging stopped up secretory glands, and removing calcium casts that form in the glands—also in the tear ducts.

Red Clover is used in modern herbalism for drippy, irritable coughs, including whooping cough, where there is a thin, clear secretion that causes irritation to the cough reflex. This secretion may result from an old accumulation of toxic material which has broken open, as Dorothy Hall suggests.

I remember a friend who was suffering from a slightly drippy, irritating cough that went on for two winters. I suggested Mullein, which is good for a dry, irritating cough, but this only palliated for a few weeks. When it came back the second winter we were both discouraged. She mentioned that she thought the secretion irritating the tract came from the sinuses and I immediately thought of the idea of a cyst in the sinuses, breaking open and releasing the irritating secretion. Whether this was accurate or not, it led to Red Clover, which was Dorothy Hall's remedy for just such old leaking cysts. This permanently cured in about four weeks time.

One recent case especially sticks out in my mind. I cannot say that Red Clover was the curative agent, or even exactly what the problem was, but I was sure glad it was in the formula. The seventeen year-old daughter of a friend noticed a hard lump in one breast. She was prone to cysts that came and went and I thought her a bit of an Easter Lily constitution, with her lily-petal like complexion. This, however, was a single hard swelling and she was terrified. The doctor set up an appointment with a surgeon. She was leaving on a trip and I didn't even get to take a case history or see her, so I just sent along a mixture of Red Clover, Easter Lily and Cleavers, the great remedies for breast cysts. Within a week the tumor started to resolve and the surgeon felt much better and waited it out until it disappeared.

The Second Chance Remedy

Dorothy Hall's understanding of Red Clover also explains why it is such a beneficial remedy in cancer. The materials walled off by the body are seriously toxic. At some point in time they may become the source of an insidious cancer. Red Clover is also a mild blood thinner, breaking up the coagulated blood which is a factor in cancer, as well as the lymphatic congestion, another factor. She goes on to say that it can restore hope and confidence, where the ravages of this terrible disease have caused one to lose hope.

I always say Red Clover looks optimistic and call it "the Little Red Riding Hood" remedy; it seems to look up innocently with its red florets. It blooms in early summer and again in late summer, but the second bloom is slightly toxic and should not be picked. Innocence has turned to experience, but hope should not be lost. "I call it the second chance remedy," says herbalist Kate Gilday. "The flowers come again." Another herbalist says, "Red Clover is good for people who are not sure whether they want to live or not. It restores the desire to live."

Red Clover is probably the single most important remedy we should know about in the herbal treatment of cancer. The early Thomsonians concentrated it down to a paste and used it for skin and other cancers. Jethro Kloss speaks highly of it in *Back to Eden* (1939):

> *Red clover is one of God's greatest blessings to man. Very pleasant to take and a wonderful blood purifier. Combined with equal parts of blue violet, burdock, yellow dock, dandelion root, rock rose [Helianthemum canadense] and goldenseal, it is a most powerful remedy for cancerous growths and leprosy affections, also pellagra. Learn to use this God-given remedy effectively. Used alone it is excellent for cancer of the stomach, whooping cough, and various spasms.*

Kloss cites an instance in his childhood, when his parents gathered Red Clover blossoms for their postmaster, who had cancer of the stomach. This was in the era long before modern medicine, so we cannot be sure of the diagnosis, but it made a strong impression upon him. He continues, "Red clover is an exceedingly good remedy for cancer on any part of the body." He recommends using strong decoctions of the tea, four or five times a day.

Although Red Clover was not, apparently in the original Essiac formula, which was introduced by Rene Caisse as an herbal cancer cure, one company has included it in an updated version. It is also found in Jason Winter's Tea. I can speak highly of it from personal experience.

One time I was down in Rochester, Minnesota, the home of the Mayo Clinic. A forty-three-year-old woman came to see me who was suffering with a very slow growing cancer in the lungs. It was tucked way inside, so the doctors did not want to remove it surgically and she did not want to take drugs, so she was doing nothing at all about it. I could not help but think that she was a bit depressed. What she came to see me for, however, was not the cancer but the chronic, drippy bronchial discharge which accompanied it and this is what I set out to help. I knew that Red Clover was useful for the kind of drippy, irritating cough she had, so I sent her off with some tincture made on my farm. "Oh yeah." I remembered something as I was leaving. "Red Clover is also a cancer remedy." I didn't think anymore about it.

Three months later I got a call on my machine from a woman in Rochester, requesting more Red Clover tincture. I called her back and left a message on her machine, telling her it was unnecessary to use my tincture; she could use any that she found down there. She called back and this time I answered the phone. "Do you remember me?" she asked. No, I didn't. She explained that I gave her Red Clover for bronchitis, but the cancer tumor had totally disappeared! I was shocked. "You'd better use exactly that same tincture," I agreed. I sent her more and she has since been fine.

Preparation and Dosage

The flowers should be picked in the full sun, when they are full and beautiful, dried in light shade and stored in a glass bottle. If it is desirable, a tincture can be made from the fresh or dried flowers.

One thing that is most distinctive about Red Clover is that it usually needs to be given consistently for about six weeks. I usually recommend three drops, three times a day, for that length of time.

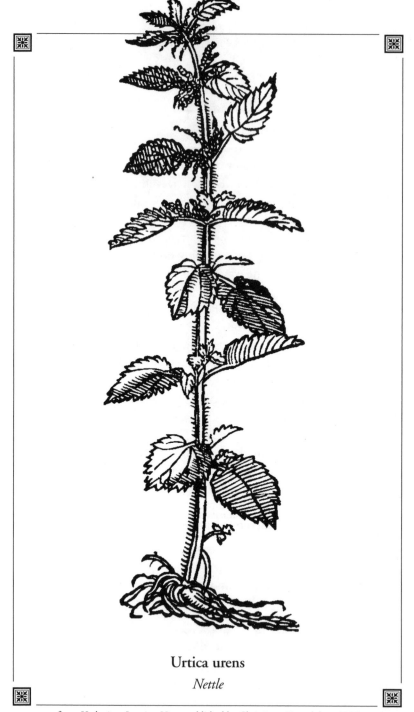

Urtica urens

Nettle

from *Herbarium Imagines Vivae*, published by Christianus Egenolphus, 1535

Urtica urens

Nettle

Various kinds of Nettle are found in waste places and woods throughout the world. They are recognized—even in the dark, as Culpeper notes—by the sting they produce on contact. Little hairs break open and exude an acid which produces stinging welts. This substance quickly breaks down, however, so that only the fresh plant stings. Nor does the itch persist very long in most people. The large European Nettle (*Urtica dioica*) or its smaller cousin (*U. urens*) or hybrids of the two are commonly used. Generally, the young leaves and the root are the part used. The young greens are eaten as a potherb in the spring. They have a taste like cooked spinach greens and are very nutritious. Nettle contains more protein than any other native plant, large amounts of iron, trace minerals, fat, and chlorophyll.

Mature Nettle stalks have fibers running through them which have been used to make cloth, rope, and netting. Nettle linen is of the finest quality and lasts for a long time. Ancient burials unearthed in the steppes of western China have brought to light two-thousand-year-old nettle clothing in a perfect state of preservation. One of the interesting things about the burials is that the occupants had blond, red and brunette hair, showing them to be the furthest eastern extension of the caucasian race.

Nettle is very much an ancestral plant associated with white people. Burial sites in the peat bogs of northern Europe also of ancient date, yielded clothing and rope made from Nettle fiber. Dr. James Compton Burnett, who used Urtica extensively as we will shortly see, writes, "I have read that its original habitat is somewhere in Asia, whence supposedly started the wanderings of the peoples," more particularly, the Indo-Europeans, or Aryans. During both World Wars, when Germany was cut off from cotton sources, uniforms were made from Nettle fiber. As one herbalist pointed out in a practical vein, "If you go to a gun show, you won't find much in the way of old American uniforms, but the Nazi uniforms are in beautiful shape." Nettle linen is not currently produced, because it is too labor intensive.

Urtica was given considerable attention by the early professional physicians and writers. Dioscorides gives a rather fractured account, but even here we begin to see its traditional uses well mapped out and a suggestion of how the remedy works. He says that Nettle "fetcheth up ye stuff out of ye Thorax," curing pleurisy and pneumonia. It is also "splenicall," dissolving "windiness" in the bowels and moving urine. It stops "fluxes of blood from ye nostrils" and treats "inflamed Uvula." The seed "doth incite to conjugation & do unstop ye womb," also promoting menstruation. It cleanses away gangrene, malignant cancers, foul ulcers, tumors, parotid apostumations, and is good for dog bites. Especially in the reference to deficient sexual energy, we already begin to see the Nettle personality emerging: it is a remedy for debility, when the system needs to get moving again.

It is, however, as a folk remedy that Nettle is most famous. It is widespread around farms and settlements in Europe and naturalized in similar places in the New World. Susun Weed speaks of Nettle as one of the half dozen basic remedies of the European "wise woman" tradition. It is widely used as a spring potherb, a general cleanser and activator, and a nutritive substance.

Nettle is not, on the other hand, a characteristically American Indian medicine, though it is not unknown to native peoples. The Anishinabe doctors said that Nettle was a remedy brought to them by Nanabojo, the Trickster. This seems appropriate for an herb that rewards the unobservant bumbler in the woods with a sting.

The Spirit of Nettle

Perhaps the first thing I noticed about Nettle, years ago, was that it likes to grow downstream from a septic system, outhouse or feedlot. It is clear that it flourishes in soil that has been contaminated—or enriched—

with nitrates and uric acid waste products. Evidently, it uses these byproducts of protein deterioration to build up the high degree of protein found in the plant. I originally concluded from this observation that Nettle should be beneficial in removing uric acid from the system. It should, therefore, be a highly rated kidney remedy. Although it does have an effect on the kidneys in some people, this insight proved to be misleading and it was years—decades, really—before I came to understand my mistake and what Nettle really does.

Nettle contains high levels of protein because it articulates these nitrogenous waste products into proteinacious structures. It removes uric acid waste products from the system, not by stimulating the kidneys, not even by sweeping waste products out of the corners of the organism, but by using protein building-blocks and not allowing them to pass uselessly into the general economy of the system. Nettle is a remedy that gets the job done. It works with complicated protein building-blocks to build some of the most complicated molecules used by the body. It is a highly nutritious food which supplies these materials, but it also supplies the know-how, the intensity, to use them.

I often visualize the Nettle spirit as an older lady with a broom or a switch exhorting people to get going, get a move on, don't just sit around, do something. In fact, Nettle is used to treat inactivity, as in impotence, but more generally, of any organ. Susan Weed mentions a case where a woman had her thyroid removed with radioactive iodine, but regretted it afterwards. The function of the organ was restored by using Nettle! Charles Millspaugh (1898) wrote, "The most ancient use of the Nettle is flagellation or urtication, a practice of whipping paralyzed limbs [with the fresh plants], to bring the muscles into action. This practice extended also to a stimulation of impotent organs, and to bring into action dormant energies. It was also resorted to in apoplexy, general cerebral and portal congestion, to bring blood to the surface and relieve more vital organs."

Dr. Dorothy Shepherd captured the essence of Nettle nicely in *A Physician's Posy*, through an allusion to history. "Some of you may remember the momentous visit of Neville Chamberlain," to Hitler at Munich in 1938. Chamberlain had been appeasing "the disturber of the peace of the world," but at this time he finally realized that Britain would be inevitably drawn into a war against a foe vastly superior in strength of arms. He acquiesced to the annexation of Czechoslovakia, in order to buy time to build up an arsenal at home. When he returned, he quoted Shakespeare, "Out of this nettle, danger, we pluck this flower, safety." In the scant few years purchased by the sacrifice of central Europe, Britain was able to manufacture enough airplanes to save itself from invasion in the great air war fought above its shores. Later it provided the beachhead, both in Europe and North Africa, through which Hitler was eventually destroyed on the western front. Meanwhile, Hitler's aroused soldiers wore uniforms made from nettle linen, fitting for this most Aryan of wars.

The Stinging Nettle

When fresh, the hairs on the stalks and leaves contain formic acid, the cause of the famous itch and nettle rash. However, formic acid quickly deteriorates and recently picked Nettles loose their itch in a number of minutes. In order to gain the benefit of the formic acid, Nettle must either be used as it was in the past (by urtication) or preserved almost immediately after picking. One company introduced the excellent idea of freeze-drying Nettle, in order to keep it in its most active state. Nettle can be kept in the freezer by the attentive householder.

Although the use of Nettles by urtication seems like an old and unwieldy practice, I have known several people who used this method with great success. While I was teaching a class in Canon Falls, Minnesota, several hours south of my place, I met a man who had used urtication. After a serious back injury as a young man, the doctors told him he would never walk again. Through alternative medicine (acupuncture and herbs) combined with sheer willpower, he managed to get back on his feet. At this point, his legs were still numb. He took walks in Nettles patches and this brought back sensation. Today, he walks like a regular person, though still subject to pain and limitation of some activities.

I knew of another case in Rochester, Minnesota, where a woman used urtication to clear up allergies and irritation of the skin. She had an angry, reddish cast to her skin. I saw her after about four or five summers during which she had romped in Nettles patches and her conditions were completely cleared up; her skin looked very pleasant.

The Nutritive Nettle

There are a good many herbalists, on the other hand, who emphasize that Nettle is for pale, anemic people. Dorothy Hall especially considers it useful for pale, anemic people who have low blood pressure and are better after exercise and activity. Herbalist William LeSassier refers to the doctrine of signatures: Nettle is beneficial for anemia, especially in tall, slender persons (as compared to the more mesomorphic people who respond better to cooked *Rehmannia* root.) Nettle has a nutritive influence, as well as a stimulating effect.

Nettle contains more protein than any other plant common in the temperate regions. Since proteins are complicated molecules which quickly breakdown, they also need to be preserved quickly. However, Nettles are still very nutritive, if they have been picked and dried or preserved with reasonable care. The old authors noted the nutritive effect on farm animals. Cows fed on Nettles give good milk and butter, horses are smart and frisky, and fowl lay more eggs. It was also found to stimulate milk production in nursing women and improves the hair and blood.

Dr. Urtica

As we have seen, Nettles have long been used to remove uric acid wastes from the body. This includes gouty deposits, eczemas and skin rashes (especially with elevated bumps, itching, or swelling), and gravel in the kidneys. Nettle extract, fresh juice, or tea is used to leech uric acid from the tissues, bring it into the bloodstream, and cause it to be taken up by the kidneys and excreted. It also probably prevents proteins from breaking down as quickly and cluttering up the system. These symptoms were called the "uric acid diathesis" in nineteenth century medicine.

One spring I was visited by an old friend who was having trouble with swelling of the fingers and red, itchy eczema on them—a capital indication for Nettle. He also felt tenderness and swelling over the kidneys. Nettle tincture quickly cured. The next week I saw a woman with the same problem, only she had no trouble in the kidney region. I knew to give Nettle again and it cured again.

Burnett used *Urtica urens* as his "sheet anchor" for gout and gravel (see *Gout and Its Cure*, 1895.) He first learned about the remedy as a good medicine for intermittent chill, later associated it with the spleen (which sometimes gets very swollen with these intermittents or agues), and then saw how it cleaned urates out of the system. When he observed many who, "under the influence of *Urtica urens,* passed grit and gravel pretty freely for the first time in their lives, I came to the conclusion that the *Urtica* possesses the power of eliminating the urates from the economy."

Following these observations, "I then proceeded to employ *Urtica urens* in the classic attacks of genuine gout, and that with very great satisfaction indeed. Within a few hours after beginning its use the urine becomes fairly free, of a high color, and the bottom of the vessel is often found more or less covered with urates in the form of grit and gravel, and simultaneously herewith the gouty attack begins to subside."

The colorful Burnett treats us to many fun case histories, of which I select one.

> *A middle-aged gentleman of position was down with an attack of gout that had relapsed over and over again, and he had then been in and out of these attacks for nearly six months. He had been swamped with alkalis and Colchicum, and mercilessly purged and lulled with narcotics most alarmingly. He thought he would 'try homeopathy,' and sent for the writer. I put him on Urtica urens as already described [the tincture in frequent doses], and he was out and about in a fortnight. In a couple of days of the treatment his urine became dark, plentiful, and loaded with uric acid gravel. His enthusiasm knew no bounds, and he declared that no remedy he had ever taken ... had nearly touched his gout like the Urtica. With him and his club intimates I became known as Dr. Urtica.*

Burnett also liked the influence of Nettle over kidney stones and pain. "Only yesterday morning I was called to see a gentleman 78 years of age suffering from 'his old enemy,' viz., pains in his left kidney region. I prescribed *Urtica* every two hours, and called again late in the evening." He was then informed, "Oh, the pain is gone, and I have passed a lot of gravel." Modern research supports the conclusion that Nettle Root is effective in some cases of benign swelling of the prostate.

Nettle is also used to help remove stagnant mucus. As a stimulating herb it may be supposed that it arouses inactive mucosa, also opening the lungs through its cleansing action on the kidneys, allowing better waste product removal. However, it also builds tissue strength as a nutritive. Culpeper advanced his own reasons why Nettle removes mucus. It is an herb of Mars because it is hot. "You know Mars is hot and dry, and you know as well that winter is cold and moist; then you may know as well the reason why nettle-tops, eaten in the spring, consumeth the phlegmatic superfluities in the body of man, that and coldness and moistness of winter hath left behind." Nettle is also "a safe and sure medicine to open the pipes and passages of the lungs, which is the cause of wheezing and shortness of breath, and helpeth to expectorate tough phlegm, as also to raise the imposthumed pleurisy, and spend it by spitting: the same helpeth the swelling of the almonds of the throat, the mouth and throat being gargled therewith."

Nettle also stimulates the large intestine to greater activity and has long been used when mucus is found in the stools. Dr. John Scudder, the great eclectic, writes, "An old practitioner informs me, that in chronic disease of the large intestine with increased mucus secretion, he has never found anything so beneficial as this remedy." Scudder was always on the lookout for specific symptoms. A later eclectic gives more detail. "Profuse choleraic and excessive mucus discharges, as in cholera infantum and dysentery," relates Harvey Felter. "It also has a restraining effect in gastric affections with excessive gastric secretion, and eructations, and vomiting." It also removes mucus from the renal system. "Chronic cystitis, with large mucus diuresis."

Just as it reins in profuse discharges of mucus, Nettle is useful for postpartum hemorrhage, bleeding piles, bloody diarrhea, bloody urine, and excessive menstrual flux. Indeed, it is not only used to increase lactation, but to stop it when children are weaned. (Here it is more friendly than the cruelly bitter Wormwood, which laid upon the breast would leave a bad taste in any child's mouth.)

The use of Nettle to remove cold and damp conditions, as noted by Culpeper, may explain its influence over intermittent fever, with alternating chills and heat. It probably operates here also by a gentle stimulation of the liver, portal circulation, lymphatics and spleen. Many obscure intermittents are associated with liver tension or blockage in the liver, spleen and intestinal areas. We should remember that both Culpeper and Burnett, who used Nettle for intermittents, were inhabitants of that famously cold and damp city, London.

Burnett used *Urtica* tincture extensively for intermittent fever.

Although he was a prestigious London homeopath, his knowledge of Nettle originated in very humble quarters. "I was treating a lady for intermittent fever of the mild English type," he writes. "One day my patient came tripping somewhat jauntily into my consulting room and informed me that she was quite cured of her fever, and wished to consult me in regard to another matter. I at once turned to my notes of her case, and inquired more closely, into the matter of the cure, in order to duly credit my prescribed remedy with the cure, and the more so as ague is not always easily disposed of therapeutically. 'Oh.' said the lady, 'I did not take your medicine at all, for when I got home I had such a severe attack of fever that my charwoman begged me to allow her to make me some nettle-tea, as that was a sure cure of fever. I consented, and she at once went into our garden, where they are plenty of nettles growing in a heap of rubbish and brickbats, and got some nettles, of which she made me a tea, and I drank it. It made me very hot. The fever left me, and I have not had it since."

Burnett realized that such a fine cure indicated a remedy that was homeopathic to the case, and not simply something masking symptoms. He noted that *Urtica* had produced fever, as well as curing it. Here we see the stimulating side of the remedy in a different, homeopathic sense.

That it produces symptoms is well known to anybody who has stepped in its way, but *Urtica* has not received a thorough homeopathic proving. Although he considered it homeopathic, Burnett did not use it in homeopathic doses, but in rather herbal ones—ten drops, two times a day was typical. We see here that there is not any substantial difference between the herbal and the homeopathic uses of Nettle.

After his case with the lady and the charwoman, Burnett forgot about Nettle for a while. "The thing escaped my mind for years, but one day being in difficulty about a case of ague [intermittent fever], I treated with a tincture of nettles and cured it straight away, and my next case also, and my next, and almost every case ever since, and with very nearly uniform success. Some of my cases of ague cured with nettle-tincture were most severe ones, invalided home from India and Burma. And quite lately a patient living in Siam, to whom I had sent a big bottle of nettle-tincture, wrote me:- 'The tincture you sent us has very greatly mitigated the fever we get here. Please order us another bottle.' I say *almost* every case has yielded to *Urtica urens;* every case, of course, has not."

Burnett recommended *Urtica* particularly for gout with slight or moderate fever, heat and cold flushes, passage of grit and gravel, uneasiness of the left rib region, indicating a splenic complication, and great restlessness. Urtica is more apt to produce a feverish reaction in the evening, than in the morning, and this is when the fever of gout is most common.

Finally, Burnett gives one case where many of the symptoms are seen together. "A gentleman of 50 odd years of age, now resident in London, consulted me for gout in the fall of the year 1890." He had long lived in India and suffered much from malaria, the root of many intermittents and agues. He suffered from gout, diarrhea, poor digestion, and fever. "After a few weeks of *Urtica,* 10 drops in a wine-glassful of water night and morning," he was free from the gout, the digestion was better, the diarrhea gone, "and my skin is much cleaner."

Burns

The doctrine of "like treats like" suggests the use of Nettle to cure burns. Margaret Tyler, a prominent London homeopath of the generation succeeding Burnett, was much impressed with his use of the remedy, but she liked it best for its qualities as a burn medicine. Applied externally, it gives "almost instant relief of pain, and rapid healing," she says. At least in burns of the first and second degree it will prevent vessication, inflammation and scarring. It is also beneficial in old burns. "One small boy came up with terrible scars and contractions on the thigh, and with considerable areas still ulcerated. These began to heal rapidly when compresses of *Urtica* were applied. And a cottage woman, one remembers, where an old burn just above the wrist had refused to heal, *did* heal promptly under the magic touch of a stinging nettle compress."

Margaret Tyler got such excellent results with this medicine, that she developed a reputation as a fanatic about it. "A doctor who could not believe the fairy tales told him regarding this power of *Urtica,* was advised to 'burn his finger and try.' He did accidentally burn it a few hours later, and was convinced."

Dr. Dorothy Shepherd relates a similar story. "The late Dr. Tyler was the first to tell me about the miraculous effect the stinging nettle tincture had on superficial burns. I must acknowledge to my shame that I was skeptical; I thought she was somewhat of a fanatic and exaggerated some of the actions of the drug. It seemed incredible." However, she gave it a try one day on a case which was especially suited to experiment, since the man had burned both ankles about evenly. She tried the conventional homeopathic treatment (Picric acid) on one, and the Nettle tincture on the other. The results so impressed her and the patient that she had to change the other dressing over to Nettle the following day. She then gives a truly horrendous case history, with remarkably happy results.

"A young, healthy male, working on our estate, came to the house about eleven o'clock one morning in great agony, hardly able to speak for shock." His right upper eyelid, right cheek and chin, arms from fingers to elbows had been badly burnt by scalding fat. "He could hardly stand, there was a strong smell of scorched hair from his body, and cold sweat pouring from his face." She dressed the wounds on the arms with a "thick cozy layer of surgical cotton wool," painted the facial burns with the white of an egg and gave *Urtica urens* 30x homeopathically every seven minutes until the pain became easier, then every fifteen minutes. There was no Nettle tincture in the house. "The result astonished the patient as well as other onlookers." The pain disappeared rapidly, there was no redness, the inflammation left the burns by 8:30 that night. "Indeed he was able to drive a motor car without any discomfort that same evening. By next morning there was no trace left of any burn."

The three burn medicines I have used are Sweet Leaf, Agrimony, and Nettle. I have less experience with the latter, but here is a case history from my own records. The parents of a four-year-old boy called me with concern. The mother had accidentally spilled a cup of hot tea on his arm. By the time she had turned up the sleeve of his pajamas, the skin was already coming off. She raced him to the emergency room where the burn was dressed. She was informed that he would have to be brought to the burn center to change the dressings regularly for the next six weeks. That afternoon she brought him to see me. Although he had been clammy right after the burn, now he was not at all sweaty. That tended to mitigate against Sweet Leaf. Although he had been holding his breath from the pain, he was now on some kind of pain reliever from the hospital, so he was not in pain. I gave her Agrimony to use if the pain came on and Nettle to rub in as close to the dressing as possible. The next day they examined him at the hospital and were surprised to see how well the burn was healing. Now they said he only needed to come into the hospital for two weeks. He healed up fine and last saw them after ten days.

Preparation and Dosage

Nettle leaves should be picked in the spring and early summer, before they become tough. The dew should be burned off and it should be a warm, dry day, as they need to be dried quickly. The plants may be bundled and tied up to dry in an open, dry, shaded part of the house. Or Nettles may be tinctured quickly in brandy or vodka. The longer the period of storage, the most persistently the material must be used.

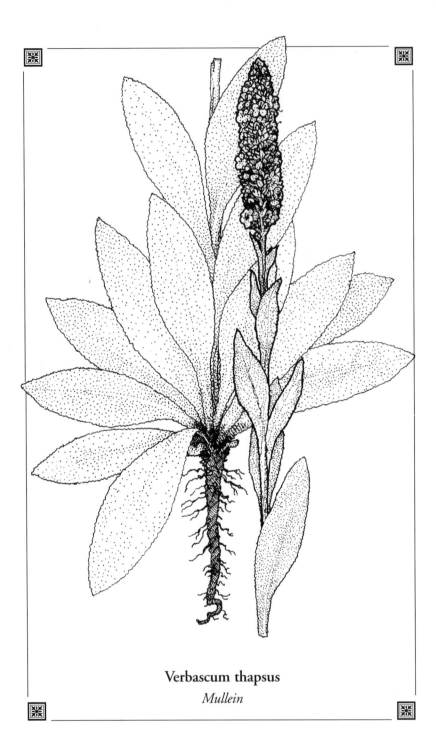

Verbascum thapsus

Mullein

Verbascum thapsus
Mullein

This is a common wayside plant which is easily recognized by the tall flower stalk. It is native to the Old World, but has been naturalized in all corners of the globe. Mullein likes disturbed soils, especially slopes. It is a biennial. The first year a rosette of soft, downy leaves appear near the ground. These are superseded the second year by a tall, staff-like flower stalk. With this the life cycle is over. Next year, new plants will be found a short distance away. Mullein seldom grows in the same place twice. It is a member of the *Scrophularia* family.

Mullein is one of those plants which strongly appeal to the folk imagination, like Yarrow. It finds a niche in the folk lore of many lands. Ulysses took it with him to protect himself against the enchantments of the sorcerer Circe. The long stalks, dipped in suet, were used as torches in religious processions in medieval Europe. In India, it is used to guard against evil spirits. The American Indians adopted Mullein after it arrived in North America. They use it for ceremony, smoking, and medicine. I have heard it recommended "by the Grandfathers," so thoroughly has it been adopted into Native American culture.

Mullein likewise has an extensive history of use as a medicinal plant. The soft, mucilaginous leaves suggested virtues to traditional healers. Although soothing to the skin and mucosa when prepared as a tea or poultice, they are actually irritating when fresh. The roots and flowers contain aromatic volatile oils. The flowers are used to soothe earache. The seeds are not used in herbal medicine because they are toxic. Mullein is chiefly used for acute respiratory diseases, congestion and dry-

491

ness of the mucosa, coughs, hoarseness, asthma, intestinal catarrh, dysentery, hemorrhoids, retained urine, loss of appetite, ulcers, rheumatism, and menstrual disorders.

Mullein was mentioned by the classical authors such as Hippocrates, Plinius, Dioscorides, and Galen. Most of the standard uses were already known at this time. Plinius and Dioscorides both noted that food wrapped in the leaves took longer to putrefy. A natural extension of this is the statement by Galen that it helps digest and cleanse corrupted tissue. Dioscorides says it will heal old coughs and eating ulcers, edema and flux, ruptures and convulsions, toothaches, and inflammations of the eyes.

The use of oil distilled from the flowers, a more sophisticated "chymical" preparation, dates from the Renaissance. Today the tea, extract, poultice, or salve made from the leaves and the oil from the flowers are commonly used in herbal medicine.

Traditional European uses are summarized by Gerard (1597.) "Mullein is of temperature drie," he reports. The leaves "boiled in water, and laid vpon hard swellings and inflammations of the eies, cureth and ceaseth the paine." They also assist the cure of hemorrhoids. The root "stoppeth the laske and bloudy flix" and "is good for them that are broken and hurt inwardly [hernia], and preuaileth much against the old cough." He goes on to quote some interesting folk practices. "The leaues worne vnder the feet day and night, in manner of a shoe sole or sock, bringeth down in yong maidens their desired sicknesse." Also, "the Countrey people, especially the husbandmen in Kent, doe giue their cattell the leaues to drinke against the cough of the lungs, being an excellent approued medicine for the same, whereupon they doe call it Bullocks Lung-woort." It is principally as a cough remedy that Mullein figures in domestic medicine. However, it has also long been popular as a hemorrhoid salve. "The later Physitions commend the yellow floures, beeing steeped in Oile and set in warme doung vntill they bee wasted into the Oile and consumed away, to bee a remedie against the piles." Martin Blochwich says Elder and Mullein salve is a specific for painful hemorrhoids.

Culpeper (1653) repeats most of these uses and adds some more. He classifies Mullein under Saturn, the dry planet. It is "a most excellent remedy for the gout," helps stiff sinews to loosen up, "openeth obstructions of the bladder and veins," and dissolves "swellings, or inflammations of the throat." Some curious uses are cited as well. "The juice of the leaves and flowers being laid upon rough warts, as also the powder of the dried roots rubbed on, doth easily take them away, but doth no good to smooth warts." The seed and leaves boiled in wine and applied to the skin "draw forth speedily thorns or splinters gotten into the flesh, ease the pains, and heal them." The same, "laid on any member that hath been out of joint, and newly set again, taketh away all swelling and pain thereof."

Verbascum was proved by Hahnemann, and an extensive list of symptoms were generated. These confirmed the traditional uses and added additional indications. However, *Verbascum* just did not quite click upon the homeopaths. It is well known to the herbalist, but individualizing symptoms calling for a specific use for the plant have not been established and it is too often used in a vague sort of way. Hopefully, the following account will contribute to a more specific concept of Mullein in both homeopathy and herbalism.

Soft and Hard

The stalks are tall, slender, and strong—we used to sword-fight with them when I was a boy. In the nineteenth-century, the soft, downy leaves were rubbed on the cheeks by girls. The slightly irritating property caused reddening. Because Quaker girls were proscribed from using makeup in those days, Mullein gained the name "Quaker Rouge." I guess this plant has a special relationship to Quakers—they were proscribed from taking up weapons as well!

The two qualities of sharpness and softness capture the spirit of Mullein. It is a remedy for conditions where sharpness has impinged on softness (rough, brutal coughs wearing down the villa of the lungs), or when the sharpness has lost its edge (edema and mucus congestion.)

The flavor of the leaf is mildly bitter and pungent, the temperature is slightly cool and definitely dry; there is a mucilaginous quality in the leaves and a slight aromatic quality in the flowers and roots. This indicates that Mullein will soothe irritated membranes (as a mucilage), reduce fever and increase secretion (as a bitter), and open the lungs (pungent, aromatic). In short, it is useful for harsh, racking coughs with a dry, irritated membrane and irritated cough reflex, where there is a lack of secretion.

There is a mutual weakness of the lungs and kidneys with this remedy. The lungs do not send water down to the kidneys and they lose the capacity to drain the lungs. The result is retention of urine and edema. Mullein has an affinity for the lungs, kidneys, and nerves.

Mullein is useful in patients who have been hit hard by a bronchial infection, in the recent or remote past. The cough reflex is irritated and hyper-reactive so that there is a painful, dry, irritative cough. The patient may complain of pain in the diaphragm, lower ribs, or abdomen—from the force and frequency of the cough. With every outburst the frame is shaken. The cough tends to develop a deep, hollow sound. The mucus membranes tend to be dry and very little phlegm is raised.

The soft, hairy, downy leaves of Mullein are similar to the villa, or hairs lining the mucus membranes of the lungs. Harsh coughing and dryness of the membranes wear down the villa. Mullein should be remembered when a cough progresses from a more superficial condition to a sub-acute condition where there is an overactive cough reflex.

There is a relationship between the lungs and the skin. Clerks in herb stores (not the most numerous vocational group) know well that powdered Mullein leaves cause irritation to the skin. A fine, miliary rash breaks out for, say, half an hour. This irritation of the skin is analogous to the irritation of the mucus linings. It is an overlooked, but characteristic symptom.

Dr. William Cook (1869) cites *Verbascum* as a major remedy for edema. "Only a few articles of the Materia Medica exert a decided influence on the absorbents, and the mullein is one of the most reliable of these," he writes. The leaves have a "peculiar and reliable power over the absorbent system, to which they seem a specific relaxant; and their power in promoting absorption in cellular dropsy, chronic abscesses, pleuritic effusions, and similar accumulations of fluid, is truly remarkable. For these purposes, the better method is to make a strong decoction of the leaves, and wilt other leaves in this and bind them over the part. They may be employed to similar purpose in synovial dropsy, and scrofulous and other swellings; though it is not proper to use them on carbuncles, buboes, cancers and other swellings from which it would be injurious to have a deposit absorbed."

Soothes the Nerves and Sets Bones

Mullein has a strong affinity for the nervous system and neuralgia. It has been used for pain relief since antiquity. Mullein flower oil is an old German folk remedy for earache. Dr. Constantine Hering brought it with him to America—it was one of the few herbal remedies the "father of American homeopathy" is known to have used. Mullein flower oil is placed in the ear to soothe earache when there is pain and a sense of obstruction. It soothes the nerves, lubricates the passages, and helps to clean out deposits of material. Mullein root is a standard remedy among herbalists in the Northeast to settle acute pain.

Mullein is particularly well indicated when there are nerve pains in the zygomatic arch related to ear pains and problems. There may also be dryness in the larynx and bronchi. The temporal-mandibular joint is sometimes the focus of difficulty. All of these symptoms have been brought out in the homeopathic provings and confirmed in practice. I have seen epidemics when these symptoms were common and Mullein was suited to a string of cases. My belief is that these symptoms occur after cold winds in fall and winter. They may also be related to some trauma to the nervous system.

Verbascum has also produced—and cured—symptoms of nerve pain in the extremities. Homeopathic literature mentions cramp-like pains in the soles, right foot, and knee. A feeling of heaviness in the lower extremities. Thumbs feeling numb. Neuralgic pains in the left ankle. Stiffness and soreness of joints in the lower extremities. This remedy may have important uses in the relief of injuries to the nerves. Experiments have been undertaken in burn-units with the external application of the leaves. They have given pain relief in major burns.

The large, downy leaves of Mullein look somewhat like those of Comfrey, and have been used in herbal medicine as an external wound-wort. They have been placed on burns, injuries and broken bones to promote healing and soothe nerve-pain. Gerard mentions the use of Mullein to ease pain after setting a joint. I find that it is excellent for stubbed or broken fingers and toes. It also is good for setting the bone.

My friend Susan was working as a professional carpenter one time when she fell forward and hit her ribs against a 2x4 that was sticking out, breaking a rib. She could feel one end protruding out against the skin, while the other jabbed inward against the viscera. In a few days this set up a nice little cough. Because Mullein cures a cough which is so violent as to break ribs, I thought perhaps it would cure a broken rib causing a cough. Besides, Mullein looks kind of like a 2x4. Susan put a Mullein leaf on her rib that night. The next morning the ends of the rib were correctly aligned with each other and the cough was gone. The break started to drift apart a week later and she had to put the leaf on again, but she never felt the pain or inconvenience of the broken rib as it healed up neatly. Later Susan helped a friend of hers who had broken his rib falling off a roof.

Although I have a penchant for weird uses of herbs, I was initially afraid to write about this property of Mullein—it seems too outlandish. It wasn't until one of my students heard the story and tried it in a similar case that I felt I could write about it. I do believe that "Mullein has the intelligence to set bones." It is especially indicated when it is hard to set a bone correctly or difficult to make an adjustment.

Here's a case which demonstrates the use of the plant in this way. A thirty-eight-year-old woman had a herniated disk in the neck (C6) which was causing severe pain and inflammation. There was fever, red complexion, warm forehead and hands. The pain was causing nausea and lack of appetite. Already thin, she looked emaciated from the loss of eight pounds. A rapid, nonresistant pulse indicated that "heat was having its way with her system." The neurologist thought there was only a "minuscule chance" that surgery could be avoided. Her chiropractor was encouraging, but not hopeful. I recommended St. John's Wort tincture until she could come in to see me the next day. It reduced the fever within five minutes. The next day the pulse was no longer fast, but sharp-edged. I recommended the following: (1) continue St. John's Wort tincture externally for the pain, fever, and irritable, torn parts of the disk, (2) Goldenseal externally because it seals clean wounds such as torn disks, (3) Mullein externally to help get the bulging disk back in place without forceful manipulations and also for the nerve pain, (4) Prickly Ash externally on the wrist for tingling in the left arm and hand, and (5) Blessed Thistle internally for her lost appetite and weight loss from nausea connected with nerve pain. She especially felt the last three remedies. Five days later the neurologist reversed his prognosis: surgery was no longer indicated. She was almost well in two weeks. In a month she was completely well. Three years later she had a slight relapse, the neck became irritated, and she had to take the Goldenseal again.

496

Several years afterwards I was reading in Dr. Christopher's *School of Natural Healing* that Mullein is beneficial for stopping the flow of fluids from "ruptured vessels." It is therefore possible that Mullein also helped seal the herniated disk.

Preparation and Dosage

Mullein leaves should be picked during the first year of their growth, before the stalk begins to shoot upward and rob nutrients from the rosette of leaves. They are still good through the winter following the first growing season. Indeed, Mullein leaves are often still alive under the snow. Once the stalk appears the medicinal potency switches to the flowers. The traditional method of preparation was to put Mullein stalks and flowers in a bottle in the sunshine and let the oil drip down to the bottom. Generally, they are now extracted in olive oil.

The leaves should be used when the condition involves the lungs and kidneys; the flowers are better for the nerves. I like to use the tea made from the leaves, the tincture of the leaves or flowers, and the oil of the flowers. Dose, one to ten drops of the tincture; one drop of the oil in the ear.

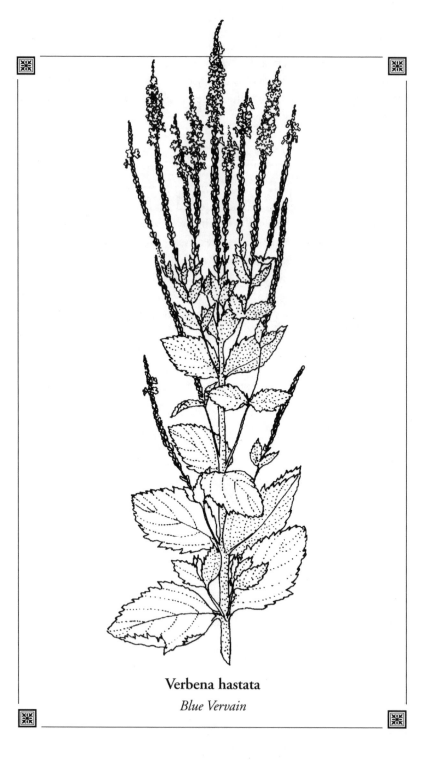

Verbena hastata

Blue Vervain

Verbena hastata
Blue Vervain

The Vervains are common weeds throughout the northern temperate region. In traditional European herbalism the officinal species is *Verbena officinalis* (Vervain), a spindly, radiating plant with mauve flowers. When the colonists came over to America they noticed the native species, *Verbena hastata*. This is a tall, more noble and erect plant with an intense blue flower top. The two plants have similar uses, but the Blue Vervain is more remarkable in appearance and is considered the better one by American herbalists. There are cousins growing in the western part of the United States as well. They are members of the Verbenaceae family.

European Vervain

Verbena officinalis has a long history of use in European folk culture. It is one of those plants around which extensive magical and religious associations attached themselves in ancient times. Both the good guys and the bad guys (apostles, priests, druids, and witches) were supposed to use Vervain in various ways. This is the most important medicine plant used by the Druid priests, second to Mistletoe.

Vervain was also mentioned by the classical writers as a medicine. Dioscorides gives a few stray uses. It cures foul ulcers, "breaks ye crusts round about which are in the tonsillae," resolves jaundice and "oedemata of long continuance." The salve is "of force against serpents."

One of the most prominent associations of Vervain in folk lore is with iron. Smiths would quench their ironwork in Vervain water, in order to give it strength. The plant was known in Germany as *Eisenkraut* (Iron Herb), *Stahlkraut* (Steel Herb), or *Eisenhard* (Iron Hard). The buoyant stalks of the plant convey the idea of tensile strength. One of the many strange beliefs attending the herb is that, "whoever carries vervain in his hand will not be barked at by dogs wherever he goes." This, according to Macer in the eleventh century.

The Renaissance herbalists demythologized the literature they had inherited. Otto Brunfels (1523) gives a typical account of Vervain for that period. He says that "for all wounds, fresh or foul," it is a most important remedy. In addition, "Iron Herb water, drunk morning and evening, opens up the stopped liver, drives out worms, purifies the kidneys, breaks up stones, calms fever, and heals inward ulcers. It is good for poisoning, fever, oppression of the chest, ulcers in the lungs, dizziness, stomach pains, jaundice and bloody urine."

Culpeper gives the astrological perspective. He associates Vervain with Venus, the planetary ruler of the sexual-urinary tract. "Above all," he wrote in 1658, "the herb of Venus, called Vervain, gathered in the hour of Venus, when the Moon is with her in Libra, is medicinal for all diseases of the reins." He also says in his *Compleat Herbal* (1653) that Vervain "is an herb of Venus, and excellent for the womb, to strengthen and remedy all the cold disorders of it, as plantain does the hot."

Because it is a simple, nontoxic plant, Vervain was ignored by professional physicians. It did not receive a homeopathic proving and is barely touched upon in homeopathic literature, though it managed to become official in the U.S. homeopathic pharmacopoeia based on a few stray indications. However, it remained for Dr. Edward Bach to bring out the genius of the plant.

The typical Vervain patient, says Dr. Bach, has an intense attitude towards life. He or she is strong-willed, enthusiastic, and generally not able to relax. This drives the person to overexertion, both mental and physical. "They refuse to be beaten and will carry on long after others would have given in. They go their own way. They have fixed ideas and are very certain that they know right. They may be obstinate in refusing treatment until compelled. They may be carried away by their enthusiasm and cause themselves much strain."

Case histories given by Bach and his followers also yield important physical indications which correspond with the mental state he describes. These show the relationship to muscular spasm, especially of the neck and shoulders, but also of the stomach and intestines, giving rise to indigestion and constipation. The traditional use in kidneystone colic is also verified. Although Dr. Bach did not attempt to link the mental symptoms to the physical ones, they show an excellent correspondence.

Bach provides a case which verifies the relationship of Vervain to the muscles of the neck. "A farmer suffered from paralysis of the neck so that the head fell forward. Besides there was weakening of the eye and mouth muscles. He was intensely strong-willed, would go about his work as usual, for months refused treatment. Vervain effected a complete cure in about two weeks."

One of Dr. Bach's friends in the homeopathic community, Dr. F. J. Wheeler, provided another case. The patient was a middle-aged man, "a very tense person, energetic and opinionated." He suffered for years from a painful spasm in the lower back. "The original diagnosis was flatulence, but an X-ray examination revealed a stone in the left kidney." The patient refused to be operated upon. By the time Wheeler saw him, he was having three severe attacks of pain a week, had to remain in bed, and was missing work. "I gave him Agrimony for his mental torture, and Impatiens for the tension. These relieved the pain, and he was able to return to work. Five days later, there was a recurrence of the pain, and he was in great distress during the night. This time I added Vervain for his tension and his strong will and his determination not to give up." An hour and a half after receiving the first dose, he passed a large kidney stone. He was back at work later that day! He experienced only a few transient afterpains.

Philip Chancellor, author of the *Handbook of the Bach Flower Remedies,* reports a case of severe mental tension accompanied by hyperacidity and pain in the stomach cured under the influence of Vervain and Pine flower essences. In another case, a migraine headache of over fifty years duration were cured by Vervain and Willow.

Dr. V. Krishnamoorty, in the *Beginner's Guide to Bach Flower Remedies* (1979), gives several striking case histories. One patient suffered from severe tension which "resulted in nervous indigestion from a tense colon," difficulty getting to sleep, tension in the muscles of the chest, and nervous exhaustion. The patient explained, "This nervous strain makes me wake early as though an express train has to be caught." Another patient used an arresting phrase: "My driven feeling seems to be growing, and I feel as if I were at the point of a bayonet; it leaves me feeling breathless." Another complained of pain "at the top of my spine which affects my whole arm and shoulder," another of "rheumatic pains in her shoulders and knees, poor sleep and chronic constipation." All of these conditions cleared up with Vervain flower essence. Krishnamoorty generalized, "If muscles and joints cannot be relaxed, they become stiff and tense and there is great tiredness and strain."

Dr. Bach gave a case history in which he used Vervain flower essence for a badly sprained ankle. It was better in a remarkably short time. The mental state of the patient led to his selection of the remedy: he was an enthusiastic person, prone to overwork. This case history is given by Nora Weeks in *The Medical Discoveries of Edward Bach.* Vervain has a tradition of use in strains and sprains in folk medicine. This is again an instance in which the physical symptoms correspond to and validate the mental symptoms.

American Blue Vervain

Blue Vervain is used by Indian practitioners as a nervine and antispasmodic. It is one of the most important remedies known to the Eastern Woodland Indians.

The intense blue flowers and the square stems are a signature indicating nerves. It was also used as an emetic for fever and stomach troubles. Blue Vervain first gained prominence in medical literature during the Revolutionary War. American army surgeons, bereft of foreign drugs, were forced to use local plants, so they drafted Blue Vervain as an emetic. Samuel Thomson considered it to be second only to Lobelia in this capacity.

In the old days, emetics were usually used to treat acute febrile conditions. Thus, we hear of Blue Vervain used to induce sweating, relieve fever, evacuate and settle the stomach and bowels, and restore suppressed menses. Blue Vervain was often compared to Boneset which is used in similar conditions, but it was generally considered inferior to this plant. By the middle of the nineteenth century *Verbena hastata* occupied but a small niche in the pharmacopoeia of American medicine, while Boneset had grown to prodigious use in popular and professional medicine. This is really as it should be: Boneset is a much more useful remedy in acute diseases.

We often have to wait for the appearance of a single individual who resonates with a particular herb in order to have a "revelation" of its properties. In the case of Blue Vervain, our revelator is Dr. O. Phelps Brown, of Jersey City, New Jersey. In *The Complete Herbalist* (1867) he explains, "The great—very great—medicinal value of this plant was brought to my attention by an accidental knowledge of the good it had effected in a long standing case of Epilepsy. Its effects in that case were of the most remarkable character, and I was, therefore led to study most carefully and minutely its medicinal peculiarities." He used Blue Vervain for disorders of the stomach, liver, and menstruation, but particularly for epilepsy. "A more valuable plant is not found within the whole range of the Herbal pharmacopoeia."

Brown preferred to use Blue Vervain in a compound with Boneset, Smartweed, and Chamomile, which he called "The Magic Assimilant." Despite the use of several ingredients, "the principal article in this reme-dy is the Blue Vervain." He tested various members of the Vervain clan, concluding that only the *hastata* was a reliable cure for epilepsy. As a par-tisan of the doctrine of signatures, Brown suggested that the difference was due to the intense blue color of the flowers.

The use of Blue Vervain as a remedy for epilepsy dates from the appearance of Brown's book. As an astrological herbalist of the Nicholas Culpeper tradition, Brown was not credited by conventional doctors as the source for the information. (He probably had an inferior medical license, as he practiced in Jersey City rather than New York.) Despite these disadvantages, the use of *Verbena hastata* in treating epilepsy even-tually seeped into eclectic and homeopathic literature. An eclectic author with some experience, Dr. French, gave praise for the remedy in restrained terms. "Verbena is of great value in some cases of epilepsy, while in others it is of no value whatever." This is, of course, what we should expect.

The slight mention of *Verbena hastata* and *V. officinalis* in homeo-pathic literature does not go much beyond eclectic and botanical sources. Boericke gives a short account of each one.

Epilepsy

Brown's graphic description leaves us in no doubt about the nature of the disease he was referring to. "In most of the cases of Fits, which have come under my notice and treatment, the first effect of the spasms has been a twisting of the neck, the chin being raised and brought round by a succession of jerks towards the shoulder, while one side of the body is usually more strongly agitated than the other. The features are greatly distorted, the brows knit, the eyes sometimes quiver and roll about, sometimes are fixed and staring, and sometimes are turned up beneath the lids, so that the cornea cannot be seen, but leaving visible the white sclerotica alone; at the same time the mouth is twisted awry, the tongue thrust between the teeth, and caught by the violent closure of the jaws, is often severely bitten, reddening by blood the foam which issues from the mouth. The hands are firmly clenched and the thumbs bent inwards on the palms, the arms are generally thrown about, striking the chest of the patient with great force. Sometimes he will bruise himself against surrounding objects, or inflict hard knocks on the friends and neighbors who have hastened to his assistance. It frequently happens that the urine and excrements are expelled during the violence of the spasms, and seminal emissions sometimes take place. The spasmodic contraction of the muscles is occasionally so powerful as to dislocate the bones to which they are attached. The teeth have thus been fractured, and the joints of the jaw and of the shoulder put out or dislocated." This is the most severe form of epilepsy. Brown had also seen the lesser grades, where there was but "a totter, perhaps, a look of confusion, but the patient does not fall." For all of these conditions, he recommended Blue Vervain alone or in the "Magic Assimilant." When taken for two the three months, "the spasms generally grow lighter and lighter, and finally disappear altogether." He claimed that over seven hundred people had been cured in this manner.

When I read this description I was surprised because I had once helped a patient who suffered from severe jerking of the neck with *Verbena hastata*. The case was a comical one that remained engraved upon my mind. A man in his early thirties used to come into Present Moment Herbs, talking in a loud, almost shouting and demanding voice. It seemed like there would always about fifteen customers swarming around the front counter when he would appear to demand help in his loud, unceasing manner. One day he was particularly difficult. In addition to his ordinary mannerism, his neck was jerking uncontrollably to the left every few seconds. He was on psychiatric drugs. Finally, just to conduct business, we were forced to help the poor soul. I sat down with him and asked him to describe the problem. "Impotence," he shouted. There were people milling all around us. I bent over my little notebook. From what cause? "Too much masturbation," he shouted, as his head jerked uncontrollably. I sank deeper into my chair. As the interview continued, the words "Blue Vervain, Blue Vervain" kept coming to my mind. (This has only happened one other time—see Milk Thistle.) I had never used Blue Vervain before and knew nothing about it. I gave him a single dose. He sighed with relief, the neck-jerking stopped (and never occurred again), his voice came down a few octaves (he is still an intense talker), and the sexual function was restored in a few days. I gave Lady's Slipper a week later to help build up the nervous system. I cannot report that he became a paragon of normalcy.

The Stiff-Necked Remedy

The cases of epilepsy which Dr. Brown felt he was most successful in treating were those where the spasm started in the neck. Through experience, I have come to appreciate that tension centered at the nape of the neck is a top-notch indication calling for *Verbena hastata*. The remedy will seldom fail when this symptom is present. A twenty-five-year-old woman, strong-willed and intense, was suffering from tension, anxiety and sleeplessness. "Whenever I have tension, it settles in my neck and shoulders," she said. I suggested Blue Vervain. "Oh, I already take that as a relaxant." She just needed someone to remind her to start taking it again. Another woman hyperextended one of her fingers. I gave her Blue Vervain tincture, externally and internally. It helped the finger, but also got rid of a chronic tension in the neck.

Dr. Brown felt as strongly about the usefulness of Blue Vervain in dyspepsia, as in epilepsy. His choice of words in describing this disease gives us some clue as to the type of patient requiring Blue Vervain. "There is something so harassing in Dyspepsia—the distress is so eccentric and erratic." Dr. Bach and Dr. Krishnamoorty give case histories for dyspepsia using the European species. The digestive distress associated with *Verbena* often involves the intestines as well as the stomach, and I do not believe that the word dyspepsia is really adequate.

The tensile, erectile strength of the flower stalk is a signature pointing to the use of *Verbena* in impotence. However, it has a more general application as a sexual remedy. Dr. Brown writes, "There is no herb so well adapted to cure all sexual derangements as the Blue Vervain, as it produces a brisk circulation of the natural secretions, thereby throwing off all impurities and curing internal ulcerations and other morbid difficulties of the parts." The mental state of the idealizing and hard-driven Vervain type, described by Dr. Bach, is one which would encourage binding up sexual energy. It should also be pointed out that the Vervains are cousins of Chaste Tree (*Vitex agnus-castus*). This small Mediterranean tree was originally used as a sexual suppressant during the late classical period. Modern scientific research and clinical experience shows that it is a hormone regulator.

Blue Vervain is an important remedy in menstrual and menopausal problems. I know quite a few practicing herbalists who have discovered that Blue Vervain is an important remedy in these kinds of problems, yet this information is not widely known or advertised in the herbal marketplace. William LeSassier gave an excellent case history during a lecture. A woman came to see him who was driven to eat just before her period, so much so that she had to starve herself the rest of the month to make up for the binge. She said she was driven to eat, "like a pack of piranhas." William, noting Dr. Bach's association of Vervain with driven impulses, gave her Blue Vervain. The condition was removed. He also points out that Blue Vervain is a specific for women who suffer flu-like symptoms just before or during their period. Remember, this is an old influenza remedy.

Blue Vervain is also a remedy of importance in menopausal conditions where there is nervous tension, flushes of heat, and the ever present driven character. Recently I helped a fifty-three-year-old woman who had been suffering from hot flashes, vascular headaches, and an excessive sexual drive. This had been driving her crazy for over a year, but she was so embarrased, I don't think she'd told anybody else about the condition. I knew she was a high-minded, driven person. Blue Vervain tincture cured all of these problems in about a week.

In Traditional Chinese Medicine, hot flashes are sometimes seen as evidence that the kidney *yin* is weak and incapable of sedating the heat and energy, which tends to move upwards. Blue Vervain seems to give this support.

The concept of "liver wind" in Traditional Chinese Medicine is also useful in understanding the pathology of Vervain. Remember from our account of Agrimony that the liver maintains flowing and spreading. When the liver is deeply affected the muscles start to go into uncontrollable spasm. This is called "liver wind." The principle symptoms are tremor, tic, numbness, dizziness, convulsions or paralysis. This may come on suddenly, as stroke, or result from emaciation or high fever.

Blue Vervain is particularly suited to the kind of liver wind resulting from "deficiency of liver *yin* with rising of liver *yang*." The principle symptoms of this kind of liver wind are sudden unconsciousness, convulsions, deviation of the eye and mouth, one-sided paralysis, aphasia or indistinct speech, dizziness, a dried red, peeled, deviated tongue, and a superficial, empty, or tense, fine, and rapid pulse. This condition can be caused by severe fever injuring the *yin* and causing uprising of *yang*.

From what has just been said, we should expect *Verbena hastata* to be useful as a remedy for severe fever which diminishes the fluids of the body, resulting in spasm. The following case history bears this out. Dr. J. N. White of Queen City, Texas, reported on a patient he cured with *Verbena hastata* around 1900. After six weeks of whooping cough, a five-year-old boy developed epileptic seizures, as many as twelve in twenty-four hours. After two months of unsuccessful treatment with every remedy he could think of, Dr. White gave *Verbena hastata*, twelve minims every four hours, except at midnight. "From the first dose of the *Verbena hastata* the boy began to improve. He would have contractions of the muscles of the arms and legs and look wild for a minute or more for the first week, but after that he never had another symptom. We kept him on the medicine, as above, for six weeks, and now he takes twelve drops three times a day. He has not had any symptoms in over two months, and all that wild vacant look is gone, and he plays, eats, sleeps, etc., as if he had never been troubled with epilepsy." This story may be found in Dr. E. P. Anshutz' *New, Old, and Forgotten Remedies* (1900).

Preparation and Dosage

The Cherokee use the mature seeds, the leaves and the roots (Hamal and Chiltowsky, *Cherokee Plants,* 1975.) My custom is to use the mature flower tops, since I learned about Vervain from Dr. Edward Bach, of flower essence fame. The flowers are picked in middle to late summer, dried for use as a tea or made into a tincture. The leaves and flowers have a bitter taste and probably have identical properties. I make a tincture by macerating the flower tops in alcohol for a few days or weeks. This gives a bitter, mauve colored preparation. The dose is one to three drops. This is sufficient when Blue Vervain is well indicated.

Herbal Repertory

This list of herbal remedies and uses has grown out of the clinical experiences of myself and several trusted friends and colleagues. Although the selection of remedies is relatively small, it is a useful bunch. A number of medicinal plants not listed in this book have been included.

In my practice I supplement this selection of medicines with most of the commonly used homeopathic remedies and some flower essences. Many of the other practitioners who have contributed knowledge to the development of this repertory use other supplementary methods and remedies as well. Thus, this repertory does not represent all that a person could or would need in order to carry on a comprehensive practice.

The repertory is arranged along the simple lines of "organ-specificity," so that it will be easy to think from the general seat of the disease to the remedy. The especially good remedies are set in italics. Highly characteristic symptoms are given in parenthesis.

I would like to thank and acknowledge the following herbal practitioners for their contributions to the material in this repertory: Lise Wolff, William LeSassier, 7Song, Margi Flint, David Winston, Michael Tierra, Amanda McQuade Crawford, Wade Boyle, ND, Keewaydino-quay, and Kate Gilday. I also consulted the excellent repertory in David Hoffmann's *New Holistic Herbal* to catch my omissions and mistakes.

Fever

With Little or No Sweat. Achillea (red, flushed face; rapid, nonresistant, full pulse; red tongue), Arctium, Asclepias (dry internal membranes and skin), Hyssopus, Nepeta (infantile fever), Sambucus (parched, dry, red skin).

With Sweat. Arctium (excessive perspiration with worry), Asclepias tuberosa (pleurisy, arthritic fever), Lobelia (high fever with profuse sweat), Monarda (cool, clammy skin), Sambucus (excessive perspiration).

Debilitating Sweat, Hectic Fever. Arctium (malar flush, profuse sweat), Lobelia (profuse sweat, collapse), Lycopus (rapid, tumultous pulse, nervousness), Nymphaea, Salvia (night sweats with fever), Solidago (malar flush, weakness following fever), Verbena (spasms from loss of fluids).

Influenza, Intermittent Fever, Chills and Heat. Achillea (sudden intense fever, with chills), Agrimonia (pain in the joints), Angelica (influenza, often with respiratory involvement), Asclepias, Capsicum, Chamomilla, *Eupatorium perfoliatum* (influenza, chills, crushing pain in bones), Sambucus (beginning of influenza, with dry skin), Tilia (nervous tension associated with flu), Verbena.

Low-grade, Septic Fever. Achillea (phlebitis, boils, abscesses), *Baptisia* (low fever with putrid discharges, swollen glands, necrosis), Calendula (low immunity, infections, boils), Carthamus (low grade fever with skin eruptions), *Echinacea* (low immunity, exhaustion, low fever, swollen veins; infected wounds, boils, abscesses), Eupatorium purpureum (abscesses, purulent matter in system), Hyssopus (low-grade infection and fever), Plantago (external on boils and infected wounds, draws out pus, infection and materials; infected roots of teeth), Sambucus (boils), Solidago (low-grade fever, sores, tired kidneys following fever).

Eruptive Fever. See Skin.

Injuries

External Application

Cuts. *Achillea* (excessive bleeding, bruises with bleeding, painful cuts), Alchemilla, Allium sativa (local dressing), Althaea officinalis (external), *Calendula* (red, sore, infected cuts, cat scratches, cuts worse from exposure to water, purulent, infected), Equisetum, Hydrastis (excessive bleeding, clean cuts; contra-indicated for dirty, infected wounds), *Hypericum* (cuts with nerve damage, inflammation and pain, loss of parts; heals slowly and closes the flesh from the inside), *Plantago* (dirty, infected cuts, puncture wounds, without much bleeding), Prunella, Stachys palustris, Stellata (external), Symphytum (old wounds slow to heal; generates flesh from the outside inwards and can cause overgrowth of tissue).

Bruises. *Achillea* (red and blue color; bruise with bleeding; blood blister), *Arnica* (red and blue; bruise without bleeding), Bellis perennis (bruises to deep tissues; obstetric bruises), Carbo vegetablis (Charcoal; blue and yellow color, old stagnant bruises), Carthamus (red and blue color; septic undertone), Hypericum (to areas rich in nerves), Sambucus (blue and swollen, ankles and wrists), Sassafras (black and blue color; old people), Stellata (external), Symphytum (black-eye).

Burns. Achillea (deep burns), *Agrimony* (pain which causes holding of the breath), Aloe vera, Chamomilla, Hypericum (pain, sunburn), Iris (scalds, sunburn), *Monarda* (with cold sweat), Plantago (herpes, shingles, blisters, burns), Polygonatum, Sambucus, Symphytum, Urtica (burning, stinging pain).

Nerve Injuries. Achillea (lacerations with pain), Agrimonia (pain, tension, holds the breath), Betonica (torture, pain, hysteria, frenzy, head injury), Chamomilla (irritable), *Hypericum* (torture, pain, inflammed nerves), Lactuca (blow to the testicles), Osmorhiza longistylis (numbness, pain, peripheral neuralgia, debility), Zanthoxylum (torture, pain).

Broken Bones. See Muscular and Skeletal System.

Drawing Agents. Allium cepa (Red Onion), Pinus strobus, Plantago, Prunella.

Mind and Emotions

Depression. Achillea (cut to the bone), *Artemisia absinthium* (brutalized, deadened, insensitive; gregarious but depressed), Artemisia vulgaris, Avena, Calendula (winter depression), Ceanothus (artistic funk, melancholy), Cimicifuga (stuck inside, brooding, withdrawn), Gentiana (doubt), *Hypericum* (depression), Iris (little addictions, sugar craving, depression), *Lactuca* (harsh experience, lost track of goal), Melissa, Pulsatilla (emotional instability), Quercus (broken-down, defeated; alcoholism), Verbena.

Nervousness and Anxiety. Arctium (worry, with sweaty brow), Betonica (lack of groundedness, hysteria, frenzy), *Gentiana* (self-doubt), Lactuca, Leonurus, Lycopus (feels like a hunted animal), Monarda (nervousness centered in the stomach), Scutellaria (nervous fear, nightmare), Valeriana (temporary palliative), Verbena (neurotic, uptight, puritanical).

Anger. *Agrimonia* (pretends not to be angry), *Chamomilla* (expresses anger; whining, peavish, complaining), Galium (annoyed, fussy), *Hepar sulphuris* (homeopathic; rage), *Nux vomica* (homeopathic; turbulent, angry personality), Smilacina racemosa (mean-spirited; alternately, flipped-out, crazy), Staphysagria (homeopathic; inability to express anger), Valeriana (hysterical anger).

Direction, Lack of, or Needs a New One. Apocynum androsaemifolium (dominated by another; change or die), Betonica (addictions), Ceanothus (artistic funk; can't think their way out of a problem), Chicorium (self-centered, childish), Crataegus (too materialistic; would like to believe in fairies, but can't), Dipsacus (feels useless), Eriodictyon (Yerba Santa; hidden obstructions), Iris (petty addictions and self-indulgence), Juglans (dominated by another), *Lactuca* (aimless), Phytolacca (lazy, apathetic), Polygonatum (needs something new in life), Quercus (broken-down, defeated, struggles on).

Food Cravings. Betonica, Iris (sugar, hypoglycaemia), *Verbena* (PMS cravings).

Loss of Memory. Arctium, Betonica (old age), Ginkgo (old age), Lycopodium (premature aging; can't grasp the right word).

Sleeplessness and Dream-disturbed Sleep. Aesculus hippocastanum (obsessive thinking), Artemisia absinthium (night-terrors, seizure during sleep), Betonica, Chamomilla (can't relax), Crataegus, Hypericum, Lactuca, Lycopus (fearful, alert), Paeonia officinalis (nightmare), Passiflora (circular thinking), Scutellaria (sleeplessness, nightmare), Tilia, Valeriana (a temporary, nonaddictive sedative).

Head

Head Injuries, Concussion, Stroke. Achillea (bruises, bleeding, pain; stroke, hematoma), Apocynum androsaemifolium, Betonica (concussion, hysteria, frenzy, stroke), Hypericum (pain), Zanthoxylum (pain).

Headache. Agrimonia (migraine, tension), *Betonica* (general headache remedy; pain to a frenzy, hysteria), *Chelidonium* (migraine, cluster headache, eyes sensitive to light), Cimicifuga (pain in the orbits of the eyes; tight traps), Eupatorium perfoliatum (crushing pain in head), Iris (hypoglycaemic migraine, from not eating), Polygonatum (occipital), Rosmarinus, Tanacetum parthenium, Verbena (tension in nape of neck connected to headache).

Vertigo, Dizzyness. Betonica, Ginkgo (dizzyness, tinnitis), *Monarda* (tinnitis, Ménière's disease).

Epilepsy, Convulsions. Artemisia absinthium (night-terrors), Hypericum (tetanus; preventative and curative), *Paeonia* (epilepsy; almost a specific; hang a fresh Peony Root around the neck), Verbena (seizures start in the nape of the neck; after fever).

Eyes, Ears, Nose, and Throat

Conjunctivitis, Eye Infection, Congestion, Redness. Calendula, Chamomilla, Euphrasia (mucus and redness), Foeniculum, Hydrastis (mucus and redness), Pulsatilla (mucus and redness), Rubus idaeus, Solidago (allergies, no mucus, irritation, watering, redness).

Ear Infections, Congestion, Pain. Alchemilla, Chamomilla (pain with whining and complaining in young children), Galium (old, lingering infections and swollen glands), *Pulsatilla* (pressure and infection without complaining), Verbascum (pain, wax stuck in ear).

Rhinitis, Sinusitis, Head-cold, Hayfever. Allium cepa (Onion; runny nose with excoriated nostrils), Allium sativa, Ambrosia (Ragweed; chew a leaf for allergy), Angelica, Betonica, Capsicum, Ceanothus (chronic sinus discharge, runny), Equisetum (hayfever, great irritation of membrane), Plantago (due to dental infection), Sambucus, *Solidago* (hayfever, cat allergy; irritated eyes; very dilute doses).

Mouth and Gums. Agrimonia (sores on tongue, canker-sores), Alchemilla, *Commiphora myrrha* (gum disease), Hydrastis (sores on tongue, canker sores, ulcers, gum disease), *Plantago* (abscessed teeth, infection after dental surgery, root canal), Propolis (sores, infections, bad breath), *Quercus* (dilapitated gums, deteriorating jaw bones), Taraxacum (infection in jaw bones).

Sore Throat, Swollen glands. *Baptisia* (mononucleosis), Calendula, Ceanothus (broad, swollen tongue coated dirty white), Echinacea, Galium, Phytolacca (homeopathic), Trifolium (mumps; swollen glands in back of neck, under and around ears).

Laryngitis. *Acorus calamus* (tracheitis, loss of voice), Agrimonia, Althaea officinalis, Baptisia, Chamomilla, Echinacea, Hydrastis, *Propolis* (instantaneous voice-producer), Quercus.

Nosebleed. Achillea, Alchemilla, Calendula, Hamamelis.

Tinnitis. Cimicifuga, Hydrastis, Lycopodium, *Monarda.*

Toothache. Echinacea.

Lungs

Cough, with Fever. Achillea (flushed face, fever, bronchitis; rapid, non-resistant, full pulse), Arctium (excess or lack of perspiration), *Hyssopus, Lobelia* (half of tongue red or half coated; high fever; prenzeling up of lungs; asthma and bronchitis), Lilium (mucus stuck, with fever), *Monarda* (clammy, cold sweat; bronchitis and bronchial asthma), *Propolis* (hot, raw bronchitis), Sambucus (young children and old age; bluish complexion).

Cough, Dry, Irritable. Agrimonia (tension, holds breath, gasps to catch breath; bronchitis, asthma, whooping cough), Betonica (weak cough reflexes), Lactuca (tightness of chest muscles, asthma without mucus), Lobelia (prenzeling up of the lungs; spasm of the vagus with heartburn and nausea; worse from cigarette smoke), Marrubium (incipient cough), Pimpinella anisum, Plantago

514

(coughs like a fiber is caught in the lung; dry, irritable cough), Polygonatum, Osmorhiza longistylis, Prunus serotina, Rumex (dry, irritable cough), Symphytum (worn down hairs of lungs, ulceration from chemicals, fever; under sternum), *Thymus* (dry, irritated membranes, coughing jags), Trifolium (irritable, drippy, sputtery cough), Tussilago, Ulmus fulva (weak respiration, unable to breath deeply), *Verbascum* (harsh, racking cough, breaks a rib; dry membranes, worn down hairs of lungs), Verbena (tense, irritable cough, dried out membranes; whooping cough).

Cough, Wet. Angelica (congestion, with influenzal symptoms; old bronchial infections cloyed with mucus), Asclepias (pleuritic stitches from old infections; dry in top of lungs, wet down below; pneumonia, congestive heart failure), Capsicum, Cimicifuga, Grindelia (bronchitis; clinging, dried out mucus), Hydrastis (thick, yellow mucus), *Inula* (green globular mucus; acute bronchitis, ripened bronchial discharge, post-nasal drip, digestive upset from swallowing mucus), Lilium (mucus dried out and stuck in the periphery of the bronchial tree), Marrubium (with salivation), Pinus strobus (green, viscid, saplike mucus, difficult to raise), Plantago (draws out mucus), Polygala senega (broncho-pneumonia), Populus tremuloides (lack of tone, allergies), Sambucus (children; croup; waking at night), Solidago (old infections, mucus), Urtica (inactive congestion).

Cough, Spasmodic. Agrimonia (trouble catching the breath), Drosera (whooping cough), Lactuca (tight chest), *Lobelia* (twisted tubes), Prunus serotina, *Thymus* (whooping cough), Trifolium (drippy, sputtery; whooping cough), Tussilago, Verbena (dried out, spasmodic).

Stomach

Digestion, Weak. Betonica (weak solar plexus with stomach problems, gastritis, gastralgia), Gentiana, Hydrastis (atonic mucosa, stomach membranes, debility, weakness; large, swollen, atonic tongue), Hypericum (irritable, weak stomach, hyper- and hyposecretion), Lycopodium (weak, dry stomach; narrow, withered tongue).

Bloating and Gas. Acorus calamus, Angelica (bloating, gas, cold), Betonica (weakness, gas), Carum (bloating, gas, heat), Chamomilla (painful distention), Foeniculum, Gentiana, Lycopodium (bloating during the meal; dry, withered tongue), Monarda, Zingiber officinalis.

Nervous Stomach, Colicky. Betonica (anxiety, lack of groundedness), Chamomilla (whining, complaining), Hypericum, Mentha piperita (Peppermint), Monarda (tension held in stomach, chest, shoulders), Nepeta.

Burning and Ulceration. Betonica (weakness, pain, burning, mild ulceration), Hydrastis (almost a specific for ulcers), Hypericum (irritation), Lobelia (heartburn, hiatal hernia, spasm), Ulmus.

Heart

Cardiovascular System

Blood. Achillea (thins the blood; thrombosis; coagulated blood, cold extremities), Capsicum (thins the blood; equalizes the circulation), Sassafras (thins the blood; coagulated blood, cold extremities; pulse feels thick like oatmeal).

Circulation. Aesculus hippocastanum (mental tension; high blood pressure; venous congestion), Agrimonia (tension), Capsicum (unequal distribution of blood; sluggish capillary circulation; flabby, middle-aged persons), Prunus serotina (histaminic irritation of capillaries), Quercus (venous atony), Rosmarinus, Ruta (venous tension and blockage).

Heart. Alchemilla (weak muscles), Asclepias (congestive heart failure; water in lungs), Cactus (pains like an iron band around heart; valve deterioration), Capsicum (strain on heart from unequal circulation; floppy valves; as a stimulant rub on hands and feet during heart attack to open the peripheral circulation), Crataegus (weak and poorly nourished heart muscle; irritability and palpitation; clogged coronary circulation; high blood pressure; cholesterol), Hydrastis (general weakness of nerves and muscles which can affect the heart), Liriodendron, Quercus (lack of tone in venous circulation and heart), Rosmarinus (cardio-pulmonary edema in old people), Sambucus (congestive heart failure; blue, swollen complexion and tissues), Tilia.

Heart Palpitations. Crataegus (weakness and irritability of cardiac muscles), Leonurus (nervous palpitation), Lycopus (fever with wild pulsation), Tilia (nervous palpitation).

High Blood Pressure. Achillea, Agrimonia (tension), Allium sativa, Crataegus, Melissa (depression), Polygonatum, Tilia, Viburnum opulus, Viburnum prunifolium, Viscum.

Low Blood Pressure. Urtica.

Arteriosclerosis. Crataegus, Tilia, Viscum.

Liver and Gallbladder

Incomplete Metabolism of Waste Products (Toxic Liver, Liver Fire). Arctium (skin rashes, acne, scalp), Berberis aquifolium (dry skin, constipation), Berberis vulgaris (low-grade bacterial infections, chronic ill-health, shattered physically and mentally, dull-minded), Solidago (skin rashes, acne, scalp), Rumex crispus (red and yellow complexion), Taraxacum (heat, swollen tissue; mapped tongue).

Jaundice. Agrimonia (tense, pinched, yellow-grey complexion), Betonica (wan, leaden complexion with weakness of gallbladder reflexes), Chelidonium (yellow; gallbladder congestion; pain under right shoulder blade), Hydrastis (infection, weakness and congestion in the gallbladder), Monarda fistulosa (bloated and yellow complexion with gallbladder congestion), Taraxacum (long term gallbladder congestion).

Liver Damage, Swelling, Pain. Agrimonia (pain), Chelidonium (congestion), Chelone, Chionanthus (pancreatic and hepatic problems), Silybum (low enzymes, damage, poisoning), Taraxacum (heat and swelling).

Gallstone Colic. Agrimonia (tension, gasping for breath), Betonica (weak gallbladder reflexes, hysteria), Chelidonium (thins bile, cuts inflammation, removes stones), Hydrastis (anti-inflammatory and cuts bile), Malus (Apple products; break down the edges of the stones), Monarda fistulosa (nervous tension), Taraxacum (slowly cleans heat and congestion in liver and gallbladder).

Pancreas

Hypoglycaemia. Iris (sugar craving, hypoclycaemic headaches, depression, blood sugar ups and downs).

Diabetes mellitus. Achillea, Curcuma (tissue regenerative), Hydrastis (a stimulant externally on ulcers and neuropathy of extremities), Oplopanax (adult onset), Osmorhiza longistylis (stabilizes sugar levels and reduces symptoms, usually does not cure; deterioration of eyesight, neuropathy), Taraxacum, Vaccinium (juvenile onset; palliative).

Lymphatics

Swollen, Congested. Calendula (red protuberances scattered about the edges of the tongue; pain in left chest from congestion of the thoracic lymphatic ducts), Ceanothus (large, dry coated tongue), Chimaphila (indurated glands), Galium (small swollen glands and cysts), Helianthemum canadense, Phytolacca (hurts to stick out the tongue; swollen and inflammed glands; mastitis), Scrophularia (enlarged, indurated glands), Trifolium (single hard, swollen cysts; encysted glands).

Intestines

Appendicitis. Agrimonia, Monarda.

Colic. Acorus calamus, Angelica, Chamomilla, Dioscorea, Foeniculum, Gentiana, Nepeta, Sambucus, Valeriana, Viburnum opulus.

Colitis. *Achillea* (bleeding), Agrimonia, Althea officinalis (palliative), Curcuma (tissue regenerative), Geranium maculatum, Myrica (mucus), Polygonatum, Quercus, Ulmus fulva, Urtica (mucus and blood in stool).

Constipation. Aloe vera, Arctium (dry stool; poor secretion and lubrication), Berberis aquifolium (dry skin, intestines), *Juglans* (torpid intestine), Monarda (gallbladder congestion; nervous stomach), *Rumex crispus* (sluggish bowels with lower back pain), Ulmus fulva (weakness).

Diarrhea. Agrimonia (with tension), Alchemilla, Carum (acute), Geranium maculatum, Iris (yellowish diarrhea), Juglans (infection, bacteria), Monarda (nervous stomach), Myrica, Polygonatum, Polygonum bistorta, *Quercus* (chronic; dilapitated intestine), *Rubus* (acute), *Spirea ulmaria* (in children).

Diverticulitis. *Achillea,* Althaea officinalis, Chamomilla, *Dioscorea,* Symphytum, Ulmus fulva.

Fissure. Agrimonia (pain), Hypericum (pain), Symphytum, Ulmus fulva (lubricates the passage).

Hemorrhoids. Achillea (bleeding), *Aesculus hippocastanum* (externally; with mental tension), Agrimonia (painful), Bidens (bleeding), *Collinsonia* (almost a specific in recent cases), Geranium maculatum, Hypericum (painful), Polygonum bistorta, Quercus (large, swollen), Scrophularia (chronic), Ulmus (lubricates passage of stool), Verbascum (highly sensitive).

"Leaky Gut Syndrome," Candidiasis. Eupatorium purpureum, Malva neglecta, Monarda (systemic candida), Myrica (inactive canal, mucus in stool), Polygonatum, Urtica (mucus in stool).

Parasites. Allinum sativa, Artemisia absinthium (homeopathic doses only; subactive gallbladder, solar plexus), Berberis vulgaris (long infection), Cucurbita pepo, Granatum, Juglans.

Kidneys and Bladder

Bladder Infection. Achillea, Agrimonia (pointing pains in the kidneys), Berberis vulgaris (low grade, chronic infection, ill-health, radiating pains), Galium (acute or relapsing; burning, pain, straining), *Monarda* (cold, clammy skin; burning pain, tension, straining), Petroselinum (cloudy urine), Triticum, Uva ursi, Zea maiz.

Kidney Stones. Agrimonia (pains in the kidneys; pain from passage, holds breath due to pain, dribbling after passage), Collinsonia, Dauca, Equisteum (stones), *Eupatorium purpureum* (stones), *Hydrangea, Parietaria,* Taraxacum, Ulmus fulva (lubricates the passage).

Dribbling of Urine. Agrimonia (connected with tension), Betonica (general weakness), Equisetum, Lycopodium (general weakness).

Female Sexual System

Menstruation, Excessive. *Achillea* (red complexion), *Alchemilla* (weakness, hemorrhage, pallor), *Capsella* (heavy, clotted bleeding), Geranium maculatum, Pulsatilla (changeable timing and moods), Trillium (pelvic weakness).

Menstruation, Lack. Achillea (red complexion), Alchemilla (anemic, pale), Betonica (weak and nervous), Caulophyllum, *Cimicifuga* (congestion, brooding, lack of flow), Helonias, *Pulsatilla* (irregular moods and cycles), Vitex.

Menstrual Cramping, Pain and Moods. Achillea (from congestion of blood), Agrimonia (hides the pain), Artemisia vulgaris, Caulophyllum, Chamomilla (complains about the pain; irritable), Cimicifuga (brooding, withdrawn; better from onset of flow), Dioscorea, Lactuca, Lilium longiflorum (feels crazy), Pulsatilla (changeable, happy/sad; tearful; nervous, on edge), Verbena hastata (food cravings, feels driven), Viburnum opulus, Viburnum prunifolium, Zanthoxylum (torture, like ovaries ripped out by wires).

Yeast Infection, Vaginitis, Discharge. Alchemilla, Berberis vulgaris (chronic, low-grade infection), *Monarda* (almost a specific), Taraxacum.

Cysts. Achillea (blood-filled ovarian cysts), Galium (fibrous breasts, numerous cysts), *Lilium longiflorum* (breast and ovarian cysts, one or two at a time, swells with the period), Stellaria (fatty cysts), Trifolium (hard cysts).

Uterine Fibroids. *Achillea* (sitz bath), Capsella, Fraxinus, Quercus, Trillium.

Prolapsed Uterus. Alchemilla, Fraxinus, Quercus.

Endometriosis. Achillea, *Dauca carota*, Dipsacus.

Infertility. Achillea (fibroids, bleeding, congestion), Alchemilla (sensitive, weak, blue-veined, pale women), Artemisia vulgaris (cold, hard uterus; after abortions, miscarriages, setbacks; stiff lower back), Dauca carota (take until regular, discontinue to get pregnant), Lactuca (tight lower back, cold uterus).

Pregnancy, Tonic. Ballota (nausea), Capsicum (poor muscle tone; flabby, needs stimulant; heart murmurs of pregnancy), Dipsacus (restless fetus; muscular pain), Helonias (nausea), Mitchella (last two months), Monarda (nerve relaxant, nutritive), Polygonatum (tones ligaments, tightness; nutritive), *Rubus* (astringent, nutritive; tones uterus, mother and fetus; third to sixth month), Scutellaria (restless fetus; gestational diabetes), Urtica (nutrient, anemia), Spirea ulmaria (nausea).

Pregnancy, Labor. Betonica (anticipation, hysteria, weak contractions; last three weeks), Caulophyllum (delayed; erratic and exhausted contractions; last few days), Cimicifuga (descends the cervix; congestion and brooding; last three weeks), Dipsacus, Lobelia (releases severe spasm; last few days); Myrica (eases labor; last few days), Sambucus (blue complexion, stagnation, inactive featus; last three weeks), Scutellaria (nervous fear, anticipation), Ulmus (lubricates passages; last few days).

Pregnancy, Postpartum. Achillea (hemorrhage, injury), Alchemilla (blood loss, anemia, weakness, atonic tissues), Bellis perennis (internal bruising), Dipsacus (torn muscles), Hypericum (injured nerves; pain in coccyx), Ulmus (convalescent nutrient).

Lactation. Foenum-graecum (stimulates milk), Silybum (stimulates milk), Trigonella, Urtica (stimulates milk, nutritive).

Breast Infection, Mastitis, Abscess. Calendula (congestion, pain deep in lymphatic ducts), Chimaphila (indurated glands), *Phytolacca* (pain during breast feeding; mastitis; indurated glands), Trifolium (encysted gland).

Menopause. Cimicifuga, Leonurus (palpitations, hot flashes), Smilacina racemosa (moods), *Verbena* (hot flashes, tension), Vitex.

Male Sexual System

Impotence. Arctium, Betonica (weakness), Lycopodium (weakness), Verbena (neurosis).

Prostate. *Arctium,* Ceanothus (swollen), Chimaphila (swollen, indurated), Monarda (inflammed), Populus tremuloides, *Sabal serrulata* (swollen).

Testicles. Lactuca (blow to testicle with pain, inflammation), Galium, Trifolium (swollen, inflammed; mumps).

Muscular and Skeletal System

Muscles, Injured, Painful. *Achillea* (bruise), Agrimonia (pinched nerve, muscle), *Arnica* (bruise), Carthamus (taken after exercize, reduces soreness), Chamomilla (complains about pain), *Cimicifuga* (muscular rheumatism; whiplash; tightness in the traps), Dipsacus (torn, wrenched; adhesions and scar tissue), Lactuca (tightness, tight lower back), Lobelia (torsion; spasm), Taraxacum (affinity to SCM; inflammed, swollen muscles), Verbena (tight nape of neck), Zanthoxylum (weakness with pain).

Muscles, Weak. Alchemilla (hernia; weak muscles and membranes), Betonica (weakness), Capsella, Glechoma hederacea (lead-poisoning), Hydrastis (weakness; swollen, pale, scalloped tongue), Panax quinquifolius (weakness), Polygonatum (convalescence), Rubus (tones and nourishes), Ulmus (convalescence), Zanthoxylum (weakness, pain).

Joints, Injured. Agrimonia (pinched tissues), *Arnica, Dipsacus* (pulled, torn, wrenched, incapacitated), Equisetum (cartilage damage), *Polygonatum* (ligaments tight or loose), Symphytum.

Arthritis. Agrimonia (inflammation, pain), Asclepias (acute inflammation, bursitis, lack of lubrication, clicking in joints), Cimicifuga (rheumatism in the belly of the muscle), Dipsacus (severe arthritic incapacity, Lyme Disease), Eupatorium purpureum (removes deposits in joints), Phytolacca (apathetic people with lazy habits), Polygonatum (pain relief in all kinds of arthritis, lack of lubrication), Sassafras (tonic preventative, warms the joints, increases circulation to extremities), Urtica (gout), Zanthoxylum (weak-nerved older people with painful joints).

Spine. Agrimonia (pinched tissues), *Cimicifuga* (bunching up of cerebralspinal fluid; whiplash with tightness in attachment of traps to scapulas on both sides), Dipsacus (torn, wrenched, pulled muscles), Eupatorium perfoliatum (compresion fracture of disk), *Hydrastis* (externally; seals torn disks, strengthens weak ones), *Hypericum* (nerve pain and inflammation, shooting pain, coccygeal pain; pain from torn disk), Lactuca (lower back tight, cold constitution), Lobelia (whiplash with torsional spasm), Polygonatum (adjusts tensions on vertebra; TMJ), Sambucus (back pain and colic), Verbascum (helps set the spine straight), Verbena (tension in nape of neck); Zanthoxylum (writhing in agony from pain of torn disk).

Bones, Broken. Achillea (bruising, bleeding, and pain connected with), Eupatorium perfoliatum (crushed and broken bones; heals slowly with good result), Eupatorium purpureum, Equisetum (weak skin, hair, nails; poor bone-healing), Polygonatum (removes bruising, sets the bones in the right place, heals quickly), Symphytum (old, difficult, slow-healing broken bones; heals quickly but causes callous and overgrowth), Verbascum (sets the bones in the right place; externally on broken ribs and toes that cannot be set; especially good for digits).

Infection in Bones. Capsicum (mastoid infection), *Taraxacum* (infection in marrow, bones, mastoid; recalcifies).

Osteoporosis. *Calcium phosphate* (homeopathic or supplement), Eupatorium perfoliatum, Quercus (recalcification), Ulmus (recalcification).

Skin

Abscess, Boils. Allium sativa (external), Altaea officinalis, *Arctium,* Baptisia, Commiphora, *Echinacea,* Galium, Iris (external), Phytolacca (external), *Plantago* (abscess of tooth or skin; external), Sambucus, Stellata (external).

Acne. Arctium (big, single pimples), *Lactuca* (chronic, pitting, scarring), Lilium longiflorum (cyst-like acne), Paeonia officinalis (pimples on chin related to period), Sambucus (opens pores on cheeks), Solidago (sheets of small pimples on checks).

Eczema and Psoriasis. Alnus rubra (Tag Alder), Arctium (dry, red skin near joints), Betula sp. (Birch), Galium, Grindelia (itching rash like poison ivy), Rumex crispus (dry, irritable, rusty patches turning to running eczema), Quercus (running eczemas, externally), Sambucus (dry, red skin over meaty areas), *Stellata* (external for a long time), Solidago (scalp, lower extremities).

Eruptive Disease. Arctium, Carthamus (low, septic fever with rash), Cimicifuga (chickenpox; to bring out the rash), Galium (measles), Malus (Apple; eat when the rash feels unclean), Pulsatilla (chickenpox), Sambucus (toxic heat).

Herpes, Shingles. Glycyrrhiza (deglycorrhinized Licorice externally),

Monarda, Osmorhiza longistylis (externally herpes, shingles), Plantago (externally on herpes, shingles), *Prunus serotina* (herpes inside mouth, shingles; red, angry), *Ranunculus bulbosus* (homeopathic dose).

Poison Ivy. (External Application). *Grindelia,* Monarda, Plantago, Polygonatum, *Quercus,* Rosmarinus (use in vinegar).

Bibliography

Allen, Timothy Field. *The Encyclopedia of Pure Materia Medica; a Record of the Positive Effects of Drugs upon the Healthy Human Organism.* 10 vols. New York: Boericke & Tafel, 1874-79.

Anderson, Hans Christian. *The Complete Hans Christian Anderson Fairy Tales.* Edited by Lily Owens. New York: Gramercy Books, 1984.

Anshutz, E. P., M.D. *New, Old and Forgotten Remedies.* Philadelphia: Boericke and Tafel, 1900.

Bach, Edward, M.D. *Collected Writings.* Edited by Julian Barnard. Hereford, U.K.: Bach Educational Program, 1987.

Banckes, Rycharde. *An Herbal [1525].* Edited and Transcribed into Modern English with an Introduction by Sanford V. Larkey, M.D., and Thomas Pyles, Ph. D. New York: Scholars' Facsimiles and Reprints, 1941.

Bartram, William. *Travels through North & South Carolina, Georgia, East & West Florida.* 1791. Reprinted as *Travels of William Bartram.* Edited by Mark Van Doren. 1928. Reprint ed., New York: Dover, 1955.

Bensky, Dan, and Gamble, Andrew, with Kaptchuk, Ted. *Chinese Herbal Medicine, Materia Medica.* Seattle: Eastland Press, 1986.

Bergner, Paul. Article on the properties of Eupatorium perfoliatum. *Medical Herbalism.* Vol. 4, no. 3. Boulder, Co.: 1995.

Bigelow, Jacob. *American Medical Botany, Being a Collection of the Native Medicinal Plants of the United States.* 3 vols. Boston: 1817-20.

Blake, William. *The Complete Poetry and Prose of William Blake.* Newly revised edition, edited by David V. Erdman, commentary by Harold Bloom. Garden City, N. Y.: Anchor Books, 1982.

Blochwich, Martin. *Anatomia Sambuci: or, the Anatomie of the Elder: Cutting out of it Plain, Approved, and Specific Remedies for Most and Chiefest Maladies.* English translation from the Latin ed. of 1629. London: T. Sawbridge, sold by H. Brome, 1670.

Boericke, William, M.D. *Pocket Manual of Homeopathic Materia Medica.* Ninth ed., revised and enlarged. Philadelphia: Boericke & Runyon, 1927.

Boger, Cyril, M.D. *A Synoptic Key to Materia Medica.* Parkersville, W.V.: Privately published, 1931.

British Herbal Medicine Association, Scientific Committee. *British Herbal Pharmacopoeia.* London: British Herbal Medicine Association, 1971.

Britton, Nathaniel Lord, and Brown, Hon. Addison. *An Illustrated Flora of the Northern United States and Canada.* 3 vols. 1913. Reprint ed., New York: Dover Publications, 1970.

Brooke, Elisabeth. *Herbal Therapy for Women.* London: Thorsons, 1992.

Brown, O. Phelps, M.D. *The Complete Herbal, or, The People Their Own Doctor.* Jersey City, N.J.: Published by the Author, 1868.

Burnett, J. Compton, M.D. *Diseases of the Spleen And Their Remedies Clinically Illustrated.* American ed., Philadelphia: Boericke & Tafel, 1917.

_____ *Gout and Its Cure.* 1895. Fourth Indian ed., Calcutta: M. Bhattacharyya & Co., 1972.

Case, Erastus, M.D. *Some Clinical Experiences of E. E. Case, with Selected Writings.* A reissue of *Clinical Experiences,* originally published in 1916. Edited by Jay Yasgur. Greenvilee, Pa.: Van Hoy Publishers, 1991.

Chancellor, Philip. *Handbook of the Bach Flower Remedies.* London: C. W. Daniel Company Ltd., 1971.

Clarke, John Henry, M.D. *A Dictionary of Practical Materia Medica.* 3 vols. 1900-03. Third ed., Rustington, Sussex: Health Science Press, 1962.

Chishti, Hakim G. M., N.D. *The Traditional Healer, a Comprehensive Guide to the Principles and Practice of Unani Herbal Medicine.* Rochester, Vt.: Healing Arts Press, 1988.

Christopher, John R., N.D. *The School of Natural Healing.* 1976. Revised and Expanded 20th Anniversay Edition. Springville, Ut.: Christopher Publications, 1996.

Clymer, R. Swinburne, M.D. *Nature's Healing Agents, The Medicine of Nature, (or the Natura System)*. Revised ed. Quakertown, Pa.: The Humanitarian Society, 1973.

Colby, Benjamin. *A Guide to Health, Being an Exposition of the Principles of the Thomsonian System of Practice*. 4th ed. 1848. Reprint ed., Orem, Utah: BiWorld Publishers, c. 1987.

Coles, William. *Adam in Eden: or, Natures Paradise*. London: Printed by J. Streater, for Nathaniel Brooke, 1657.

Cook, William H., M.D. *The Physio-Medical Dispensatory: A Treatise on Therapeutics, Materia Medica, and Pharmacy*. 1869. Portland, Or.: Eclectic Medical Publications, 1985.

Cowan, Eliot. *Plant Spirit Medicine*. Newberg, Or.: Swan•Raven & Co., 1995.

Cowperthwaite, A. C., M.D. *A Text-Book of Materia Medica and Therapeutics*. Fourteenth ed. Philadelphia: Boericke & Tafel, 1949.

Crellin, John K., and Philpott, Jane. *Herbal Medicine Past and Present*. 2 vols. Durham and London: Duke University Press, 1990.

Cullen, William. *Professor Cullen's Treatise of Materia Medica... Including Many New Articles Wholly Omitted in the Original*. Edited by Benjamin S. Barton. 2 vols. Philadelphia: Parker, 1812.

Culpeper, Nicholas. *Culpeper's Astrological Judgment of Diseases*. 1655. Reprint ed. including Culpeper's *Urinalia, or A Treatise of the Crisis hapning to the Urine*. 1658. Tempe, Az.: American Federation of Astrologers, 1959.

_____ *Culpeper's Complete Herbal. & English Physician, Enlarged*. 1652. Reprint of the 1814 London ed. Glenwood, Ill.: Meyerbooks, Publisher, 1944.

_____ *Pharmacopoeia Londinensis: or the London Dispensatory*. London: Peter Cole, 1653.

Cutler, Manasseh. "An account of some of the vegetable productions naturally growing in this part of America, botanically arranged." 1785. Reprinted by the *Bulletin of the Lloyd Library*, No. 7. Cincinatti: The Lloyd Library, 1903.

Davenport, Guy. *Herakleitos & Diogenes*. Translated from the Greek. Bolinas, Ca.: Grey Fox Press, 1979.

Dioscorides. *The Materia Medica of Dioscorides*. Englished by John Goodyear, 1655. Edited by Robert T. Gunther. London and New York: Hafner Publishing Co., 1933.

Dunham, Carroll, M.D. *Homoeopathy, the Science of Therapeutics: A Collection of Papers Elucidating and Illustrating the Principles of Homoeopathy.* 1877. Reprint ed., Philadelphia: Boericke & Tafel, c. 1930.

Erichsen-Brown, Charlotte. *Medicinal and Other Uses of North American Plants, A Historical Survey with Special Reference to the Eastern Indian Tribes.* New York: Dover, 1989.

Ellingwood, Finley, M.D. *American Materia Medica, Therapeutics and Pharmacognosy.* 1918. Reprint ed., Portland, Or.: Eclectic Medical Publications, 1989.

Emerson, Ralph Waldo. *Collected Poems and Translations.* New York: Penquin Books USA, 1994.

Felter, Harvey, M.D. *The Eclectic Materia Medica, Pharmacology, and Therapeutics.* 1927. Reprint ed., Portland, Or.: Eclectic Medical Publications, 1989.

Felter, Harvey Wickes, M.D., and Lloyd, John Uri, Ph.D. *King's Dispensatory.* Entirely Rewritten and Enlarged. Eighteenth ed., third revision. 2 vols. 1898. Reprint ed., Portland: Eclectic Medical Publications, 1983.

Foster, Steven. *Echinacea, Nature's Immune Enhancer.* Rochester, Vt.: Healing Arts Press, 1991.

Foster, Steven, and Duke, James. *A Field Guide to Medicinal Plants, Eastern and Central North America.* Peterson Field Guides. Boston: Houghton Mifflin Co., 1990.

Fyfe, John William, M.D. *Specific Diagnosis and Specific Medication.* Cincinnati: The Scudder Brothers, 1909.

Gerard, John. *The Herball or Generall Historie of Plantes.* First ed., 1597. The Complete 1633 Edition Revised and Enlarged by Thomas Johnson. New York: Dover Publications, Inc., 1975.

Gilmore, Melvin R. *Uses of Plants by the Indians of the Missouri River Basin.* 1919. Reprint ed., Lincoln: University of Newbraska Press, 1977.

Green, Thomas. *The Universal Herbal; or Botanical, Medical, and Agricultural Dictionary.* Liverpool: Printed at the Caxton Press by H. Fisher, 1820.

Grieve, M[aude]. *A Modern Herbal, the Medicinal, Culinary, Cosmetic and Economic Properties, Cultivation and Folk-Lore of Herbs, Grasses,*

Fungi, Shrubs & Trees. Edited by Hilda Winifred Leyel. 1931. 2 vols. New York: Dover Publications, Inc., 1971.

Grigson, Geoffrey. *The Englishman's Flora.* 1955. Reprint ed., London: Hart-Davis, MacGibbon, 1975.

Hale, Edwin M., M.D. *Homeopathic Materia Medica of the New Remedies: their Botanical Description, Medical History, Pathogenetic Effects and Therapeutical Application in Homeopathic Practice.* Second ed., revised and enlarged. Detroit: Edwin A. Lodge, Homeopathic Pharmacy, 1867.

Hall, Dorothy. *Creating Your Herbal Profile.* New Canaan, Ct.: Keats Publishing, 1988.

Harris, Ben Charles. *The Compleat Herbal.* Barre, Ma.: Barre Publishers, 1972.

Harris, Thomas Lake. *Arcana of Christianity: an Unfolding of the Celestial Sense of the Divine Word.* Part II., The Apocalpyse, vol. 1. 1867. Reprint ed., New York: AMS Press, 1976.

Hartmann, Franz, M.D. *The Life of Paracelsus.* 1887. Reprint ed., San Diego: Wizard's Bookshelf, 1985.

Hemple, Charles Julius, M.D. *Jahr's New Manual, (or Symptomen-Codex).* 2 vols. New York: William Radde, 1848.

Herb Success Stories, Actual Case Histories. Springville, Ut.: Thornwood Books, 1980.

Hill, John. *The British Herbal.* London: Osborne and Shipton, 1756.

Hite, George, M., M.D. "Abridgment of Symptoms." *Annual of Eclectic Medicine and Surgery.* Edited by Finley Ellingwood, M.D. Chicago: 1890.

Hobbs, Christopher. *Echinacea; The Immune Herb!* Capitola, Ca.,: Botanica Press, 1990.

Hoffman, David. *The Complete Illustrated Holistic Herbal, A Safe and Practical Guide to Making and Using Herbal Remedies.* New York: Barns & Noble, 1996.

Hool, Richard Lawrence. *Common Plants and Their Uses in Medicine.* Lancashire: Lanchashire Branch of the National Association of Medical Herbalists, 1922.

Hoyne, Temple S., M.D. *Clinical Therapeutics.* 2 vols. 1878-80. Reprint ed. in one vol., New Delhi: Jain Publishing Co., 1974.

Hughes, Richard, M.D. *A Manual of Pharmacodynamics.* 1880. Eighth ed., revised and enlarged. Second Indian ed., Calcutta: C. Ringer & Co., c. 1960.

Hutchins, Alma R. *A Handbook of Native American Herbs.* Boston: Shambhala, 1992.

Iamblichus. *Iamblichus on the Mysteries of the Eqyptians, Chaldeans, and Assyrians.* Translated by Thomas Taylor. Second ed., London: B. Dobell and Reeves and Turner, 1895.

Jones, Eli, M.D. *Definite Medication.* 1910. Reprint ed., New Delhi: B. Jain Publishing, 1988.

Kaptchuk, Ted. *The Web That Has No Weaver, Understanding Chinese Medicine.* New York: Congdon and Weed, 1983.

Katz, Richard, and Kaminski, Patricia. *Flower Essence Repertory.* Nevada City, Ca.: The Flower Essence Society, 1994.

Kent, James Tyler, M.D. *Lectures on Homeopathic Materia Medica.* 1905. Reprint ed., Calcutta: Sett Dey & Co., 1962.

Kloss, Jethro. *Back to Eden.* 1939. Reprint ed., Coalmont, Tn.: Longview Publishing House, 1969.

Kneipp, Sebastian. *The Kneipp Cure, an Absolutely Verbal and Literal Translation of "Meine Wasserkur."* Complete American ed., translated from the fiftienth German ed. New York: The Kneipp Cure Publishing Company, 1896.

Krishnamoorty, V., M.D. *Beginner's Guide to Bach Flower Remedies.* New Delhi: B. Jain Publishers, 1979.

Kroeber, Ludwig, M.D. *Das Kraüterbuch.* Fourth ed. 3 vols. Stuttgart: Hippokrates-Verlag Marquardt & Cie., 1948-9.

Leighton, Ann. *Early American Gardens, "For Meate or Medicine."* Boston: Houghton Mifflin Co., 1970.

Lighthall, J. I. *The Indian Folk Medicine Guide.* c. 1875. Reprint ed., New York: Popular Library, 1973.

Lippe, Adolph, M.D. *Text Book of Materia Medica.* 1865. Reprint ed., New Delhi, India: B. Jain Publishers, 1984.

Locke, Frederick J., M.D. *Syllabus of Eclectic Materia Medica and Therapeutics.* Edited by Harvey W. Felter, M.D., with notes by John Uri Lloyd. Cincinnati: John M. Scudder's Sons, 1895.

Long, Max Freedom. *The Secret Science Behind Miracles.* Marina del Rey, Ca.: DeVorss & Company, 1948.

Macer, Aemilius. *Virtue of Herbs.* Translated by Daniel Patrick O'Hanlon. New Delhi: Hemkunt Press, 1981.

Messegue, Maurice. *Health Secrets of Plants and Herbs.* New York: William Morrow and Co., 1979.

Mills, Simon. *The Essential Book of Herbal Medicine.* First published as *Out of the Earth,* 1991. Reprint ed., New York: Arkana, 1993.

Millspaugh, Charles F., M.D. *American Medicinal Plants.* 1892. Reprint ed., New York: Dover Publications, 1974.

Milton, John. *Paradise Lost and Paradise Regained.* New York: Franklin Watts, Inc., c. 1970.

Mooney, James. "The Swimmer Manuscript, Cherokee Sacred Formulas and Medicinal Prescriptions." *Bureau of American Ethnology, Smithsonian Institution, Bulletin 99.* Revised, Completed, and Edited by Frans M. Olbrechts. Washington, D.C.: United States Government Printing Office, 1932.

Moore, Michael. *Medicinal Plants of the Mountain West.* Santa Fe: Museum of New Mexico Press, 1979.

_____ *Medicinal Plants of the Desert and Canyon West.* Santa Fe: Museum of New Mexico Press, 1989.

Monroe, John. *The American Botanist and Family Physician.* Compiled by Silas Gaskill. Danville, Vt.: Eben'r Eaton, Printer, 1824.

Nash, E. B., M.D. *Leaders in Homeopathic Therapeutics.* First ed., 1898. Seventh ed., 1926. Reprint. Philadelphia: Boericke & Tafel, 1959.

Pahlow, Mannfried, Apothecary. *Das grosse Buch der Heilpflanzen* Munich, Gräfe und Unzer, 1989.

Palmer, Thomas. *The Admirable Secrets of Physick & Chirurgery.* Original unpublished ms., 1696. New Haven, Ct.: Yale, 1986.

Paracelsus. *Selected Writings.* Edited with an introduction by Jolande Jacobi, translated by Norbert Guterman. Bollingen Series XXVIII. Second edition, revised. New York: Pantheon Books, 1958.

Plinius. *The History of the World commonly called The Natural History of C. Plinius Secundus, or Pliny.* Translated by Philemon Holland, 1601. Selected and introduced by Paul Turner. New York: McGraw-Hill Book Company, 1962.

Priest, A. W., and Priest, L. R. *Herbal Medication, A Clinical and Dispensary Handbook.* London: L. N. Fowler & Co. Ltd., 1982.

Rabe, R. F., M.D. *Medical Therapeutics for Daily Reference.* Philadelphia: Boericke & Tafel, 1920.

Rafinesque, Constantine S. *Medical Flora; or, Manual of the Medical Botany of the United States of America.* 2 vols. Philadelphia: 1828-30.

Royal, George, M.D. *Text-Book of Homeopathic Theory and Practice of Medicine.* 1923. Reprint ed., New Delhi: B. Jain Publishers Pvt. Ltd., 1987.

Salmon, William, M.D. *Botanologia: The English Herbal: or, History of Plants.* London: Printed by I. Dawkes, for H. Rhodes and J. Taylor, 1710.

Scott, Walter. *Hermetica: The Ancient Greek and Latin Writings Which Contain Religious or Philosophic Teachings Ascribed to Hermes Trismegistus.* Reprint ed., Boston: Shambhala, 1985.

Scudder, John M., M.D. *Specific Diagnosis, a Study of Disease with Special Reference to the Administration of Remedies.* 1874. Reprint ed., Portland, Or.: Eclectic Medical Institute, 1985.

_____ *Specific Medication and Specific Medicines.* Fifteenth ed., fourth revision. 1903. Reprint ed., Portland, Or.: Eclectic Medical Institute, 1985.

Shakespeare, William. *The Complete Works.* Edited by Peter Alexander. London: Collins, 1951.

Shepherd, Dorothy, M.D. *A Physician's Posy.* "Thornbury Edition." 1969. Reprint ed., Saffron Walden, England: Health Science Press, 1981.

Shook, Edward, N.D. *Advanced Treastise in Herbology.* 1946. Reprint ed., Beaumont, Ca.: Trinity Center Press, 1978.

Smith, Huron. "Ethnobotany of the Ojibwe." *Bull. Pub. Mus. Milwaukee* 4, no 3. (1932): 391.

Smith, Peter. *The Indian Doctor's Dispensary Being Father Smith's Advice Respecting Diseases and Their Cure.* 1812. Reprinted by the *Bulletin of the Lloyd Library.* With Biography by John Uri Lloyd. Cincinnati: Lloyd Library, 1901.

Stewart, R. J. *The UnderWorld Initiation, A Journey Towards Psychic Transformation.* Wellingborough, U.K.: The Aquarian Press, 1985.

Teste, Alphonse, M.D. *The Homeopathic Materia Medica.* Translated from the French, and edited by Charles J. Hempel, M.D. 1854. Reprint ed., New Delhi, B. Jain, 1985.

Thomson, Samuel. *Life and Medical Discoveries of Samuel Thomson, and a history of the Thomsonian Mater Medica.* Reprinted by the *Bulletin of the Lloyd Library.* Cincinnati: Lloyd Library, 1909.

_____ *The Thomsonian Materia Medica, or Family Botanic Physician.* Albany: Munsell, 1841.

Thoreau, Henry David. *The Portable Thoreau.* Edited, with an introduction by Carol Bode. Revised ed. New York: The Viking Press, 1966.

Tierra, Michael, C.A., O.M.D., N.D. *Planetary Herbology, An Integration of Western Herbs Into The Traditional Chinese and Ayurvedic Systems.* Edited and supplemented by David Frawley, O.M.D., and Christopher Hobbs, C.A. Santa Fe: Lotus Press, 1988.

Treben, Maria. *Health through God's Pharmacy.* Ninth ed. Steyr, Austria: Wilhelm Ennsthaler, 1987.

Tyler, Margaret, M.D. *Homeopathic Drug Pictures.* Reprint ed., Saffron Walden: Health Science Press, 1982.

Vaughan, Thomas. *The Works of Thomas Vaughan, Mystic and Alchemist.* Edited by A. E. Waite. 1919. Reprint. New York: University Books, 1968.

Weed, Susun. *Wise Woman Herbal, Healing Wise.* Woodstock, New York: Ash Tree Publishing, 1989.

Weeks, Nora, and Bullen, Victor. *The Bach Flower Remedies, Illustrations and Preparation.* London: C. W. Daniel Company Ltd., 1976.

Weiss, Rudolf Fritz, M.D. *Herbal Medicine.* Translation. Beaconsfield, England: Beaconsfield, 1988.

Willard, Terry, Ph.D. *Textbook of Modern Herbology.* Calgary: Progressive Publishing Inc., 1988.

Wilson, Charles, and Gisvold, Ore. *Textbook of Organic Medicinal and Pharmaceutical Chemistry.* Second ed. Philadelphia: Lippincott, 1954.

Unpublished Lectures and Communications

Michel Meir Abeshera of Los Angeles, California; Halsey Brandt of Bisbee, Arizona; Stefan Doll of Athens, Greece; Margie Flint of Marblehead, Massachusetts; Malcolm Gardener of Portland, Oregon; Kate Gilday of Coldbrook, New York; Chris Hafner of Minneapolis, Minnesota; Yolanda LaCombe of Los Angeles, California; William LeSassier of New York City, New York; Amanda McQuade of Ojai, California; Victor Rangel of St. Paul, Minnesota; 7Song of Ithaca, New York; Terry Willard of Calgary, Alberta; and David Winston of Broadway, New Jersey.

Illustrations by the author, except where indicated. The following sources have been used for old herbal illustrations.

Egenolphus, Christianus. *Herbarium Imagines Vivae.* First published Frankfurt: Christianus Egenolphus excudebat, 1535. Reprint edition, Allgau, Germany: Editions Medicina Rara Ltd., c. 1980.

Fuchs, Leonard. *De historia stirpium.* Originally published, Basil: in officina Isingriniana, 1542. Reprinted in Agnes Arber, *Herbals Their Origin and Evolution.* Originally published 1912. Reprint edition, Cambridge: Cambridge University Press, 1988.

Colby, Benjamin. *A Guide to Health.* Original edition, Milford, N.H.: John Burns, 1846. Reprint edition, Orem, Ut.: BiWorld Publishers, 1986. [The illustrations in this book are found in a number of old Americal herbals and are not original to this publication; as a consequence, they are labeled "from an old American print" in the text.]

Bibliography, Second Edition

Hamal, Paul B., and Chiltoskey, Mary U. *Cherokee Plants, their uses—a 400 year history.* [Privately published], 1975.

Janos, Elisabeth. *Country Folk Medicine.* New York: Galahad Books, 1995.

Meyer, Joseph. *The Herbalist.* Revised and enlarged edition. [Privately published], 1960.

Mooney, James, and Olbrechts, Frans M. *The Swimmer Manuscript, Cherokee Sacred Formulas and Medicinal Prescriptions.* Smithsonian Institution, Bureau of American Ethnology, Bulletin 99. Washington: United Stated Government Printing Office, 1932.

Index

Page references in *italic* denote an illustration. Page references in **bold** denote entries in the Herbal Repertory, which begins on page 509.